PRE-DESCEMET'S ENDOTHELIAL KERATOPLASTY (PDEK)

System requirement:

Windows:

- Operating System:
  - Windows Vista or above
  - Macintosh OS X or above
- Recommended Web Browser – Google Chrome & Mozilla Firefox
- Essential plugins – Java & Flash player
  - If facing problems in viewing content – enable/re-install Java plugin on your web browser setting.
  - If Videos don't show up – enable/re-install Flash Player or manage Flash setting on your web browser settings.
  - You can test Java and Flash by using the links from the help section of the CD/DVD.

Accompanying CD/DVD Rom is compatible and playable only in Computers and not in DVD player.

CD/DVD has Autorun function (*only for Windows based systems*). If Autorun feature doesn't work, then follow the steps below to access the contents manually:

Windows:

- Click on My Computer
- Select the CD/DVD drive and click open/explore – this will show list of files in the CD/DVD
- Find and double click file – "launch.html"

Mac:

Double click the file "launch.html" located on the root after inserting the CD/DVD. The Mac OSX operating system does not support an Autorun feature.

For more information about troubleshoot of Autorun click on:
http://support.microsoft.com/kb/330135

PRE-DESCEMET'S ENDOTHELIAL KERATOPLASTY (PDEK)

Editor

Amar Agarwal MS FRCS FRC Ophth
Chairman and Managing Director
Dr Agarwal's Group of Eye Hospitals and Eye Research Center
Chennai, Tamil Nadu, India

Foreword

Susan MacDonald MD

JAYPEE The Health Sciences Publisher
New Delhi | London | Panama

Jaypee Brothers Medical Publishers (P) Ltd

Headquarters
Jaypee Brothers Medical Publishers (P) Ltd.
4838/24, Ansari Road, Daryaganj
New Delhi 110 002, India
Phone: +91-11-43574357
Fax: +91-11-43574314
E-mail: jaypee@jaypeebrothers.com

Overseas Offices
JP Medical Ltd.
83, Victoria Street, London
SW1H 0HW (UK)
Phone: +44-20 3170 8910
Fax: +44(0)20 3008 6180
E-mail: info@jpmedpub.com

Jaypee-Highlights Medical Publishers Inc.
City of Knowledge, Bld. 235, 2nd Floor, Clayton
Panama City, Panama
Phone: +1 507-301-0496
Fax: +1 507-301-0499
E-mail: cservice@jphmedical.com

Jaypee Brothers Medical Publishers (P) Ltd.
17/1-B, Babar Road, Block-B, Shyamoli
Mohammadpur, Dhaka-1207
Bangladesh
Mobile: +08801912003485
E-mail: jaypeedhaka@gmail.com

Jaypee Brothers Medical Publishers (P) Ltd.
Bhotahity, Kathmandu, Nepal
Phone: +977-9741283608
E-mail: kathmandu@jaypeebrothers.com

Website: www.jaypeebrothers.com
Website: www.jaypeedigital.com

Inquiries for bulk sales may be solicited at: jaypee@jaypeebrothers.com

Pre-Descemet's Endothelial Keratoplasty (PDEK)

First Edition: **2018**

ISBN: 978-93-5270-303-6

Printed at: Ajanta Offset & Packagings Ltd., Faridabad, Haryana.

Dedication

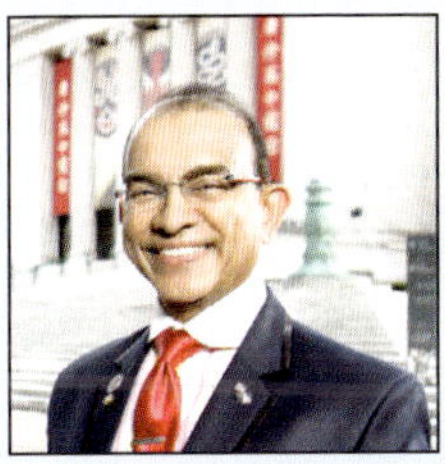

A great corneal surgeon and friend
Thomas "TJ" John
USA

Contributors

Amar Agarwal MS FRCS FRC Ophth
Chairman and Managing Director
Dr Agarwal's Group of Eye Hospitals
and Eye Research Center
Chennai, Tamil Nadu, India

Ashvin Agarwal MS
Dr Agarwal's Group of Eye Hospitals
and Eye Research Center
Chennai, Tamil Nadu, India

Athiya Agarwal MD DO
Dr Agarwal's Group of Eye Hospitals
and Eye Research Center
Chennai, Tamil Nadu, India

Patrick Conrick BA
Gavin Herbert Eye Institute
University of California
Irvine, California, USA

Adam Fox BS
Gavin Herbert Eye Institute
University of California
Irvine, California, USA

Sumit Garg MD
Vice Chair of Clinical Ophthalmology
Medical Director
Director of Technology
Associate Professor
Cataract, Corneal and Refractive Surgery
Gavin Herbert Eye Institute
University of California
Irvine, California, USA

Soosan Jacob MS FRCS DNB MNAMS
Dr Agarwal's Group of Eye Hospitals
and Eye Research Center
Chennai, Tamil Nadu, India

Carol L Karp MD
Professor of Ophthalmology
Richard K Forster Chair in
Ophthalmology
Bascom Palmer Eye Institute
University of Miami Miller School of
Medicine
Miami, Florida, USA

Dhivya Ashok Kumar MD
Dr agarwal's Group of Eye Hospitals
and Eye Research Center
Chennai, Tamil Nadu, India

Carolina Mercado MD
Bascom Palmer Eye Institute
University of Miami Miller School of
Medicine
Miami, Florida, USA

Priya Narang MS
Narang Eye Hospital
Ahmedabad, Gujarat, India

Ibrahim Osama MD
Bascom Palmer Eye Institute
University of Miami Miller School of
Medicine
Miami, Florida, USA

Elizabeth Shen MD
Gavin Herbert Eye Institute
University of California
Irvine, California, USA

Rahul Tonk MD MBA
Bascom Palmer Eye Institute
University of Miami Miller School of
Medicine
Miami, Florida, USA

Foreword

"You must live in the present, launch yourself on every wave, find your eternity in each moment."
Henry David Thoreau

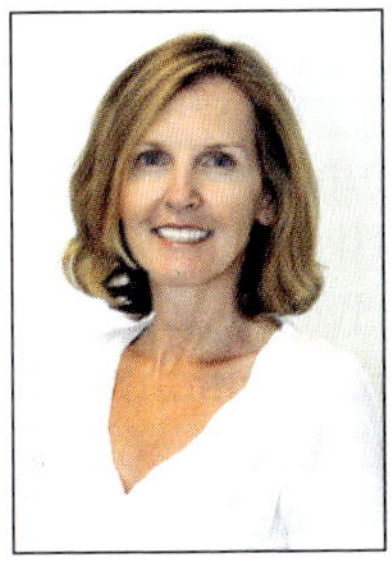

Dr Amar Agarwal is a giant in the field of ophthalmology. I am honored to have been asked to write this introduction, and feel blessed to call him my friend. I am further of hope that you, the reader, may also come to know him. When you first meet Amar, his enthusiasm towards learning and sharing knowledge will grab you and pull you in. He is a noted scientist and clinician, whose skills have improved the field of ophthalmology. A true leader, touching the lives of thousands.

As an inspirational teacher, Dr Agarwal has trained doctors from all over the world. He innovated new surgical procedures that improved our surgical techniques, and how we return sight to our patients.

What I adore most about Dr Agarwal is the way he teaches his students and apprentices, and the kindness and encouragement he radiates to those who are fortunate to be in his presence. Like all exceptional doctors, he is always looking for an opportunity to help others advance their career. He encourages their ideas, and inspires leaders to challenge themselves. To his women colleagues, he is a feminist and a constant source of strength and guidance. He is an advocate for women's education, and has provided key opportunities to advance women's training and their careers.

Dr Agarwal is happily married to Athiya Agarwal, also a brilliant doctor. Together, they have raised four beautiful sons: Adil, Ashvin, Anosh, and Ashar. All of them are talented ophthalmologists. Family is the most important thing in the lives of Athiya and Amar. Their hard work has brought eye care to many areas of the world.

What have I learned from Dr Amar?

While the world is full of physicians, what patients need is a doctor with a good heart, who never fails to give them hope; who is innovative, professional, and caring. That is how I have come to know Dr Amar Agarwal. He has inspired not only me, but the thousands he has treated and met over the course of his extraordinary life.

Dr Amar Agarwal (MS, FRCS, FRC Ophth), was born in Chennai, India in 1960, to his visionary father, Dr Jaiveer Agarwal, and mother, Dr Tahira Agarwal. Together, they founded Dr Agarwal's Eye Hospital, in their home in 1957.

After completing his MBBS from Madras University, and then his MS Ophth from Gujarat University, Amar went to the UK and earned his FRCS at the prestigious Royal College of Surgeons of Edinburgh. Later, he also received his FRC Ophth from the Royal College of Ophthalmologists.

The Agarwals have expanded the original eye hospital into a major eye hospital network with some seventy branches, across twelve countries, including: Madagascar, Ghana, Rwanda, Tanzania and the Seychelles.

A great part of the Agarwal hospitals' success can be attributed to the innovation and vision of Dr Amar Agarwal, Chairman and Managing Director. His father, Dr Jaiveer Agarwal, was awarded the country's third-highest civilian award: the Padma Bhushan. In fact, the hospital received global recognition when it was included in the Major Eye Centers of the World by the International Congress of Ophthalmology.

Dr Amar Agarwal is the pioneer of Phakonit Cataract-Removal Technology, which became popularized as Bimanual phaco; Microincision Cataract Surgery (MICS). Further innovations include the glued IOL technique for PCIOL fixation in eyes with absent or insufficient capsular support. Amar has been instrumental in developing phacoemulsifican techniques and Pre-Descemet's Endothelial Keratoplasty (PDEK). These are just a few of his numerous inventions and innovations in the field of advanced eye care.

Amar's achievements include numerous awards such as: Barraquer, Kelman, and Golden Apple awards. Dr Amar Agarwal also received the Best Doctor award from the Tamil Nadu State Government. It was awarded to him by the former (late) Chief Minister, Jayaram Jayalalithaa. Dr Agarwal's Eye Hospital has received many international accolades from the American Society for Cataract and Refractive Surgery (ASCRS).

Today, Amar's hospitals specialize in the Glued IOL procedure, to treat complicated lens problems and PDEK.

Dr Agarwal is a past President of the International Society of Refractive Surgery. He serves as Secretary General of the Scientific Committee Chairman of the Indian Intraocular Implant and Refractive Society (IIRSI).

This amazing man has further written more than 70 books, including: Phacoemulsification, Laser cataract surgery and Foldable IOL's- First edition, Lasik and Beyond Lasik and Refractive Surgery. (His many works have been translated into Spanish and Polish.)

His latest book, focuses on Pre-Descemet's Endothelial Keratoplasty (PDEK), a corneal procedure, which was first performed by Dr Agarwal himself in 2013.

The book *Pre-Descemet's Endothelial Keratoplasty (PDEK)* outlines a cutting edge procedure in which PDEK graft can be harvested from a donor of any age and grafted into adults. This means endothelial cells would have maximum regenerative capacity. Dr Agarwal's findings were crucial since results showed faster recovery, quick visual rehabilitation with minimum haziness, and very low immune rejection rates.

Dr Amar, you are an inspiration to me and countless others. Thank you for your phenomenal contribution to the ophthalmology field. I wish you a world of success in future endeavors.

Susan MacDonald MD
Associate Professor of Ophthalmology
Tufts School of Medicine
Massachusetts, USA

Preface

The main goal of writing this book was to embark upon the minute details of *Pre-Descemet's Endothelial Keratoplasty (PDEK)* procedure and its various applications and modifications adopted in the surgical technique. The aim is to provide the readers with the most comprehensive and current information on PDEK and it is hoped that this edition captures the current state of this vital and dynamic science from international perspective. PDEK being a latest iteration in the arena of endothelial keratoplasty harbors on the concept of separating the pre-Descemt's layer (Dua's layer) along with the Descemet's membrane and the endothelium layer by the creation of Type-1 bubble. The presence of pre-Descemet's layer adds an extra splint to the graft and facilitates the graft handling and unfolding inside the eye.

The book has various chapters covering various aspects of PDEK and a DVD with videos showcasing the surgical aspects of handling numerous clinical conditions related to PDEK and its nuances. I hope that this book benefits all the readers so that the knowledge is transferred in dealing successfully with our patients to enhance the visual outcomes and that it sets a framework that allows the readers to gain new information and current concepts in surgical practice in a larger context.

Amar Agarwal

Acknowledgment

Nothing in this world moves without HIM and so also this book was only written by HIM.

Contents

SECTION I: BASICS

SECTION II: SURGICAL TECHNIQUE

DVD Contents

SECTION I: BASICS

SECTION II: SURGICAL TECHNIQUE

SECTION III: SPECIAL SITUATIONS

SECTION V: MISCELLANEOUS

SECTION 1

Basics

CHAPTER 1

Corneal Anatomy and Ultrastructure

Dhivya Ashok Kumar, Amar Agarwal

INTRODUCTION

Human cornea, the anterior most transparent structure and the refractive surface is the major refractive component of the eye. The normal vertical and horizontal diameter is about 11.5 mm and 12 mm respectively. The radius of curvature is 7.8 mm anteriorly and 6.5 mm posteriorly. It measures about 0.52–0.54 mm thick in the center. Corneal ultrastructure can be divided into five different layers namely—(1) The epithelium, (2) The Bowman's layer, (3) The stroma, (4) The Descemet's membrane (DM) layer, and (5) The endothelium (Fig. 1.1).[1,2] Recently a new layer has been noted which varies from normal stroma by few histological characteristics and it has been popularly termed as pre-Descemet's layer (PDL) or Dua's layer.[3]

CORNEAL HISTOLOGY

Epithelium

The most superficial layer, present in contact with the tear film layer is made up of stratified squamous nonkeratinized cells. They are about five to six layers and in three types. The lower most cells are basal cells that are columnar type and are attached to the underlying basement membrane with hemidesmosomes. The wing cells occupy the layer above the basal cells and are usually in two to three layers thickness. The outermost layer is the layer of squamous cells which possess microvilli or plicae for its adhesion with overlying tear film.

Bowman's Layer

This is an acellular, basement membrane layer, formed by randomly arranged collagen fibrils. Constituents of this layer are believed to be synthesized and secreted by both epithelial cells and stromal keratocytes. Collagen fibrils in this layer are smaller than that of the stroma. Collagen type I, V, and VII are some of the types of collagen present in this layer along with proteoglycans.

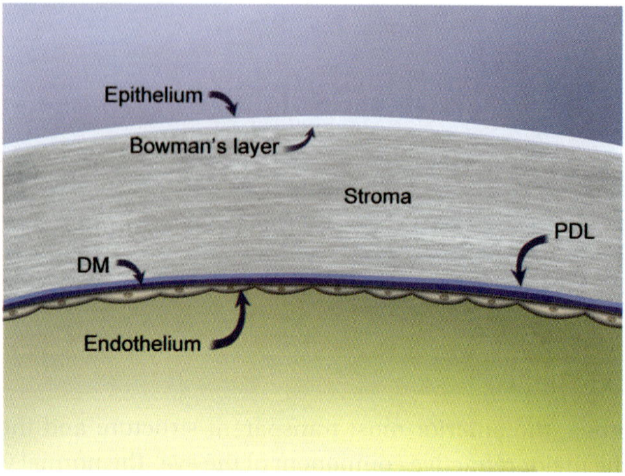

Fig. 1.1: Anatomical layers of cornea.
(DM: Descemet's membrane; PDL: pre-Descemet's layer).

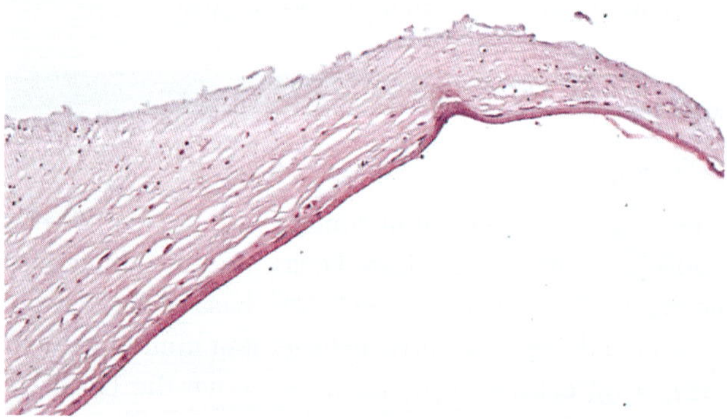

Fig. 1.2: Corneal histopathology section showing the stroma with the Descemet's membrane (DM). (*Courtesy:* Professor Harminder Dua, Nottingham, UK).

Stroma

This forms the major portion of cornea (Fig. 1.2). It is made up of regularly arranged collagen fibrils spaced by proteoglycans namely dermatan sulfate and keratan sulfate. It also contains the modified fibroblasts named keratocytes. Lumican and keratan are the core proteins of keratan sulfate proteoglycan. Collagen type I, V, VI, and XII are distributed widely in the lamellae.

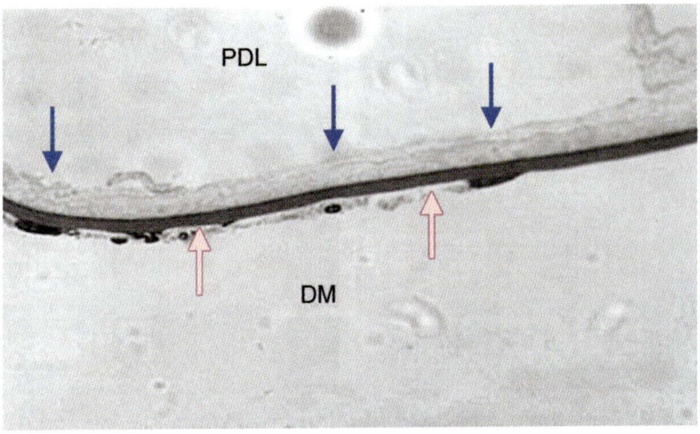

Fig. 1.3: Pre-Descemet's layer (PDL) (blue arrows) and Descemet's membrane (DM) layer (pink arrows) as seen in a corneal section by electron microscopy. (*Courtesy:* Professor Harminder Dua, Nottingham, UK)

Pre-Descemet's Layer or Dua's Layer

This layer has been recently identified by Dua et al. as it showed few differences from normal corneal stroma.[3] It measured about 10.15 ± 3.6 μm (Fig. 1.3) thick (range 6.3–15.83 μm) in his study.[3] It was observed to be made of five to eight thin lamellae of tightly packed collagen bundles which were oriented in longitudinal, transverse, and oblique directions. In immunohistochemistry staining, CD34 was negative in the PDL which showed the lack of keratocytes in this layer unlike stroma. Collagens IV and VI, seemed to be more positive for PDL compared with the corneal stroma. There has been another recent report showing the separation of PDL to be randomly arranged cleavage in collagen layers measuring 4.5–27.5 μm and variable presence of keratocytes.[4]

Descemet's Membrane

This is a defined sheet of collagen (Figs. 1.2 and 1.3) with anterior banded and posterior nonbanded zone. This is a specialized basement membrane of the endothelium that lies in front of the endothelial cells. It is about 10 ± 2 microns thick.

Endothelium

This is a monolayer of hexagonal cells arranged in mosaic pattern (Figs. 1.4A and B). The average density of corneal endothelial cells at birth is approximately 4,000 cells/mm^2. Each cell is 4–6 μm thick, 20 μm wide, and has a surface area of about 250 μm^2. There are active pumps present in the endothelial cells which functions continuously for nurturing the corneal layers and maintaining transparency.

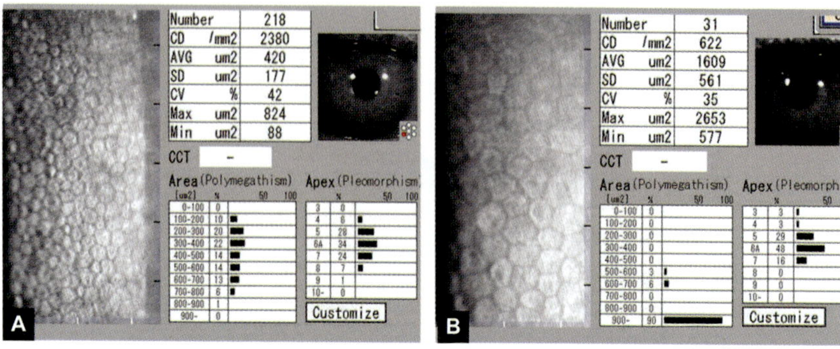

Figs. 1.4A and B: Endothelial cell layer (A) Normal hexagonal cells and (B) Endothelial cells showing polymegathism (enlarged cell area).

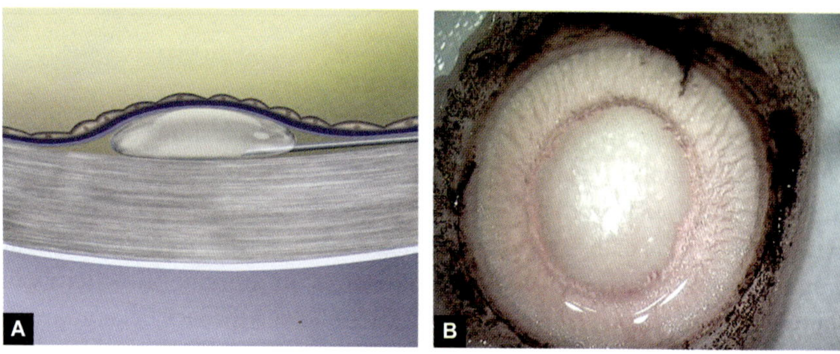

Figs. 1.5A and B: Pre-Descemet's endothelial keratoplasty (PDEK). Schematic diagram showing the cleavage plane in pneumatic dissection (A) and the type 1 bubble obtained during donor preparation (B).

ISOLATION OF PRE-DESCEMET'S LAYER

Pre-Descemet's layer can be harvested by pneumatic dissection on injecting air from the limbus into the mid-peripheral stroma of donor cornea with 30G needle. Type 1 big bubble which starts from the center, well circumscribed and thicker is the complex containing endothelium, DM along with PDL (Figs. 1.5A and B). The bubble with PDL extended to the periphery about 7–8.5 mm and do not usually go beyond 9 mm. The overlying DM layer can be peeled and still the bubble of PDL stays intact due to its fibrous nature. The type 1 bubble was known to withstand pressure up to 1.4 bars as compared to isolated DM bubble which popped at 0.6 bars. The bubble can also be separated using viscoelastic or storage medium. The findings from additional study which evaluated the cleavage plane of DM after dissection provided the evidence for the existence of a physiologic cleavage plane between the interfacial matrix, the anterior most adhesive zone of DM, and the corneal stroma, suggesting a relatively weak attachment that can be disconnected by mechanical forces.[5]

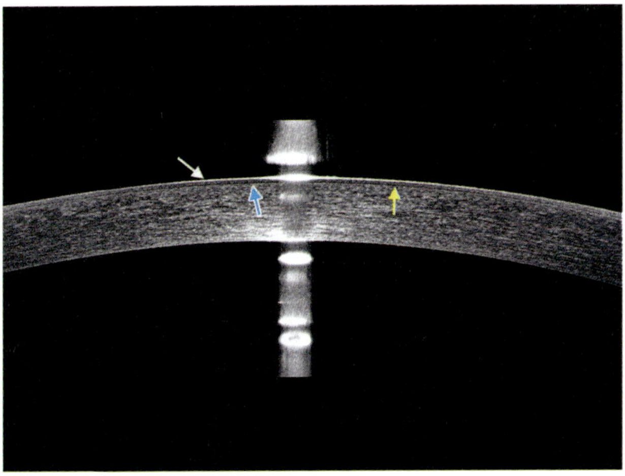

Fig. 1.6: Optical coherence tomography showing the tear film-epithelial interface (white arrow) and normal epithelium (blue arrow), yellow arrow: Bowman's layer.

CORNEAL LAYERS AND THEIR APPLIED ANATOMY

Epithelium

Epithelium's unique functions include light refraction, protection, transmittance, and survival over an avascular bed. The function of light refraction is obtained by its smooth, wet apical surface, and its extraordinarily regular thickness. The layer traverses the high sensory nerve supplies that terminate in the suprabasal and squamous cells. The epithelium has high regenerative or proliferative property and grows centripetally from the existing limbal stem cells. The layer protects the cornea from external injury, pathogens, and fluid loss. The mitogenic activity takes place in the basal cells and moves apically. Apical surface has microplicae and glycocalyx that help in tear film adhesion for forming the smooth ocular surface (Fig. 1.6). Persistent epithelial defect can happen in chronic ocular surface problems, upper eyelid, or tear film abnormalities.

Bowman's Layer

This layer has protective function between the epithelium and stroma (Fig. 1.6).

Stroma

The stroma of the human eye contains 200–250 lamellae. Lamellae in the middle and posterior regions of the stroma are arranged at approximate right angles, whereas those in the anterior stroma are arranged at less than right angles. The small diameter of the collagen fibrils and their close, regular

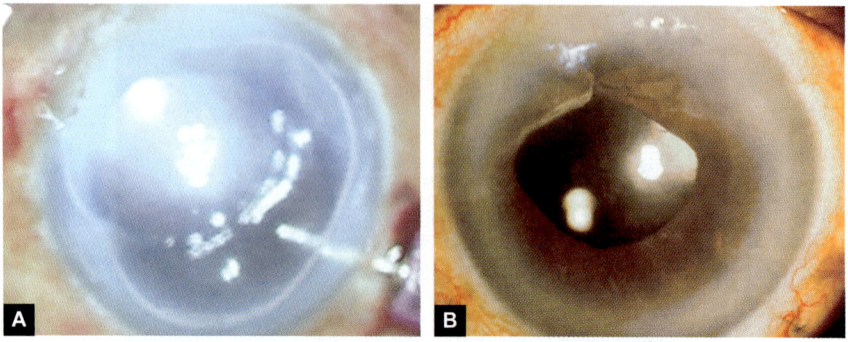

Figs. 1.7A and B: Pre-Descemet's endothelial keratoplasty (PDEK): (A) Preoperative decompensated cornea and (B) Postoperative clear cornea.

packing creates a lattice or three-dimensional diffraction grating.[6] The "lattice theory" of Maurice suggests that the ability of the cornea to scatter 98% of the falling light with equal spacing of collagen fibrils.[7] Whole of the corneal stroma or partial lamellar stroma can get damaged due to corneal trauma, inflammation, infection, or surgery leading to corneal opacity.

Keratoplasty techniques have evolved over the time period from full thickness to individual layer transplantation. Penetrating keratoplasty contain the transplantation of all the layers of stroma along with endothelium.[8] Lamellar keratoplasties popularly done involve customized corneal layers transplanted.[9-11] Deep anterior lamellar keratoplasty, posterior lamellar keratoplasty, anterior lamellar keratoplasty, and Descemet's stripping endothelial keratoplasty are some of the prevalent procedures. Since stroma is highly antigenic, the risk of rejection has been known to occur more in penetrating keratoplasties than lamellar.[12]

Pre-Descemet's Layer

The discovery and the realization of the existence of this layer has aided in the innovation of new technique of utilizing this layer in corneal endothelial disease. The plane between the PDL and stroma has been exploited in generating the pre-Descemet's endothelial keratoplasty (PDEK) surgery (Figs. 1.7A and B).[13] The additional PDL along with DM will provide strength for the graft handling during surgery. Posterior stromal pathologies like acute hydrops in keratoconus or descemetocele after chronic infection may also seemed to be related to the changes in PDL as a part of the original pathologies in progressive disease. The PDL and DM layer complex can be obtained from any age group unlike the isolated DM layer which is often retrieved from elderly corneas.[14]

Descemet's Layer

Descemet's membrane can be torn during cataract surgery (Fig. 1.8) and can remain detached which can lead to corneal edema in chronic cases.

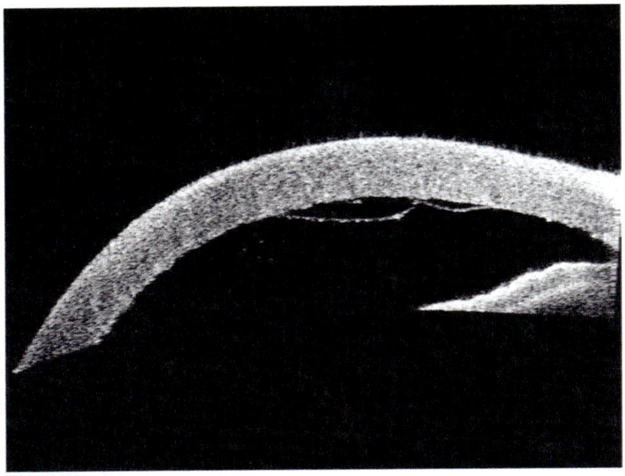

Fig. 1.8: Descemet's membrane as seen in an anterior segment optical coherence tomography (OCT) in a patient with detachment following an intraocular surgery.

DM along with endothelial monolayer can be transplanted in eyes with decompensated cornea.[15] This thin layer prevents complications of interface problems associated with thicker grafts. Descemet's membrane endothelial keratoplasty (DMEK) is a technique of replacing recipient diseased endothelium by new healthy donor Descemet's endothelium layer. DM layer is expected to have loose adhesion with posterior stroma in aged population and this helps in easy retrieval of DMEK graft in elderly.

Endothelial Layer

The endothelium is responsible for maintaining the relatively low level of stromal hydration required for corneal transparency. The endothelium has ionic pumps that draw water from the stroma, thus maintaining the highly organized collagen lamellar structure. The "pump-leak" hypothesis states that the rate of fluid leakage into the stroma is balanced by the rate of fluid pumped out of the stroma. The endothelium also secretes components for DM.[16] As such, the glucose, amino acids, vitamins, etc. needed by the epithelial cells and stromal keratocytes must traverse the corneal endothelial monolayer. Loss of endothelial cells (by trauma or dystrophy) or damage to endothelium (Figs. 1.9A and B) due to surgery can lead to bullous keratopathy or corneal decompensation. Though endothelial cells have previously known to be non-proliferative, recent investigations showed that they possess the property of slow regeneration and their ability to grow human corneal endothelial cells in tissue culture indicates that these cells retain proliferative capacity that can be harnessed under appropriate conditions.[17-19] Hence corneal pathologies involving dysfunction of endothelium are nowadays treated by endothelial

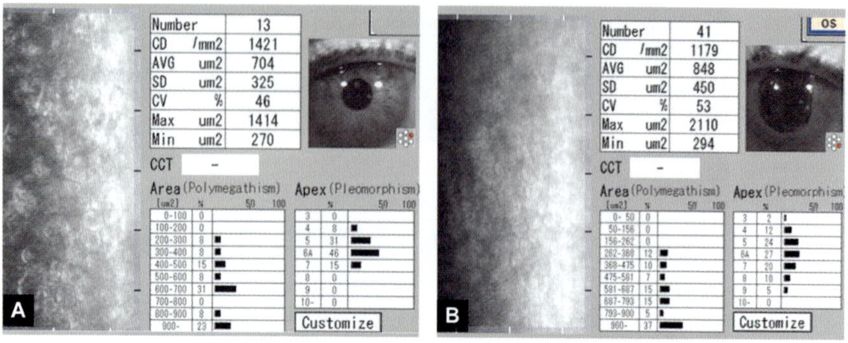

Figs. 1.9A and B: Abnormal endothelial cells. (A) Endothelium showing guttate changes and (B) Endothelium seen in patient with chronic bullous keratopathy.

replacement via donor cornea.[20,21] Cultured human corneal endothelial cells have been tried for treating corneal decompensation due to endothelial dysfunction.[22] Recently ex vivo studies have shown that corneal endothelial precursors may be an effective strategy for corneal endothelial regeneration.[23]

SUMMARY

Corneal microanatomy has been physiologically fashioned for its functional capability. All individual layers separately and together provide the optical transparency required for its very nature. Disease or disorder in the ultrastructure of any of its component is known to affect its competence. Understanding the intricate details of the fundamental microstructure of cornea is indispensable to face the upcoming newer diseases or refractory chronic disorder. Though the discussion of the entire physiology and applied anatomy of cornea is out of scope of the book, related structural differences have been detailed here. Combined with the thorough knowledge of basic anatomy and biomechanics and aided by recent technological "advancements, ophthalmologists" will surely gain the advantage of diagnosing and managing the corneal diseases at preliminary stage.

REFERENCES

1. Gipson IK. Anatomy of the conjunctiva, cornea, and limbus. In: Smolin G, Thoft RA (Eds). The Cornea. Boston: Little, Brown and Company; 1994.
2. Warwick R. Eugene Wolff's Anatomy of the Eye and Orbit, 7th edition. London: Chapman & Hall Medical; 1997.
3. Dua HS, Faraj LA, Said DG, et al. Human corneal anatomy redefined: a novel pre-Descemet's layer (Dua's layer). Ophthalmology. 2013;120(9):1778-85.
4. Schlötzer-Schrehardt U, Bachmann BO, Tourtas T, et al. Ultrastructure of the posterior corneal stroma. Ophthalmology. 2015;122(4):693-9.
5. Schlötzer-Schrehardt U, Bachmann BO, Laaser K, et al. Characterization of the cleavage plane in Descemet's membrane endothelial keratoplasty. Ophthalmology. 2011;118(10):1950-7.

6. Berman E. Cornea. In: Berman E (Ed). Biochemistry of the Eye. New York: Plenum; 1991.
7. Maurice DM. The structure and transparency of the cornea. J Physiol. 1957; 136(2):263-86.
8. Nanavaty MA, Wang X, Shortt AJ. Endothelial keratoplasty versus penetrating keratoplasty for Fuchs endothelial dystrophy. Cochrane Database Syst Rev. 2014;(2):CD008420.
9. Cursiefen C, Schaub F, Bachmann B. Update: Deep anterior lamellar keratoplasty (DALK) for keratoconus. When, how and why. Ophthalmologe. 2016; 113(3):204-12.
10. Chen G, Tzekov R, Li W, et al. Deep Anterior Lamellar Keratoplasty Versus Penetrating Keratoplasty: A Meta-Analysis of Randomized Controlled Trials. Cornea. 2016;35(2):169-74.
11. Acar BT, Akdemir MO, Acar S. Visual acuity and endothelial cell density with respect to the graft thickness in Descemet's stripping automated endothelial keratoplasty: one year results. Int J Ophthalmol. 2014;7(6):974-9.
12. Abudou M, Wu T, Evans JR, et al. Immunosuppressants for the prophylaxis of corneal graft rejection after penetrating keratoplasty. Cochrane Database Syst Rev. 2015;(8):CD007603.
13. Agarwal A, Dua HS, Narang P, et al. Pre-Descemet's endothelial keratoplasty (PDEK). Br J Ophthalmol. 2014;98(9):1181-5.
14. Agarwal A, Agarwal A, Narang P, et al. Pre-Descemet endothelial keratoplasty with infant donor corneas: a prospective analysis. Cornea. 2015;34(8):859-65.
15. Ham L, Balachandran C, Verschoor CA, et al. Visual rehabilitation rate after isolated descemet membrane transplantation: descemet membrane endothelial keratoplasty. Arch Ophthalmol. 2009;127(3):252-5.
16. Gipson IK, Joyce N. Anatomy and cell biology of the cornea, superficial limbus, and conjunctiva. In: Albert D, Miller J, Azar D, Blodi B (Eds). Albert & Jakobiec's Principles & Practice of Ophthalmology, 3rd edition. Philadelphia: Elsevier Saunders; 2008. pp. 423-9.
17. Joyce NC. Proliferative capacity of the corneal endothelium. Prog Retin Eye Res. 2003;22(3):359-89.
18. Joyce NC, Zhu CC. Human corneal endothelial cell proliferation: potential for use in regenerative medicine. Cornea. 2004;23(8 Suppl):S8-19.
19. Engelmann K, Böhnke M, Friedl P. Isolation and long-term cultivation of human corneal endothelial cells. Invest Ophthalmol Vis Sci. 1988;29(11): 1656-62.
20. Boynton GE, Woodward MA. Evolving Techniques in Corneal Transplantation. Curr Surg Rep. 2015;3(2).
21. Ple-Plakon PA, Shtein RM. Trends in corneal transplantation: indications and techniques. Curr Opin Ophthalmol. 2014;25(4):300-5.
22. Mimura T, Yamagami S, Yokoo S, et al. Cultured human corneal endothelial cell transplantation with a collagen sheet in a rabbit model. Invest Ophthalmol Vis Sci. 2004;45(9):2992-7.
23. Mimura T, Yamagami S, Amano S. Corneal endothelial regeneration and tissue engineering. Prog Retin Eye Res. 2013;35:1-17.

CHAPTER 2

Preoperative Assessment, Indications and Contraindications in Endothelial Keratoplasty

Dhivya Ashok Kumar, Amar Agarwal

INTRODUCTION

Endothelial keratoplasty (EK) has enormously overtaken the full thickness penetrating keratoplasty surgery in the last 2 decades without doubt.[1-6] It is known from the terminology as selective transplantation of the endothelium-Descemet's membrane complex with or without the posterior stroma. As compared to the whole corneal transplantation, it has its specific clinical advantages. Early visual recovery, less suture-related complications, and minimal postoperative complications have made EK widespread. Since the introduction of the posterior lamellar keratoplasty, various modifications have occurred in EK which includes Descemet's stripping endothelial keratoplasty (DSEK), Descemet's stripping automated endothelial keratoplasty (DSAEK), Descemet's membrane endothelial keratoplasty (DMEK), and recently pre-Descemet's endothelial keratoplasty (PDEK).[7-11] Even though EK is typically performed in eyes with the decompensated cornea as a result of abnormal endothelial function, patient selection is highly vital to acquire the best postoperative outcome. Thus, the current chapter has been solely dedicated for the preoperative examinations, indications, contraindications, and evaluations for an ideal patient selection for EK.

INDICATIONS

Endothelial keratoplasty is the treatment of choice for any patient with corneal endothelial dysfunction that has become visually disabling. The indications can be broadly classified into:

- *Primary or intrinsic endothelial disorders:*
  - Fuchs endothelial dystrophy
  - Posterior polymorphous corneal dystrophy
  - Congenital hereditary endothelial dystrophy
  - X-linked endothelial corneal dystrophy
  - Iridocorneal endothelial syndrome.
- *Secondary or acquired endothelial disorders:*
  - Postsurgical

- Cataract
  - Pseudophakic bullous keratopathy
  - Aphakic bullous keratopathy
  - Toxic anterior segment syndrome
  - Chronic Descemet's membrane detachment (after failed attempts of air injection).
- Keratoplasty
  - Immunologic rejection
  - Endothelial decompensation in an existing graft.
- Glaucoma
  - Postfiltration surgery (tube shunt)
  - Chronic topical medication toxicity
  - Congenital glaucoma.

▪ Trauma
  - Birth forceps injury
  - Blunt injury.

CONTRAINDICATIONS

Endothelial keratoplasty is contraindicated in conditions like keratoconus, corneal ectasia, stromal opacity or scarring (posttrauma/viral infection/interstitial keratitis), stromal (granular or lattice) or epithelial dystrophy, and borderline hypotony (results in poor clearing of graft).

PREOPERATIVE ASSESSMENT

Careful and elaborate preoperative assessment is mandatory to ensure that each patient will visually benefit from the surgery.

Clinical History

Preoperative clinical history is obtained from all the patients during their initial assessment and it is crucial in identifying any previous viral illness, dystrophic conditions, familial predisposition, and trauma. Previous surgical history, comorbidity treatment, and systemic ailments have to be documented. Patients on antiglaucoma medications or antiuveitis drugs should be obtained. Patient's history on antiglaucoma of an already failed keratoplasty, graft rejection, and dry eye has to be acquired because they will not only let us know the risk of complications but also in postoperative prognosis and management.

Assessment of Visual Potential of the Affected Eye

Visual potential assessment is the basic test for any preoperative corneal surgical workup. Snellen's distant acuity chart or Early Treatment Diabetic

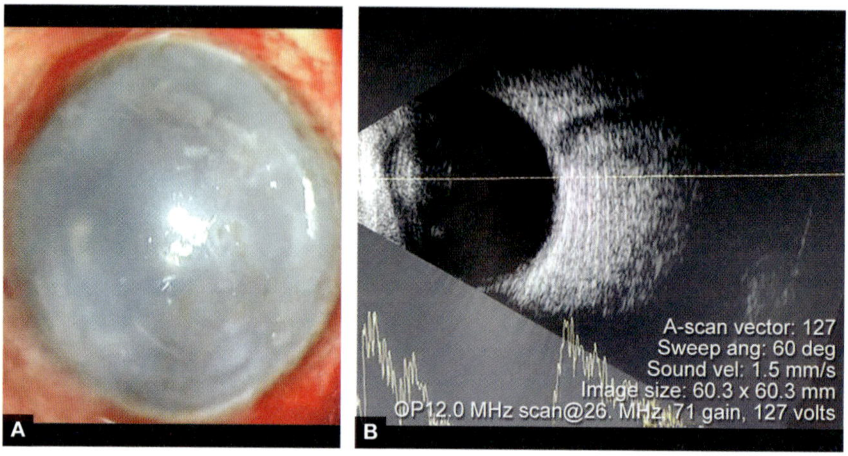

Figs. 2.1A and B: (A) Clinical picture of an eye with severe corneal edema hindering fundus examination; and (B) Ultrasound examination for evaluation of posterior segment.

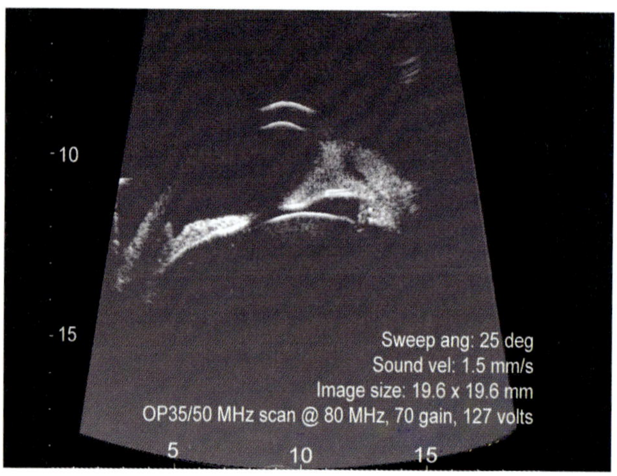

Fig. 2.2: Ultrasound biomicroscopy in an eye with iridocorneal endothelial syndrome showing peripheral anterior synechiae.

Retinopathy Study (ETDRS) chart for distance vision and times Roman or J-type near acuity charts for near vision by can be used. Visual acuity not correlating with the corneal opacity has to be confirmed by pinhole visual acuity, potential acuity meter, laser interferometry, or retinal acuity meter. In cases, where visualization of posterior segment is difficult because of corneal edema or scarring, patients should be tested for four-quadrant light projection; thus denoting bedside analysis of retinal and optic nerve function. Ancillary investigations such as B scan can be used for posterior segment (Figs. 2.1A and B) and ultrasound biomicroscopy (Fig. 2.2) for anterior

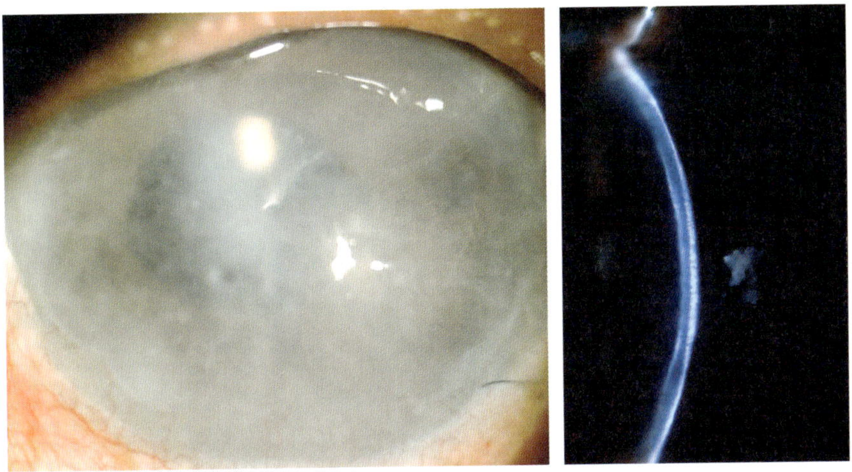

Fig. 2.3: Slit lamp examination of preoperative status of an eye with corneal endothelial decompensation.

segment in cases of hazy cornea. Optical coherence tomography of macula or optic nerve and electrophysiological studies may also be required to evaluate the visual potential of eye.

Slit Lamp Biomicroscopy

A careful slit lamp examination is required as a preliminary assessment for all eyes undergoing EK. Corneal opacity grade, corneal thickness, level of scar, nature of epithelium (presence of bullae, hypertrophy, microvesicles, edema), subepithelial scar, and epithelial defect have to be noted (Fig. 2.3). Staining can be done in specific cases if required. Anterior chamber (depth, inflammation if present), pupil reaction, and lens status (phakic or pseudophakic) should be observed and has to be noted in the case file. In pseudophakic eyes, one has to look for the centeration of intraocular lens (IOL), tilt, capsule defect, pseudophacodonesis, and synechiae. The IOL-related (Fig. 2.4) complications (malpositioned IOL, tilted IOL) and pupil damage had to be corrected in the same sitting or prior to EK procedure. Examination of the fellow eye has to be performed without fail in all eyes with unilateral involvement. It can give clues like early guttata, or other dystrophic changes. Thus, slit lamp examination has to be performed meticulously not only to evaluate the existing primary corneal pathology but also to identify the etiology.

Adnexa Examination

Attention should be paid to the regularity of lid margins, position of lids, adequacy of lid closure, and blink rate. Lid abnormalities such as trichiasis,

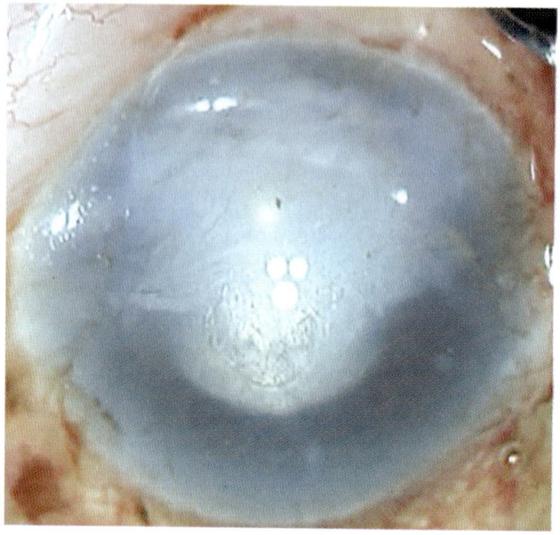

Fig. 2.4: Preoperative image of an eye showing decompensated cornea and malpositioned intraocular lens.

lagophthalmos, entropion, and ectropion should be corrected prior to the surgery. Globe position and extraocular movements should also be assessed in preliminary examination. Lacrimal system obstruction has to be checked in all eyes before surgery by examining the sac region, looking for regurgitation from sac on pressing the sac region, punctum status, and syringing. Any preexisting nasolacrimal duct obstruction has to be treated by appropriate procedure like dacryocystorhinostomy before EK.

Tear Film

Diminished tear production and dry eye may predispose to ocular surface problems and prevent normal epithelial growth postoperatively. Schirmer 1 and 2, tear film breakup time, and tear meniscus examination can help in tear film analysis. An intact trigeminal and facial nerve is necessary for ensuring adequate corneal protection and lid closure.

Intraocular Pressure

Eyes after any keratoplasty will require prolonged topical steroids. Therefore, one has to rule out any predisposition conditions for rise in intraocular pressure (IOP) or glaucoma prior to surgery. This will let the surgeon inform the patients about the surgical outcomes and risks. Goldmann applanation tonometer is the standard method in IOP evaluation. Any eyes with ocular hypertension have to be evaluated for glaucoma. Additional evaluation like gonioscopy and visual field analysis has to be performed in specific cases. Optimization of IOP is a prerequisite before surgery.

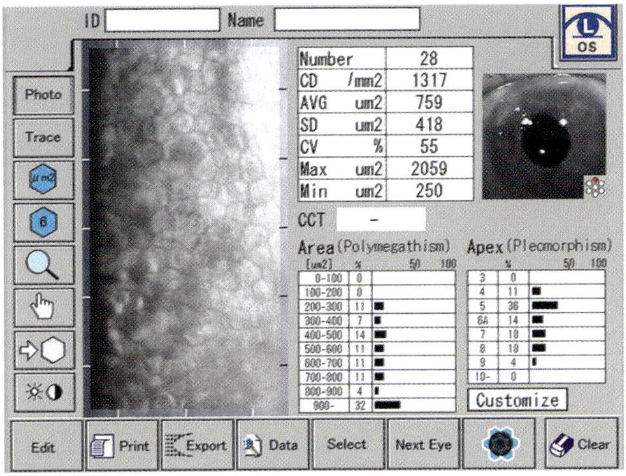

Fig. 2.5: Specular microscopy showing polymegathism.

Control of Inflammation

Patients with previous uveitis have the risk of recurrent inflammation after EK. Especially with autoimmune conditions like rheumatoid arthritis or systemic collagen diseases; there is added risk for ocular inflammation. The anterior chamber cellular grading may be hindered in the patients with coexisting corneal haze and uveitis. Hence one can use optical coherence tomography to assess the cellular reaction in such eyes.[12] Preexisting inflammation should be controlled before surgery with adequate steroids. Preliminary treatment with topical steroids prior to surgery improves outcome in eyes that are chronically inflamed.

Ancillary Investigations

- *Specular microscopy*: Specular microscopy is helpful in confirming the morphological changes of endothelium. It provides endothelial cell count, presence of polymorphism or polymegathism (Fig. 2.5), and as well as takes a photographic record. Wide-field specular microscopy can be performed throughout the entire cornea thus allowing the study of regional variability.
- *Confocal microscopy*: Confocal microscopy is used to study individual cell layers of cornea even in cases with edema and scarring. It provides more spatial resolution and magnification of image.
- *Anterior segment optical coherence tomography*: This is a noncontact imaging device that can provide intrinsic details of the corneal layers. It provides analysis of endothelial guttate changes, integrity of Descemet's membrane endothelial complex (Fig. 2.6), depth and size of scars or

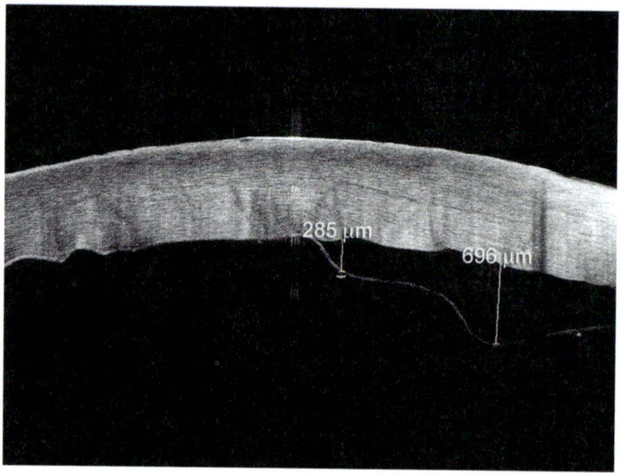

Fig. 2.6: Spectral domain optical coherence tomography showing detached Descemet's membrane and endothelial complex.

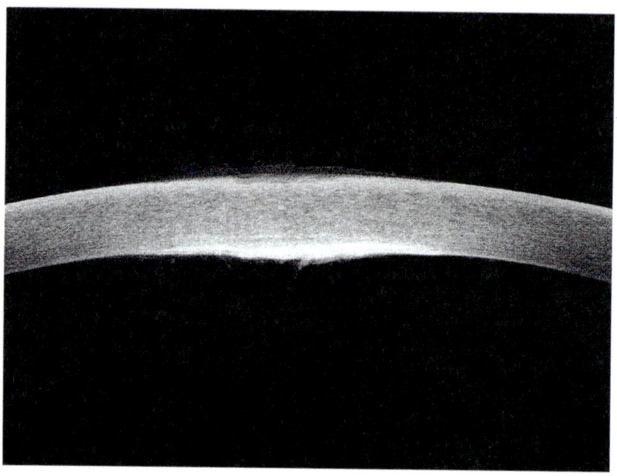

Fig. 2.7: Spectral domain optical coherence tomography showing dense Descemet's membrane scar.

opacity (Fig. 2.7), and is also useful in assessing presence of corneal bullae or edema.

- *Corneal pachymetry*: Pachymetry measures the corneal thickness, which is a sensitive indicator of endothelial physiology. Normal cornea has an average central corneal thickness of about 530–540 μm. Folds in Descemet's membrane are first seen when corneal thickness increases by 10%. Pachymetry can be measured by ultrasound method or by optical coherence tomography.

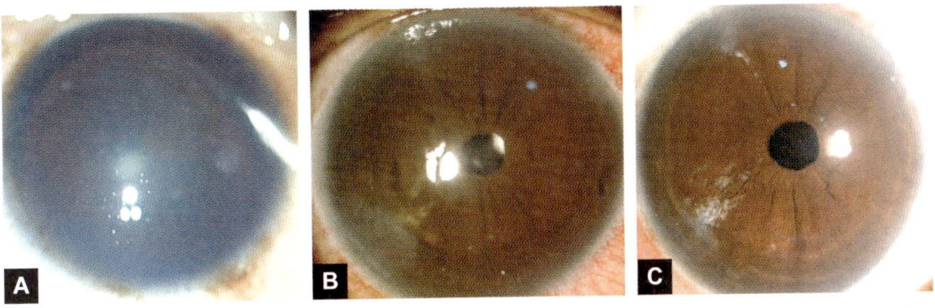

Figs. 2.8A to C: (A) Serial photograph showing clinical improvement from preoperative Fuchs dystrophy (PDEK phaco and IOL done) to postoperative period; (B) 1 month; and (C) 6 months (vision 20/20).

- *Clinical photography*: Serial clinical photography of the cornea may add additional information for the surgeon in planning for management and follow-up (Figs. 2.8A to C). Improvement of corneal clarity from preoperative to postoperative period, preoperative scar status, postoperative epithelial toxicity, and progression or regression of neovascularization can be documented.
- *Conjunctival microbial swab*: Conjunctival microbial analysis is required in an eye which has shown previous recurrent conjunctival infection or inflammation. Especially in one-eyed patients it is mandatory before ocular surgery. If the conjunctival fornix swab is noted to have bacterial growth, it has to be treated with appropriate antibiotics and rechecked after 3 days. EK can be performed only after the swab becomes negative for growth. Patients with prior nasolacrimal duct obstruction and those with fellow eye prosthesis are the other candidates who will require preoperative conjunctival swab analysis.
- *Corneal topography and aberrometry*: Corneal topography will be required in some eyes with coexisting thinning and especially for academic reasons if the surgeon wants to follow-up the corneal topography post-surgery.[13] Corneal haze will hinder aberrometry analysis in majority of patients preoperatively; however postoperatively aberration profiles can be documented and assessed for research purpose.
- *Biometry*: Ocular biometry including IOL power calculation details (Fig. 2.9) are required in all eyes undergoing EK or for that matter any keratoplasty. The simple reason is that whenever there is intraoperative requirement of exchange of IOL, the IOL power calculations have to be there for the surgeon to use it.
- *Donor graft assessment*: Donor cornea evaluation is the important preoperative assessment in EK. Slit lamp examination for grading of corneal status (epithelium, stroma, endothelium) and endothelial cell count to assess the viability of the cornea for EK has to be determined before

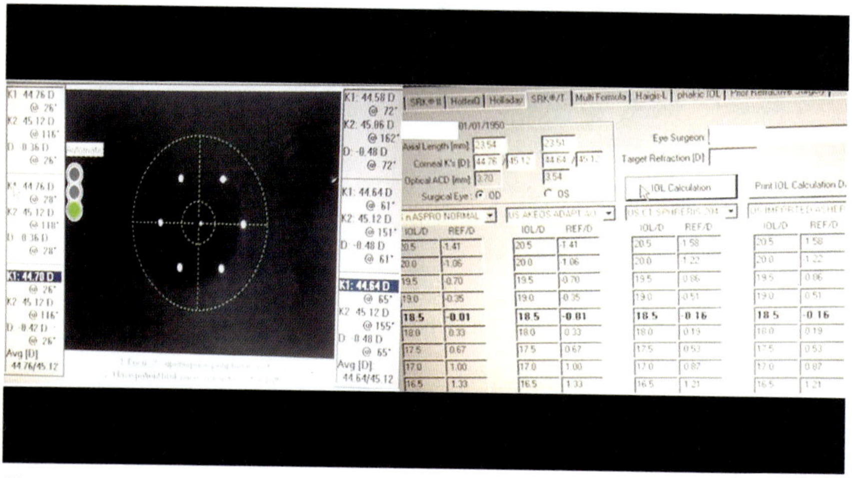

Fig. 2.9: Ocular biometry being performed for intraocular lens power calculation.

surgery. Endothelial cell count more than 2,500 cells/sq. mm can be utilized for EK procedures. Culture and microbial analysis of the donor graft is required in all cases to confirm the absence of infective source before transplantation. Donor corneas with preexisting Descemet's fold, damaged endothelium, and scar are not ideal for EK.

General Medical Evaluation

Medical evaluation by a physician is required to assess the patient's anesthetic risks and stabilization of the any medical conditions is necessary if general anesthesia is planned. Systemic morbid conditions like diabetes, hypertension, and other ailments need to be managed before corneal surgery. Patients on blood thinning drugs require few days of clearance before surgery. For repeat grafts requiring systemic immunosuppression, one should exclude the diseases that contraindicate its use such as active infection, tuberculosis, and viral hepatitis.

SUMMARY

The objective of any keratoplasty is to provide the best visual potential and less postoperative complications to the patient. Unless the initial assessments are meticulously performed in terms of correct diagnosis, proper control of comorbid ocular pathology, and ideal selection of procedure, the postoperative outcome becomes affected. Therefore, the clinical history, routine examination, and appropriate ancillary tests in specific patients are vital in good preoperative evaluation to provide the desired functional and anatomical results.

REFERENCES

1. Fuest M, Ang M, Htoon HM, et al. Long-term visual outcomes comparing Descemet stripping automated endothelial keratoplasty and penetrating keratoplasty. Am J Ophthalmol. 2017. pii: S0002-9394(17)30309-4.
2. Price MO, Gupta P, Lass J, et al. EK (DLEK, DSEK, DMEK): New frontier in cornea surgery. Annu Rev Vis Sci. 2017. [Epub ahead of print]
3. Singh A, Zarei-Ghanavati M, Avadhanam V, et al. Systematic review and meta-analysis of clinical outcomes of Descemet membrane endothelial keratoplasty versus Descemet stripping endothelial keratoplasty/Descemet stripping automated endothelial keratoplasty. Cornea. 2017. [Epub ahead of print]
4. O'Brien PD, Lake DB, Saw VP, et al. Endothelial keratoplasty: case selection in the learning curve. Cornea. 2008;27(10):1114-8.
5. Price FW, Price MO. Descemet's stripping with endothelial keratoplasty in 50 eyes: a refractive neutral corneal transplant. J Refract Surg. 2005;21(4):339-45.
6. Engelmann K, Bednarz J, Valtink M. Prospects for endothelial transplantation. Exp Eye Res. 2004;78(3):573-8.
7. Hosny MH, Marrie A, Karim Sidky M, et al. Results of femtosecond laser-assisted Descemet stripping automated endothelial keratoplasty. J Ophthalmol. 2017;2017:8984367.
8. Nahum Y, Mimouni M, Madi S, et al. Visual Outcomes of repeat versus primary Descemet stripping automated endothelial keratoplasty: a paired comparison. Cornea. 2016;35(5):592-5.
9. Busin M, Madi S, Santorum P, et al. Ultrathin Descemet's stripping automated endothelial keratoplasty with the microkeratome double-pass technique: two-year outcomes. Ophthalmology. 2013;120(6):1186-94.
10. Jardine GJ, Holiman JD, Galloway JD, et al. Eye bank-prepared femtosecond laser-assisted automated Descemet membrane endothelial grafts. Cornea. 2015;34(7):838-43.
11. Agarwal A, Dua HS, Narang P, et al. Pre-Descemet's endothelial keratoplasty (PDEK). Br J Ophthalmol. 2014;98(9):1181-5.
12. Agarwal A, Ashokkumar D, Jacob S, et al. High-speed optical coherence tomography for imaging anterior chamber inflammatory reaction in uveitis: clinical correlation and grading. Am J Ophthalmol. 2009;147(3):413-6.e3.
13. Gupta R, Kinderyte R, Jacobs DS, et al. Elimination of anterior corneal steepening with Descemet membrane endothelial keratoplasty in a patient with Fuchs dystrophy and keratoconus: implications for IOL calculation. Cornea. 2017;36(10):1260-2.

CHAPTER 3

Classification of Descemet's Membrane Detachment

Soosan Jacob, Amar Agarwal

INTRODUCTION

Corneal damage could be secondary to various surgeries, vitreous loss, manipulations by the surgeon, difficult and prolonged surgery or even following minimal manipulations in a patient with low endothelial counts to start with.[1-32]

DESCEMET'S MEMBRANE DETACHMENT

Descemet's membrane (DM) detachment is a complication occasionally faced after surgery.[7,8] It has been treated by various means including observation,[9] viscoelastic injection,[10] air injection, the use of long-acting intracameral gas,[11,12] and insertion of transcorneal mattress sutures.[13] A detached Descemet's membrane can be diagnosed on slit-lamp examination as a clear optical space between the stroma and the Descemet's membrane.

During surgery, trypan blue can be used to stain the DM. Excess dye is washed away and the AC is irrigated to study DM motility and its clinical characteristics (Fig. 3.1). An air bubble is then injected to appose the Descemet's membrane to the corneal stroma. Gases, such as sulfur hexafluoride (SF_6) or perfluoropropane (C_3F_8), can also be used in more severe or long-standing cases.

NEW CLASSIFICATION OF DESCEMET'S MEMBRANE DETACHMENT

Based on pathological features, Descemet's membrane detachment had been classified in 1928 by Samuels as active (pushed back), or passive (pulled back and torn away), due to difference in elasticity between the parenchyma and the glass membrane.[6] Samuels also stated that this classification was more relevant pathologically and no great importance could be ascribed to these forms of detachment from the surgical standpoint. Descemet's membrane detachment has also been previously classified as planar (<1 mm gap between Descemet's membrane and stroma) or nonplanar (>1 mm gap between Descemet's membrane and stroma) based on morphology.[7]

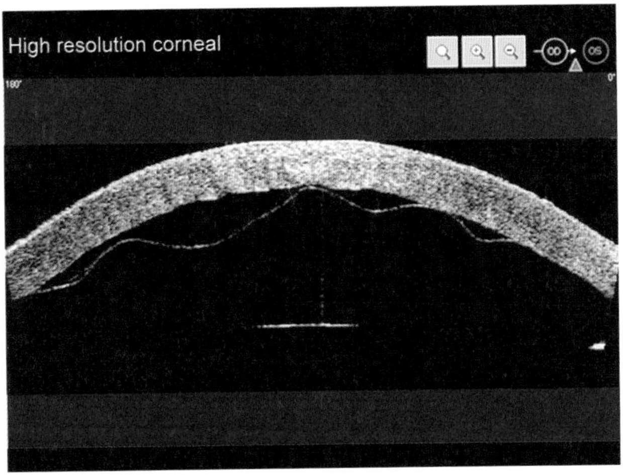

Fig. 3.1: A stripped Descemet's membrane is seen on ASOCT. It typically lies loose, floating free in the anterior chamber.

Dr Soosan Jacob proposed a new classification of Descemet's membrane detachment based on the clinicomorphological, etiological, tomographic, and intraoperative features, and also a new treatment algorithm for Descemet's membrane detachment based on its classification. This classification of Descemet's membrane detachment is analogous to the classification of retinal detachment. The Descemet's membrane is a vital layer of the cornea and is necessary for maintaining the clarity of the cornea, just as the neurosensory retina is required for visual perception. As a retinal detachment can be rhegmatogenous retinal detachment [RRD (secondary to hole, tear, or dialysis)], tractional retinal detachment (TRD), or bullous/exudative retinal detachment, Descemet's membrane detachment can also be clasisfied as rhegmatogenous Descemet's detachment (RDD), tractional Descemet's detachment (TDD), bullous Descemet's detachment (BDD), or complex Descemet's detachment (CDD) (Table 3.1).

An RDD generally occurs as an intraoperative event when there is a break in the Descemet's membrane, with fluid accumulation between the Descemet's membrane and overlying stroma. Analogous to an RRD, an RDD can be secondary to a hole (e.g. a double anterior chamber following perforation during deep anterior lamellar keratoplasty) or a tear (e.g. Descemet's membrane detachment occurring during insertion of blunt instruments or IOL implantation during phacoemulsification). RDD can also occur secondary to a dialysis of the Descemet's membrane from its attachment at the Schwalbe's line, a complication that is sometimes seen during trabeculotomy, insertion of instruments at the limbus, uncontrolled DM stripping during Descemet Membrane Endothelial Keratoplasty (DMEK) etc.

Table 3.1: Differentiating features of types of Descemet's membrane detachments.

	Rhegmatogenous Descemet's detachment (RDD)	*Tractional Descemet's detachment (TDD)*	*Bullous Descemet's detachment (BDD)*	*Complex Descemet's detachment*
Onset	Occurs during surgery	Postoperative	During surgery, postoperative or secondary to disease process	Intra- or postoperative
History	History of surgery	History of inflammation/ trauma/ surgery	History of surgery or history specific to underlying etiology	Generally history of surgery
Cause	Tear, hole or dialysis	Incarcerated DM	Intraoperative complication, e.g. blood or accidental injection of viscoelastic/ disease process, infection or inflammation	Poorly positioned DMEK graft Combination of other Descemet's detachments (DDs)
Clinical findings	Undulating membrane freely floating in AC with folds	Stretched out DM between points of attachment No folds	Slightly convex/ bulging membrane seen in the AC with no break	Complex configurations or combination features of others
Anterior segment OCT	Undulating linear hyper-reflective signal in the AC	Straight taut linear hyper-reflective signal between two points of attachment	Convex hyper-reflective signal bulging into AC from overlying stroma	Complex configurations or combination features of others
Prognosis	Good if residual endothelial function adequate	Good if residual endothelial function adequate	Prognosis depending on cause	Depending on cause

The Descemet's membrane may also become detached secondary to an inflammatory/fibrotic process, resulting in TDD. This could be secondary to incarceration of the Descemet's membrane in an inflammatory process (e.g. in peripheral anterior synechiae or within the graft host junction in large diameter grafts) or secondary to incarceration in a wound or suture with subsequent contraction, resulting in a TDD. A long-standing RDD could also sometimes adhere to intraocular contents with secondary fibrosis, thus becoming a TDD. A BDD can occur secondary to accidental hydroseparation of the DM from the overlying stroma during stromal hydration of paracentesis. This is more likely to occur if the cannula is unintentionally placed too posteriorly. It may also more rarely occur secondary to a disease process, such as posterior corneal abscess, tumor, infection, or inflammation (analogous to bullous retinal detachment). In this type of Descemet's membrane detachment, a separation and convex bulging of the Descemet's membrane into the anterior chamber occurs in the absence of a break in the Descemet's membrane. The space in between the stroma and the Descemet's membrane is filled with fluid, pus, exudates, viscoelastic, or air, depending on the cause of BDD. This configuration of Descemet's membrane can also be seen as part of the Anwar's big bubble technique in deep anterior lamellar keratoplasty, which detaches the Descemet's membrane from the stroma and sometimes occurs from accidental injection of viscoelastic into the pre-Descemetic space. Clinically, an RDD is usually seen as an undulating membrane lying loose in the anterior chamber. It may also be scrolled or crumpled, depending on the extent of detachment. It has folds and is mobile, similar to an RRD. On the other hand, a TDD is stretched out tight, like a trampoline, between the points of attachment. It has no folds and is not mobile. A BDD is seen as a convex membrane bulging into the anterior chamber, similar to a bullous retinal detachment. A CDD shows complex folds or scrolls or shows combination features of others and can be seen sometimes in a poorly attached DMEK graft.

ANTERIOR SEGMENT OPTICAL COHERENCE TOMOGRAPHY FEATURES

Overlying corneal epithelial and stromal edema makes visualization difficult in the presence of DM detachment. Anterior segment optical coherence tomography (ASOCT) is therefore immensely useful for diagnosis, as well as differentiating between various types of DM detachment. An RDD is seen as an undulating linear hyper-reflective signal in the anterior chamber, whereas a TDD is seen as a straight, taut linear signal between two points of attachment (Fig. 3.2). In TDD, the arc length of the cornea, if measured, is found to be more than the length of the detached Descemet's membrane, unlike in RDD, where the arc length of the overlying corneal stroma is similar to the length

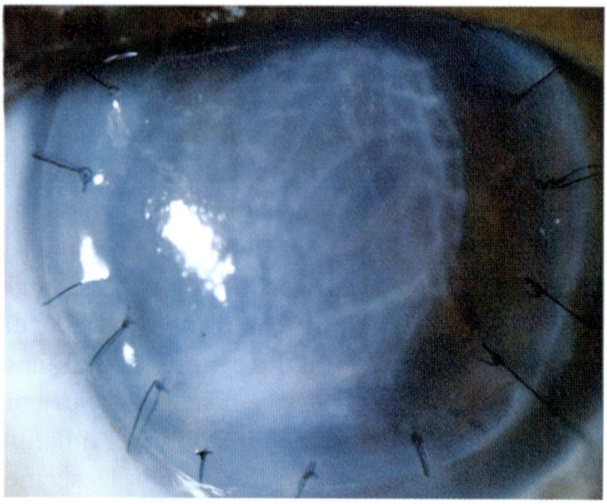

Fig. 3.2: A localized DD seen in eye with corneal graft.

of the detached Descemet's membrane. A BDD is seen as a convex, hyperreflective signal bulging into the anterior chamber from the overlying stroma, with the space in between filled with fluid exudate, pus, or air, depending on the cause of Descemet's membrane detachment. A CDD shows complex configurations on anterior segment OCT.

RELAXING DESCEMETOTOMY

Relaxing retinotomy is used in vitreoretinal surgery for treating periretinal traction and retinal foreshortening that does not allow the retina to settle down. Similar traction on the DM secondary to inflammation or fibrosis or the Descemet's membrane becoming incarcerated in a wound or suture leading to a TDD may not respond to the classic management strategies for Descemet's membrane detachment. Injecting air or long-acting gas into the anterior chamber in an eye with TDD will not appose it to the corneal stroma because of the foreshortening.[33] Similarly in BDD, pneumdescemetopexy cannot drain the supra-Descemetic fluid as there is no break in the DM for the fluid to escape out completely through. An ab externo relaxing descemetotomy may be done for BDD secondary to hydroseparation following stromal hydration. This is done simply by making a keratome entry at the limbus that goes past the BDD and also creates an incision on the DM thus providing an exit wound to allow fluid drainage. Ab externo and ab interno relaxing Descemetotomy techniques have been described by Dr Jacob.

TREATMENT FOR DESCEMET'S MEMBRANE DETACHMENT BASED ON CLASSIFICATION

The treatment of the aforementioned conditions also differs from each other. Although both RDD and TDD require internal gas tamponade or pneumodescemetopexy and supra Descemet's fluid drainage, TDD also requires an incision to be made on the taut DM to allow it to settle onto the stroma. Prior to performing this, however, the condition of the endothelium must be assessed as reattachment may not occur in all cases, depending on the extent of damage to the endothelium. In such cases, the patient may require a posterior lamellar or full-thickness graft instead. Therefore, in very fibrotic, opaque or thickened RDD, an endothelial keratoplasty may be preferred. If however, relaxing Descemetotomy is opted for this can be done by ab interno relaxing descemetotomy incisions.[33] Supra-Descemet's fluid drainage is carried out by injecting air or gas from the side opposite to the tear (internal drainage) or, in some cases, by making a small stab incision in the cornea overlying the Descemet's membrane detachment to drain the fluid externally. Ab interno relaxing Descemetotomy may also be carried out for BDD that is not close to the limbus.

Ab interno relaxing descemetotomy may be performed with an anterior chamber manitainer connected to pressurized air inserted into the AC. The tip of a 26-gauge needle is bent in the reverse direction to a capsulotomy needle, and is introduced into the anterior chamber to make the relaxing descemetotomy incisions (Figs. 3.3A and B). The extent of the incision is determined during surgery by assessing the degree of foreshortening that still remains. If foreshortening is not completely relieved, the incisions are further extended until the Descemet's membrane is able to lie fully apposed against the stroma. These incisions are made in the peripheral cornea avoiding the visual axis. Postoperative tamponade with either air or nonexpansile concentration of C_3F_8 (14%) or SF_6 (12%) is administered with face-up positioning of the patient for 1 hour. Ab externo relaxing Descemetotomy for accidental hydroseparation secondary to stromal hydration has been discussed earlier.

The term *descemetotomy* was first used by Loewenstein in 1993.[21-24] It was used with reference to a procedure where the neodymium-doped yttrium aluminum garnet (Nd:YAG) laser was used in the postoperative period to perform descemetotomy in order to create communication between the anterior chamber and the supernumerary chamber after intentionally retaining the Descemet's membrane during keratoplasty for bullous keratopathy. The authors of those studies found that the membrane was resistant to Nd:YAG laser and required the use of high-energy levels and multiple pulses. Steinemann et al.[25] and Masket et al.[26] also used the Nd:YAG laser to create a central opening in inadvertently retained opacified host Descemet's membrane after penetrating keratoplasty. Chen et al.[27] surgically removed a similarly retained host Descemet's membrane after keratoplasty.

The authors had previously used the term *iatrogenic descemetorhexis*[14] for a case where accidental descemetorhexis occurred in a patient during phacoemulsification. A similar case was also reported by Pan and Au Eong.[15]

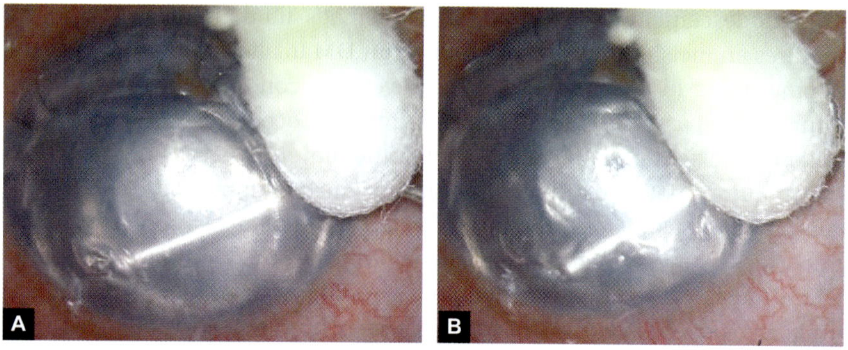

Figs. 3.3A and B: Ab interno relaxing Descemetotomy incisions are made for a taut Descemet's detachment following a corneal tear repair.

Descemetorhexis has been described as part of endothelial keratoplasty procedures, where the central Descemet's membrane is intentionally removed from the host cornea.[28-32] The term *relaxing descemetotomy* differs from these in describing a therapeutic procedure that creates an exit route for supra-Descemetic fluid in BDD or relieves the traction forces and decreases foreshortening of the Descemet's membrane in a procedure similar to that of relaxing retinotomy in RDD. The tautness of the Descemet's membrane is relieved, and an air or gas bubble is able to appose the now lax Descemet's membrane against the overlying corneal stroma.[11,12]

REFERENCES

1. Machemer R. Cutting of the retina: a means of therapy for retinal reattachment. Klin Monbl Augenheilkd. 1979;175(5):597-601.
2. Machemer R. Retinotomy. Am J Ophthalmol. 1981;92(6):768-74.
3. Machemer R, McCuen BW, de Juan E. Relaxing retinotomies and retinectomies. Am J Ophthalmol. 1986;102:7-12.
4. Alturki WA, Peyman GA, Paris CL, et al. Posterior relaxing retinotomies (analysis of anatomic and visual results). Ophthalmic Surg. 1992;23:685-8.
5. Bovey EH, de Juan E, Gonvers M. Retinotomies of 180 degrees or more. Retina. 1995;15:394-8.
6. Samuels B. Detachment of Descemet's membrane. Trans Am Ophthalmol Soc. 1928;26:427-37.
7. Mackool RJ, Holtz SJ. Descemet membrane detachment. Arch Ophthalmol. 1977;95:459-63.
8. Kim T, Sorenson A. Bilateral Descemet membrane detachments. Arch Ophthalmol. 2000;118:1302-3.
9. Minkovitz JB, Schrenk LC, Pepose JS. Spontaneous resolution of an extensive detachment of Descemet membrane following phacoemulsification. Arch Ophthalmol. 1994;112:551-2.
10. Hoover DL, Giangiacomo J, Benson RL. Descemet membrane detachment by sodium hyaluronate. Arch Ophthalmol. 1985;103:805-8.

11. Zusman NB, Waring GO III, Najarian LV, et al. Sulfur hexafluoride gas in the repair of intractable Descemet's membrane detachment. Am J Ophthalmol. 1987;104:660-2.
12. Kim T, Hasan SA. A new technique for repairing Descemet membrane detachments using intracameral gas injection. Arch Ophthalmol. 2002;120:181-3.
13. Amaral CE, Palay DA. Technique for repair of Descemet's membrane detachment. Am J Ophthalmol. 1999;127:88-90.
14. Agarwal A, Jacob S, Agarwal A, et al. Iatrogenic descemetorhexis as a complication of phacoemulsification. J Cataract Refract Surg. 2006;32(5):895-7.
15. Pan JC, Au Eong KG. Spontaneous resolution of corneal oedema after inadvertent 'descemetorhexis' during cataract surgery. Clin Exp Ophthalmol. 2006; 34(9):896-7.
16. Dirisamer M, Dapena I, Ham L, et al. Patterns of corneal endothelialization and corneal clearance after Descemet membrane endothelial keratoplasty for Fuchs endothelial dystrophy. Am J Ophthalmol. 2011;152(4):543-55.e1.
17. Jacobi C, Zhivov A, Korbmacher J, et al. Evidence of endothelial cell migration after Descemet membrane endothelial keratoplasty. Am J Ophthalmol. 2011;152(4):537-42.e2.
18. Balachandran C, Ham L, Verschoor CA, et al. Spontaneous corneal clearance despite graft detachment in Descemet membrane endothelial keratoplasty. Am J Ophthalmol. 2009;148(2):227-34.
19. Stewart RM, Hiscott PS, Kaye SB. Endothelial migration and new Descemet membrane after endothelial keratoplasty. Am J Ophthalmol. 2010;149(4):683-4.
20. Cursiefen C, Kruse FE. DMEK: Descemet membrane endothelial keratoplasty. Ophthalmologe. 2010;107(4):370-6.
21. Lazar M, Loewenstein A, Geyer O. Intentional retention of Descemet's membrane during keratoplasty. Acta Ophthalmol (Copenh). 1991;69:111-2.
22. Loewenstein A, Geyer O, Lazar M. Intentional retention of Descemet's membrane in keratoplasty for the surgical treatment of bullous keratopathy. Acta Ophthalmol (Copenh). 1993;71:280-2.
23. Loewenstein A, Lazar M. Deep lamellar keratoplasty in the treatment of bullous keratopathy. Br J Ophthalmol. 1993;77:538.
24. Loewenstein A, Geyer O, Lazar M. Descemetotomy. J Cataract Refract Surg. 1996;22(6):652.
25. Steinemann TL, Henry K, Brown MF. Nd:YAG laser treatment of retained Descemet's membrane after penetrating keratoplasty. Ophthalmic Surg. 1995;26(1):80-1.
26. Masket S, Tennen DG. Neodymium:YAG laser optical opening for retained Descemet's membrane after penetrating keratoplasty. J Cataract Refract Surg. 1996;22(1):139-41.
27. Chen YP, Lai PC, Chen PY, et al. Retained Descemet's membrane after penetrating keratoplasty. J Cataract Refract Surg. 2003;29(9):1842-4.
28. Dapena I, Ham L, Moutsouris K, et al. Incidence of recipient Descemet membrane remnants at the donor-to-stromal interface after descemetorhexis in endothelial keratoplasty. Br J Ophthalmol. 2010;94(12):1689-90.
29. Mehta JS, Hantera MM, Tan DT. Modified air-assisted descemetorhexis for Descemet-stripping automated endothelial keratoplasty. J Cataract Refract Surg. 2008;34(6):889-91.
30. Wylegała E, Tarnawska D, Dobrowolski D, et al. Outcomes of endothelial keratoplasty with descemetorhexis (DSEK). Klin Oczna. 2007;109(7-9):287-91.

31. Bradley JC, McCartney DL, Busin M, et al. Donor corneal disk insertion techniques in descemetorhexis with endokeratoplasty. Ann Ophthalmol (Skokie). 2007;39(4):277-83.
32. Nieuwendaal CP, Lapid-Gortzak R, van der Meulen IJ, et al. Posterior lamellar keratoplasty using descemetorhexis and organ-cultured donor corneal tissue (Melles technique). Cornea. 2006;25(8):933-6.
33. Jacob S, Agarwal A, Agarwal A, Saijimol AI. Recognizing and managing bullous Descemet's detachment secondary to accidental hydroseparation during phacoemulsification/cataract surgery by relaxing descemetotomy. Cornea. 2017 (In press).

CHAPTER 4

Keratoplasty Techniques for Corneal Endothelial Disease: A Comparison of Procedures

Rahul Tonk, Carolina Mercado, Ibrahim Osama, Carol L Karp

INTRODUCTION AND HISTORICAL BACKGROUND

Franz Reisinger is credited as having first conceived of keratoplasty in 1818 as the use of living corneal tissue for transplantation.[1,2] Early experiments on this concept in rabbits, chickens, and doves produced variable results. Nonetheless, these experiments did help outline the basic principles for keratoplasty surgery, including the need for similar size and shape of the donor and recipient tissues, rapid transfer of donor tissue to host, attachment of donor tissue in an atraumatic fashion, and preservation of intraocular contents.

Interest in keratoplasty resurged in the late 1800s after Arthur von Hippel performed the first successful human corneal transplant of a full-thickness rabbit cornea into a human recipient corneal lamellar bed in 1886.[3] Lamellar keratoplasty of this kind was promoted by von Hippel and his contemporaries, Dürr and Fox, who theorized it would portend a greater chance of graft survival with a lower risk of complications.[2]

Two decades later, in 1905, Eduard Zirm performed the first successful human-to-human penetrating keratoplasty (PK).[4] While this proof-of-concept work refocused attention on full-thickness corneal transplantation, it remained a procedure of last resort until the mid-20th century, whereupon advances in surgical instrumentation (including microscopes and suture), tissue preservation, and anti-inflammatory agents helped give rise to the modern era of keratoplasty.[5]

In the second half of the 20th century, PK became the dominant corneal transplantation procedure due in large part to the issues of interface haze, scarring, and epithelial ingrowth associated with nascent lamellar transplantation.[6] Nevertheless, the limitations of PK with respect to long recovery, immunogenicity, astigmatism, and impaired integrity of the host cornea soon became apparent. These realizations, along with further advances in surgical techniques and instrumentation, led to a renewed interest in selective keratoplasty: targeting different layers of the cornea for transplantation.

Barraquer and Tillett first proposed posterior lamellar keratoplasty (PLK) in the 1950s as selective replacement of the corneal endothelium for the treatment of corneal edema.[7,8] In their original approach, an anterior corneal flap was created, the posterior cornea was replaced in a partial thickness fashion, and the corneal flap was repositioned with suture fixation. In 1999, Melles and colleagues modified PLK with the use of a posterior approach.[9] This consisted of a deep, manual excision of the posterior host stroma and endothelium using curved instruments, insertion of a matching donor lenticule, and injection of air to press the donor button against the overlying recipient bed. Terry popularized a modification of this procedure in the United States as deep lamellar endothelial keratoplasty (DLEK).[10]

While PLK and DLEK were successful procedures, the manual stromal dissections were time consuming, required heightened technical skill, and resulted in optical distortions in the deep stromal interface that limited final visual acuity.[11-13] These findings prompted further modification and refinement of techniques for endothelial keratoplasty (EK), and ultimately gave rise to the techniques described below: Descemet's stripping endothelial keratoplasty (DSEK), Descemet's membrane endothelial keratoplasty (DMEK), and, most recently, pre-Descemet's endothelial keratoplasty (PDEK).

PENETRATING KERATOPLASTY

Penetrating keratoplasty is a transplant procedure in which full-thickness host corneal tissue is replaced with donor corneal tissue. This surgery enjoys surgeon familiarity and a sound success rate—defined as grafts remaining clear at 1 year—of over 90% in numerous series.[14,15] When performed for eyes with endothelial dysfunction, it can achieve excellent visual results. Indeed, a 2014 Cochrane review comparing PK with EK for Fuchs' endothelial dystrophy did not show any significant differences between procedures with respect to best-corrected visual acuity (BCVA) at 2 years.[16]

- Nonetheless, full-thickness transplantation can present a variety of challenges to the patient and surgeon, including:
- Lengthy postoperative course
- Incidence of allograft rejection (3–70%, depending on the indication/host milieu)[17]
- Suture complications: exposure, vascularization, and infection[18]
- Weak graft-host junction: Risk of traumatic wound dehiscence and globe rupture[19]
- Unpredictability of corneal toricity and degree of ametropia
- Corneal denervation and epithelial complications.[20]

In light of these challenges, a trend has emerged away from PK toward partial-thickness procedures, with the goal of maintaining healthy tissue and removing only diseased portions. Anterior lamellar keratoplasty, while beyond the scope of this chapter, is increasingly being performed for keratoconus, stromal dystrophies, and partial-thickness corneal scars.[21] Moreover,

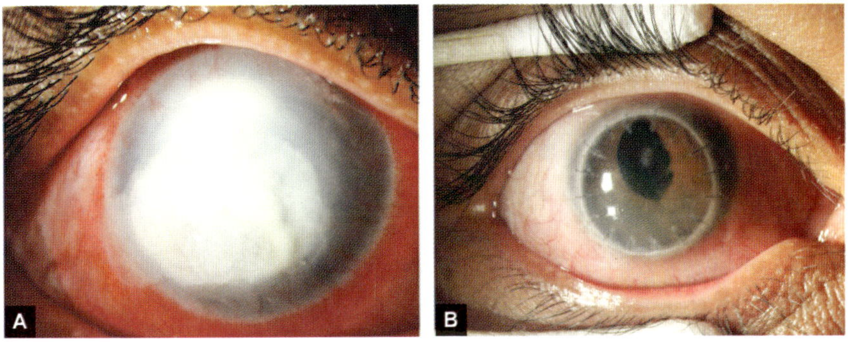

Figs. 4.1A and B: (A) A patient with severe *Fusarium* keratitis progressing to corneal perforation; (B) Four months after large-diameter penetrating keratoplasty, the patient is able to achieve a best-corrected spectacle acuity of 20/25.

EK has now supplanted PK as the procedure of choice for endothelial failure.[22-29,31] In 2015, The Eye Bank Association of America's member eye banks collectively distributed 28,394 grafts to treat endothelial failure; 81.2% of these were EK grafts and 18.8% were PK grafts.[22]

Penetrating keratoplasty may still be indicated in the following cases of corneal endothelial disease:

- Combined endothelial and stromal disease; for example, eyes with severe stromal opacity or scarring secondary to chronic bullous keratopathy,[23,24] or eyes with full-thickness infection and corneal perforation (Figs. 4.1A and B).
- Eyes with anatomy less suited for EK:
    - Poor visualization
    - Aphakia
    - Aniridia
    - Presence of intraocular hardware (glaucoma drainage implants, anterior chamber intraocular lenses, etc.)
- Patients not capable of postoperative head positioning
- Eyes with hypotony.

DESCEMET'S STRIPPING ENDOTHELIAL KERATOPLASTY

In 2004, Melles et al. proposed a modification to PLK in which manual dissection of the recipient cornea was replaced by simple stripping of Descemet's membrane and endothelium (descemetorhexis) prior to insertion of a posterior lamellar graft.[25] The new procedure became known as DSEK. Gorovoy subsequently popularized the use of a microkeratome for preparation of the donor tissue, in an adaptation that became known as Descemet's stripping automated endothelial keratoplasty (DSAEK).[26] For simplification, both procedures will heretofore be referred to as DSEK unless otherwise specified.

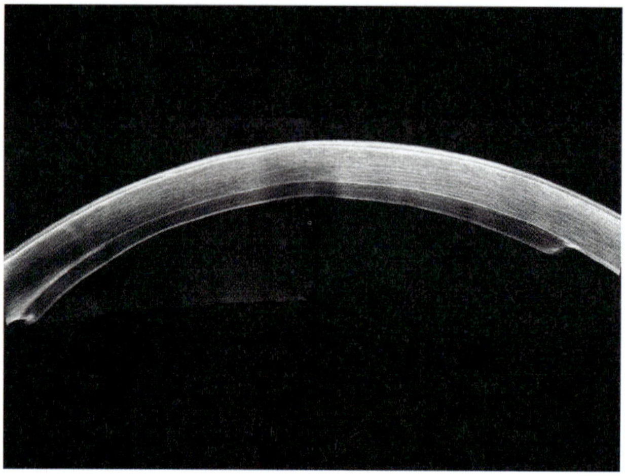

Fig. 4.2: Anterior segment optical coherence tomography showing an attached Descemet's stripping endothelial keratoplasty graft in immediate postoperative period.

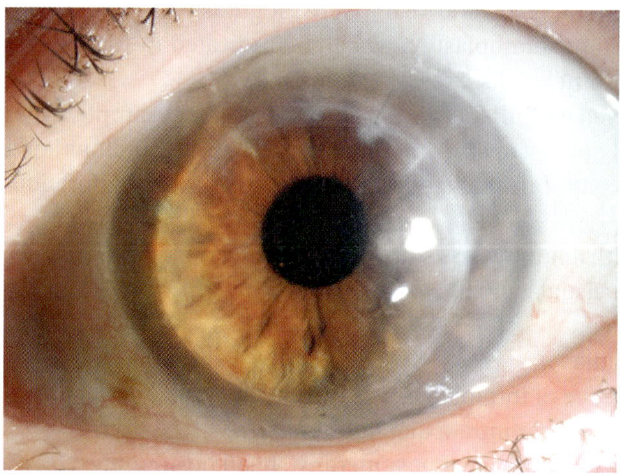

Fig. 4.3: Descemet's stripping endothelial keratoplasty graft restoring clarity to a penetrating graft which had become opaque from endothelial rejection.

In the late 2000s, Price, Chen, and Terry reported hundreds of cases of successful DSEK surgery with rapid recovery to a BCVA in the range of 20/30–20/40.[27,28] These results, combined with continued refinement of surgical technique and instrumentation, have helped EK overtake PK as the procedure of choice for visually disabling endothelial dysfunction.[29-31] This procedure can be done as a primary transplant (Fig. 4.2) or as endothelial replacement to a failed full-thickness graft (Fig. 4.3).

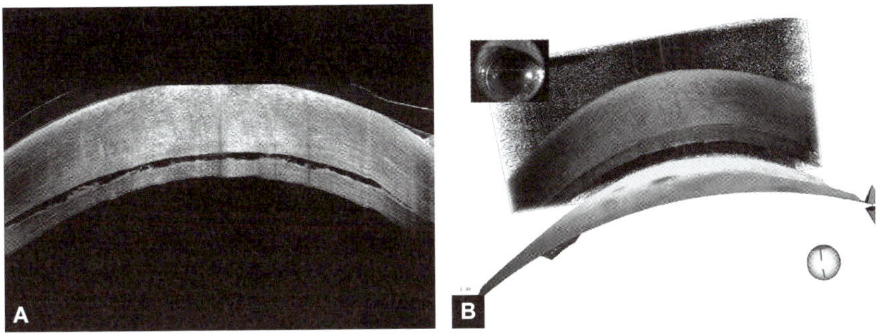

Figs. 4.4A and B: (A) Anterior segment optical coherence tomography showing shallow detachment of a Descemet's stripping endothelial keratoplasty graft in immediate post-operative period; (B) Reattachment of the graft after a rebubble procedure.

The principal advantages of DSEK over PK include:

- *Faster visual recovery*: Optimal visual outcome can be achieved in weeks to months with DSEK as compared to months to years with PK.[32]
- *Improved safety profile*: While DSEK has its own, idiosyncratic risks—such as pupillary block from the use of intracameral air—it avoids the more serious complications of open-sky corneal transplantation, including suprachoroidal hemorrhage and prolapse of intraocular contents.[33]
- *Improved postoperative refractive results*: PK can lead to unpredictable corneal topography, irregular astigmatism, and variable shifts in spherical equivalent. By comparison, DSEK induces far less topographic and refractive astigmatism, and is associated with a more predictable 0.80–1.25 diopter hyperopic shift.[28,30]
- *Decreased incidence of graft rejection*—believed to be due to decreased antigenic load.[32]
- *Retained tectonic strength of the cornea*, which can be protective in cases of globe trauma.[19,34]
- *Elimination of suture-induced complications*, such as exposure, neovascularization, and infection.[18]

DSEK's principal disadvantages include:

- *Potential dislocation of the donor corneal graft*: Incidence of this complication varies in the literature, but averaged 2–25% in large, initial case series.[26,27,35] Studies have shown that these complications occur less frequently with increasing surgical experience.[35] A number of surgical innovations, such as corneal surface massage, venting incisions, stromal roughening, and the use of intraoperative optical coherence tomography have helped to further decrease the rate of detachment to between 1% and 10%.[35-37] When needed, graft repositioning and/or rebubbling can be done, which successfully reattaches the graft in approximately 70% of cases (Figs. 4.4A and B).[35]

- *Initial endothelial cell loss*: Several initial studies of DSEK showed acute postoperative endothelial cell loss to be in the range of 24–50%, often due to traumatic pre- or intraoperative technique.[26,30,38] As with graft dislocation, studies have shown that this occurs less frequently with increasing surgical experience.[35] Long-term studies of DSEK have revealed that initial endothelial cell loss plateaus at 6–24 months, with an overall *lower* rate of endothelial cell loss in postoperative years 3–5 amongst DSEK eyes as compared with PK eyes.[32] Considerable attention has been given to improving methods of inserting the donor tissue for further reduction in intraoperative endothelial cell loss.[6]
- *Interface haze and opacification*: Visual outcomes studies of DSEK have shown that, while over 90% of patients without macular disease achieve 20/40 or better vision, only 20% are able to achieve 20/20.[27,28] Factors such as interface quality and residual recipient stromal optical impurities have been shown to have an effect on final visual outcome.[39,40]

Ultra-thin DSAEK (UT-DSAEK), a variation of DSAEK that uses donor tissue of 50–100 μm thickness as opposed to the traditional 100–200 μm thickness, has capitalized on studies showing improved visual outcomes with the use of a thinner donor lenticule.[41,42] The techniques involved for tissue preparation, insertion, and deployment are similar though somewhat more challenging than that of standard DSAEK. Initial studies demonstrate an improved visual outcome, faster visual rehabilitation, and lower immunologic rejection rate over standard DSAEK.[43]

DESCEMET'S MEMBRANE ENDOTHELIAL KERATOPLASTY

Melles et al. first performed DMEK in 2006, selectively transplanting donor Descemet's membrane and endothelial cells without the use of a stromal carrier.[44] Fundamentally, this technique involves a standard descemetorhexis, insertion of a scroll of donor tissue into the recipient anterior chamber, and unfolding and positioning of the tissue using a combination of balanced salt solution (BSS) and air. Visual outcomes from this group's first 50 DMEK cases were promising—with 75% of successful DMEK cases going on to achieve 20/25 vision or better—but there was a high regraft rate of 20% for graft dislocation or iatrogenic endothelial cell loss.[45,46] In the last several years, advances in preparation, handling, and unfolding of the delicate DMEK graft have reduced the rate of donor tissue loss and standardized the procedure for broad use among corneal surgeons.[47]

The principal advantages of DMEK over DSEK include:

- *Improved visual outcomes*: Multiple studies have demonstrated DMEK to have a one- to two-line better mean BCVA and improved contrast sensitivity as compared to DSEK, with 80% of DMEK eyes without ocular comorbidities achieving greater than or equal to 20/25.[46-49] In a study of patients

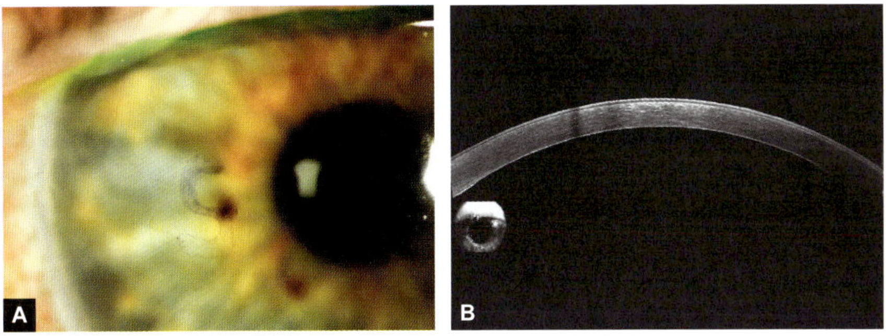

Figs. 4.5A and B: (A) Slit-lamp photograph of a cornea that has undergone Descemet's membrane endothelial keratoplasty (DMEK). An S-stamp placed on the stromal side of the graft during tissue preparation helped guide intraoperative unfolding and positioning; (B) Anterior segment optical coherence tomography in the same patient demonstrates a smooth, hyper-reflective band in the posterior cornea denoting an attached DMEK graft. The patient's final corrected visual acuity is 20/25.

who underwent DSEK in one eye and DMEK in their fellow eye, over 80% preferred the vision in their DMEK eye.[50] The difference in vision primarily relates to decreased posterior corneal surface higher-order aberrations as compared to eyes undergoing DSEK or PK (Figs. 4.5A and B).[51]

- *Faster visual rehabilitation*: DMEK typically allows for functional visual recovery within weeks, with most patients reaching their final BCVA within 1–3 months.[46,48,49] This can be helpful for patients who are monocular, active, or who have bilateral disease and desire expeditious surgery for their fellow eye.
- *Lower incidence of graft rejection*: Studies of grafts for endothelial failure have found the 2-year incidence of immune rejection to be 1–5% for DMEK, as compared to 8–12% for DSEK and 5–17% for PK.[52,53] Possible explanations for this phenomenon include decreased antigenic load as well as the general lower antigenicity of the endothelium.[32,54]
- *More predictable refractive outcome*: In one large series, the amount and range of spherical equivalent shift with DMEK (mean 0.33 D hyperopic shift, range 2.5 D) was substantially less than that typically reported after DSEK (mean 1.00 D hyperopic shift, range 4 D).[28,46]
- *Smaller incision*: The scrolled DMEK tissue can be inserted through an incision as small as 2.4 mm, about half the size of that used in DSEK. This decreases surgically induced astigmatism and may obviate the need for suture closure.

DMEK's principal disadvantages include:

- *Increased incidence of air reinjection*:[48] Initially, rates of air reinjection for partial graft detachments in DMEK were as high as 63% (Figs. 4.6A to D).[46] These rates reflected the learning curves of individual surgeons as well as

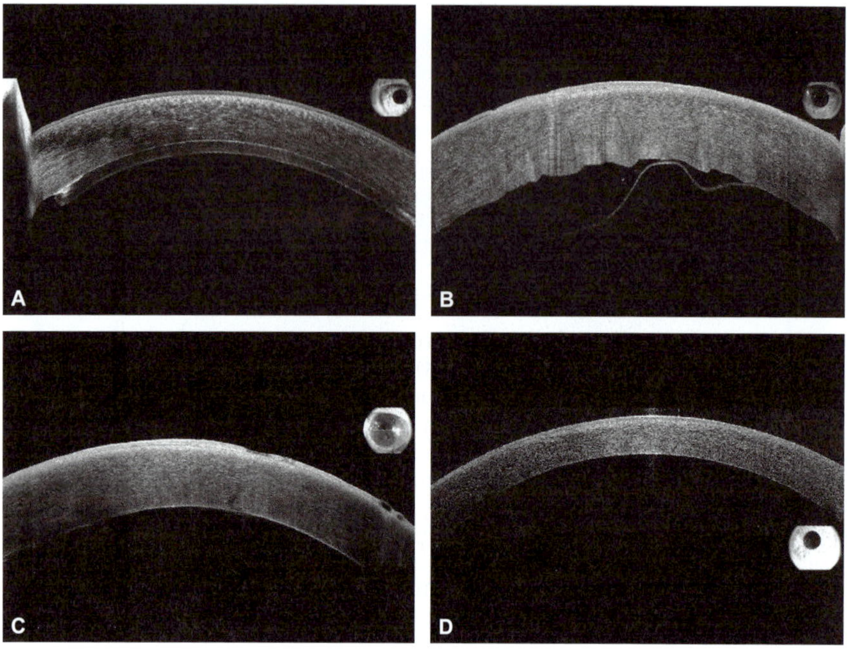

Figs. 4.6A to D: Series of anterior segment optical coherence tomography images from a patient who underwent (A) Descemet's stripping endothelial keratoplasty (DSEK) in the left eye and (B to D) Descemet's membrane endothelial keratoplasty (DMEK) in the right eye. (A) DSEK graft in situ on the first postoperative day. Patient went on to achieve corrected visual acuity of 20/40; (B) DMEK graft with a visually significant detachment on the first postoperative day involving over a third of the graft surface area including the visual axis; (C) After reinjection of air, the DMEK graft reattaches to the host cornea; (D) One month after surgery, the DMEK graft remains attached and the posterior corneal surface is smooth. Final corrected visual acuity is 20/20.

the relatively aggressive approach of air reinjection for any form of incomplete attachment. It has since been shown that small, peripheral detachments that do not affect visual acuity can safely be observed, and often spontaneously clear (Fig. 4.7).[55] As techniques and instrumentation have evolved, air reinjection rates have reduced to 0–20% in multiple studies, with more experienced surgeons achieving rates on the lower end of this range.[56,57] Techniques used to counter graft detachment include leaving a large air bubble in the anterior chamber (necessitating a peripheral iridotomy) and/or utilizing longer-lasting, nonexpansile SF_6 gas.

- *Steep learning curve*: DMEK tissue can be exceptionally fragile. Thus, graft unfolding and positioning is best achieved with a standardized, but complex, "no-touch" technique in which direct tissue manipulation is minimized.[58] This surgical approach may not be intuitive to beginning surgeons, and can be especially challenging in the event of a tight donor scroll.

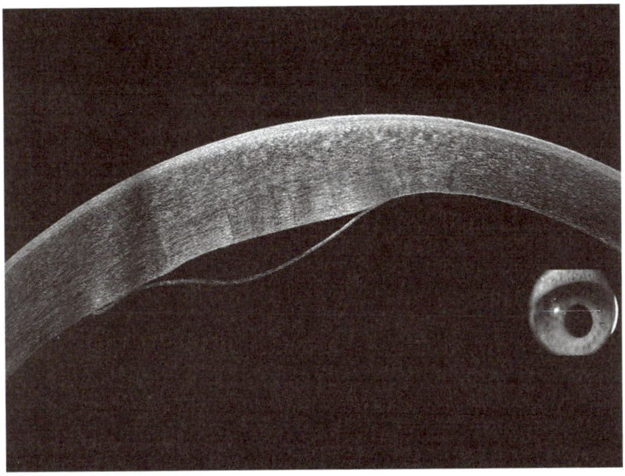

Fig. 4.7: Anterior segment optical coherence tomography 1 week after Descemet's membrane endothelial keratoplasty (DMEK) surgery reveals a shallow, paracentral detachment of the graft. The patient was observed without a reinjection of air. By 6 months after surgery, the DMEK graft is fully reattached and corrected visual acuity measures 20/20.

- *Less versatile*:[59] DMEK can be challenging or relatively contraindicated in a number of eyes with unusual anatomy:
    - Eyes with intraocular hardware (glaucoma drainage implant, anterior chamber intraocular lens), which can damage donor endothelium during unfolding.
    - Eyes with aphakia, aniridia, or other iris abnormalities through which a graft can dislocate into the posterior chamber.
    - Eyes with high myopia or prior vitrectomy, which may make it difficult to achieve the shallow chamber needed to unfold the graft.
    - Eyes with poor visualization of graft scrolling, position, and orientation.
- *Limits on donor age*: DMEK grafts from young donors can form tight scrolls in the anterior chamber that are difficult to unfold using a standard no-touch technique. To counter this phenomenon, many surgeons selectively use grafts from older donors (>40–65), which form broader graft rolls.[60] This precludes the use of young donor tissue, which has a relatively greater density and uniformity of endothelial cells.

PRE-DESCEMET'S ENDOTHELIAL KERATOPLASTY

Pre-Descemet's endothelial keratoplasty, proposed by Dua in 2013 and first performed by Agarwal in 2013, is a novel procedure in which a standard recipient descemetorhexis is followed by transplantation of a composite graft containing pre-Descemet's layer (PDL, or Dua's layer), Descemet's membrane, and endothelium.[61,62] The collagenous PDL affords a splinting effect to the PDEK graft, reducing its tendency to scroll, which in turn makes it easier than DMEK tissue to unfold, handle, and center in the eye.[63]

Pre-Descemet's endothelial keratoplasty graft preparation involves injection of air into the donor corneal stroma to create a well-circumscribed, dome-shaped central elevation of the posterior cornea (type I big bubble). This method cleaves the cornea at the histologically distinct, deep stromal PDL rather than at Descemet's membrane itself.[61,64] While Busin and others had previously described techniques to pneumodissect tissue to be used for DMEK, Dua was the first to recognize the presence and value of the PDL, and how to consistently achieve its inclusion in a PDEK composite graft.[65,66]

As with UT-DSAEK and DMEK, PDEK capitalizes on the optical and immunologic benefits of thin endothelial grafts.[41-43] Initial clinical results of PDEK are promising and comparable to DMEK, with patients on average achieving 20/30 vision within 1 month of surgery.[62,67] Nonetheless, larger studies with longer follow-up duration are still needed.

The principal advantages of PDEK over DMEK include:

- *Improved intraoperative handling*: As previously noted, the PDL splints the Descemet's membrane and reduces overall scrolling of the composite PDEK graft, making intraoperative handling, unfolding, and centration smoother.[63]
- *Freedom to use donor tissue from younger, healthier eyes*: DMEK grafts from young donors can be difficult to harvest and to unfold inside the eye.[60] By contrast, PDEK grafts are just as easily harvested from young donors as from old, and tend to form broad scrolls across all ages that unfold relatively smoothly.[63] Indeed, PDEK can be successfully performed even with infant donor tissue.[67]

PDEK's principal disadvantage is that the *graft size is limited.* The mean graft diameter in PDEK is 7.6 mm, as compared to 8.5–9 mm in other forms of EK.[62] This is due to adhesions between the collagenous layers in the peripheral cornea, which limit the size of the type I big bubble used to pneumodissect PDEK grafts.[61] A smaller graft has the inherent disadvantage of transferring fewer endothelial cells. It remains to be seen whether this effect can be compensated for by the use of younger, endothelial cell rich grafts, or by a lower rate of cell loss during graft unfolding.

CONCLUSION

Surgical treatment of corneal endothelial dysfunction has undergone exciting and dramatic change in the last 15 years, with various forms of EK now supplanting PK as the procedures of choice for this condition. Advances in instrumentation, technique, and basic science have allowed patients to achieve excellent and predictable visual results, a rapid recovery, and reduced risk of graft rejection. Nonetheless, it is clear that there is no "one-size-fits-all" procedure. Rather, the modern corneal surgeon must be adaptable and tailor his/her approach to the patient's individual anatomy and visual needs.

ACKNOWLEDGMENTS

Support from: NIH Center Core Grant P30EY014801, RPB Unrestricted Award and Career Development Awards, Department of Defense (DOD-Grant#W81XWH-09-1-0675) The Ronald and Alicia Lepke Grant, The Lee and Claire Hager Grant, The Jimmy and Gaye Bryan Grant, The H. Scott Huizenga Grant, The Grant and Diana Stanton-Thornbrough, The Robert Baer Family Grant, The Emilyn Page and Mark Feldberg Grant, The Gordon Charitable Foundation and the Richard Azar Family Grant (institutional grants).

REFERENCES

1. Reisinger F. Die keratoplastik: ein Versuch zur Erweiterung der Augenheilkunst. Bayerische Annalen. 1824;1:207-15.
2. Mannis MJ, Mannis A. Corneal Transplantation: A History in Profiles. Oostende, Belgium: JP Wayenborgh; 1999.
3. von Hippel A. Eine neue methode der hornhauttransplantation. Arch Ophthalmol. 1888;34(I):108-30.
4. Zirm EK. Eine erfolgreiche totale keratoplastik (a successful total keratoplasty). Arch Ophthalmol. 1906;64:580-93.
5. Verdier D. Penetrating keratoplasty. In: Krachmer JH, Mannis MJ, Holland EJ (Eds). Cornea: Fundamentals, Diagnosis and Management. St. Louis, Mo: Mosby/Elsevier; 2011.
6. Terry M. Endothelial keratoplasty: history, current state and future directions. Cornea. 2006:25(8):873-8.
7. Barraquer JI. Queratoplastia: problemas que plantea la fijacion del injerto. Opthalmologicum Acta. 1951;16:999-1004.
8. Tillett CW. Posterior lamellar keratoplasty. Am J Ophthalmol. 1956;41:530-3.
9. Melles GR, Eggink FA, Lander F, et al. A surgical technique for posterior lamellar keratoplasty. Cornea. 1998,17.610-26.
10. Terry MA, Ousley PJ. Deep lamellar endothelial keratoplasty in the first United States patients: early clinical results. Cornea. 2001;20:239-43.
11. Terry MA, Ousley PJ. Deep lamellar endothelial keratoplasty (DLEK): visual acuity, astigmatism and endothelial survival in a large prospective series. Ophthalmology. 2005;112:1541-9.
12. Amayem AF, Terry MA, Helal MH, et al. Deep lamellar endothelial keratoplasty (DLEK): surgery in complex cases with severe postoperative visual loss. Cornea. 2005;24:587-92.
13. Fogla R, Padmanabhan P. Initial results of small incision deep lamellar endothelial keratoplasty (DLEK). Am J Ophthalmol. 2006;141(2):346-51.
14. Vail A, Gore SM, Bradley BA, et al. Corneal graft survival and visual outcome. A multi-center study. Corneal Transplant Follow-up Study Collaborators. Ophthalmology. 1994;101:120-7.
15. Ing JJ, Nelson LR, Hodge DO, et al. Ten-year post-operative results of penetrating keratoplasty. Ophthalmology. 1998;105:1855-65.

16. Nanavaty MA, Wang X, Shortt AJ. Endothelial keratoplasty versus penetrating keratoplasty for Fuchs endothelial dystrophy. Cochrane Database Syst Rev. 2014;(2):CD008420.
17. Panda A, Vanathi M, Kumar A, et al. Corneal graft rejection. Surv Ophthalmol. 2007;52(4):375-96.
18. Dandona L, Naduvilath TJ, Janarthanan M, et al. Survival analysis and visual outcome in a large series of corneal transplants in India. Br J Ophthalmol. 1997;81(9):726-31.
19. Elder MJ, Stack RR. Globe rupture following penetrating keratoplasty: how often, why, and what can we do to prevent it? Cornea. 2004;23:776-80.
20. Martin XY, Safran AB. Corneal hypoesthesia. Surv Ophthalmol. 1988;33:28-40.
21. Anwar M, Teichmann KD. Big-bubble technique to bare Descemet's membrane in anterior lamellar keratoplasty. J Cataract Refract Surg. 2002;28:398-403.
22. Eye Bank Association of America. 2015 Eye Banking Statistical Report. [online] Available from: www.restoresight.org. [Accessed September, 2017].
23. Laibson PR. Current concepts and techniques in corneal transplantation. Curr Opin Ophthalmol. 2002;13:220-3.
24. Price MO, Price FW. Endothelial keratoplasty—a review. Clin Exp Ophthalmol. 2010;38(2):128-40.
25. Melles GR, Wijdh RH, Nieuwendaal CP. A technique to excise the Descemet membrane from a recipient cornea (descemetorhexis). Cornea. 2004;23:286-8.
26. Gorovoy MS. Descemet-stripping automated endothelial keratoplasty. Cornea. 2006;25:886-9.
27. Price FW, Price MO. Descemet's stripping with endothelial keratoplasty in 200 eyes. Early challenges and technique to enhance donor adherence. J Cataract Refract Surg. 2006;32:411-8.
28. Chen ES, Terry MA, Shamie N, et al. Descemet-stripping automated endothelial keratoplasty: six-month results in a prospective study of 100 eyes. Cornea. 2008;27(5):514-20.
29. Price MO, Price FW. Descemet's stripping endothelial keratoplasty. Curr Opin Ophthalmol. 2007;18:290-4.
30. Bahar I, Kaiserman I, McAllum P, et al. Comparison of posterior lamellar keratoplasty techniques to penetrating keratoplasty. Ophthalmology. 2008;115: 1525-33.
31. Price MO. Comparison of endothelial keratoplasty and penetrating keratoplasty outcomes. In: Price FW, Price MO (Eds). DSEK: All You Need to Know about Endothelial Keratoplasty. Thorofare, NJ: Slack, Inc.; 2008. pp. 37-52.
32. Price MO, Gorovoy M, Price FW, et al. Descemet's stripping automated endothelial keratoplasty: three-year graft and endothelial cell survival compared with penetrating keratoplasty. Ophthalmology. 2013;120:246-51.
33. Lee WB, Jacobs DS, Musch DC, et al. Descemet's stripping endothelial keratoplasty: safety and outcomes: a report by the American Academy of Ophthalmology. Ophthalmology. 2009;116(9):1818-30.
34. Terry MA. Trauma and wound rupture in endothelial keratoplasty. Cornea. 2008;27:127-8.
35. Suh L, Yoo SH, Deobhakta A, et al. Complications of Descemet's stripping with automated endothelial keratoplasty—survey of 118 eyes at one institute. Ophthalmology. 2008;115:1517-24.
36. Koenig SB, Covert DJ. Early results of small-incision Descemet's stripping and automated endothelial keratoplasty. Ophthalmology. 2007;114(2):221-6.

37. Terry MA, Shamie N, Chen ES, et al. Endothelial keratoplasty: a simplified technique to minimize graft dislocation, iatrogenic graft failure, and pupillary block. Ophthalmology. 2008;115(7):1179-86.
38. Terry MA, Saad HA, Shamie N, et al. Endothelial keratoplasty: the influence of insertion techniques and incision size on donor endothelial survival. Cornea. 2009;28:24-31.
39. Hindman HB, Huxlin KR, Pantanelli SM, et al. Post-DSAEK optical changes: a comprehensive prospective analysis on the role of ocular wavefront aberrations, haze, and corneal thickness. Cornea. 2013;32(12):1567-77.
40. Patel SV, Baratz KH, Hodge DO, et al. The effect of corneal light scatter on vision after Descemet stripping with endothelial keratoplasty. Arch Ophthalmol. 2009;127(2):153-60.
41. Neff KD, Biber JM, Holland EJ. Comparison of central corneal graft thickness to visual acuity outcomes in endothelial keratoplasty. Eye Contact Lens. 2009;35:196-202.
42. Cleynenbruegel HV, Remeijer L, Hillenaar T. Descemet endothelial automated keratoplasty: effect of intraoperative lenticule thickness on visual outcome and endothelial cell density. Cornea. 2011;30:1195-2000.
43. Busin M, Madi S, Santorum P, et al. Ultrathin Descemet's stripping automated endothelial keratoplasty with the microkeratome double-pass technique: two-year outcomes. Ophthalmology. 2013;120:1186-94.
44. Melles GR, Ong TS, Ververs B, et al. Descemet membrane endothelial keratoplasty (DMEK). Cornea. 2006;25(8):987-90.
45. Ham L, Dapena I, van Luijk C, et al. Descemet membrane endothelial keratoplasty (DMEK) for Fuchs endothelial dystrophy: review of the first 50 consecutive cases. Eye. 2009;23:1990-8.
46. Price MO, Giebel AW, Fairchild KM, et al. Descemet's membrane endothelial keratoplasty: prospective multicenter study of visual and refractive outcomes and endothelial survival. Ophthalmology. 2009;116(12):2361-8.
47. Rodríguez-calvo-de-mora M, Quilendrino R, Ham L, et al. Clinical outcome of 500 consecutive cases undergoing Descemet's membrane endothelial keratoplasty. Ophthalmology. 2015;122(3):464-70.
48. Zhu L, Zha Y, Cai J, et al. Descemet stripping automated endothelial keratoplasty versus Descemet membrane endothelial keratoplasty: a meta-analysis. Int Ophthalmol. 2017.
49. Tourtas T, Laaser K, Bachmann BO, et al. Descemet membrane endothelial keratoplasty versus Descemet stripping automated endothelial keratoplasty. Am J Ophthalmol. 2012;153(6):1082-90.
50. Guerra FP, Anshu A, Price MO, et al. Endothelial keratoplasty: fellow eyes comparison of Descemet stripping automated endothelial keratoplasty and Descemet membrane endothelial keratoplasty. Cornea. 2011;30:1382-6.
51. Rudolph M, Laaser K, Bachmann BO, et al. Corneal higher-order aberrations after Descemet's membrane endothelial keratoplasty. Ophthalmology. 2012;119:528-35.
52. Anshu A, Price MO, Price FW Jr. Risk of corneal transplant rejection significantly reduced with Descemet's membrane endothelial keratoplasty. Ophthalmology. 2012;119:536-40.
53. Hos D, Tuac O, Schaub F, et al. Incidence and clinical course of immune reactions after Descemet membrane endothelial keratoplasty: retrospective analysis of 1,000 consecutive eyes. Ophthalmology. 2017;124(4):512-8.

54. Hori J, Joyce NC, Streilein JW. Immune privilege and immunogenicity reside among different layers of the mouse cornea. Invest Ophthalmol Vis Sci. 2000;41(10):3032-42.
55. Dirisamer M, van Dijk K, Dapena I, et al. Prevention and management of graft detachment in Descemet membrane endothelial keratoplasty. Arch Ophthalmol. 2012;130(3):280-91.
56. Dapena I, Ham L, Droutsas K, et al. Learning curve in Descemet's membrane endothelial keratoplasty: first series of 135 consecutive cases. Ophthalmology. 2011;118:2147-54.
57. Rodriguez-Calvo-de-Mora M, Quilendrino R, Ham L, et al. Clinical outcome of 500 consecutive cases undergoing Descemet's membrane endothelial keratoplasty. Ophthalmology. 2015;122:464-70.
58. Dapena I, Moutsouris K, Droutsas K, et al. Standardized "no-touch" technique for Descemet membrane endothelial keratoplasty. Arch Ophthalmol. 2011;129(1):88-94.
59. Anshu A, Price MO, Tan DT, et al. Endothelial keratoplasty: a revolution in evolution. Surv Ophthalmol. 2012;57(3):236-52.
60. Heinzelmann S, Hüther S, Böhringer D, et al. Influence of donor characteristics on Descemet membrane endothelial keratoplasty. Cornea. 2014;33(6):644-8.
61. Dua HS, Faraj LA, Said DG, et al. A novel pre-Descemet's layer (Dua's layer). Ophthalmology. 2013;120:1778-85.
62. Agarwal A, Dua HS, Narang P, et al. Pre-Descemet's endothelial keratoplasty (PDEK). Br J Ophthalmol. 2014;98(9):1181-5.
63. Dua HS, Termote K, Kenawy MB, et al. Scrolling characteristics of pre-Descemet endothelial keratoplasty tissue: an Ex Vivo study. Am J Ophthalmol. 2016;166:84-90.
64. Anwar M, Teichmann K. Big-bubble technique to bare Descemet's membrane in anterior lamellar keratoplasty. J Cataract Refract Surg. 2002;28:398-403.
65. Busin M, Scorcia V, Patel AK, et al. Pneumatic dissection and storage of donor endothelial tissue for Descemet's membrane endothelial keratoplasty: a novel technique. Ophthalmology. 2010;117:1517-20.
66. Zarei-Ghanavati S, Khakshoor H, Zarei-Ghanavati M. Reverse big bubble: a new technique for preparing donor tissue of Descemet membrane endothelial keratoplasty. Br J Ophthalmol. 2010;94:1110-1.
67. Agarwal A, Agarwal A, Narang P, et al. Pre-Descemet endothelial keratoplasty with infant donor corneas: a prospective analysis. Cornea. 2015;34(8):859-65.

Chapter 5

Pre-Descemet's Endothelial Keratoplasty: Principles and Types of Big Bubbles

Ashvin Agarwal, Priya Narang, Dhivya Ashok Kumar, Amar Agarwal

BACKGROUND

The major endothelial keratoplasty (EK) techniques performed by the surgeons around the globe in the recent past include the Descemet's membrane endothelial keratoplasty (DMEK) and the Descemet's stripping endothelial keratoplasty (DSEK). The automated versions of the above procedures termed as Descemet's membrane automated endothelial keratoplasty (DMAEK) and Descemet's stripping automated endothelial keratoplasty (DSAEK) are also popularly practiced. In terms of visual output, DMEK as an EK procedure has always scored in spite of it being technically challenging as compared to other EK procedures. DMEK represents the removal of host diseased Descemet's membrane (DM)-endothelial complex and transplantation of new healthy donor Descemet's membrane (DM)-endothelial complex.[1,2]

Pre-Descemet's endothelial keratoplasty (PDEK)[3] is a new variant in the field of EK that mainly comprises the separation of pre Descemet's layer (PDL) along with DM endothelium complex from the residual donor stroma by the formation of a type-1 bubble (bb).[4] The feasibility of the PDEK procedure with both an adult and infant donor tissue[3,5] makes it highly acceptable in the era of shortage of donor tissue.

PNEUMATIC DISSECTION AND BIG BUBBLE CREATION

Pre-Descemet's endothelial keratoplasty (PDEK) is a variant of endothelial keratoplasty procedure that involves the creation of type-1 bb that is created with a 30 G needle attached to an air-filled 5-mL syringe. This procedure has a theoretical advantage of safer manipulation of tissue and greater ease of deployment than has been encountered during traditional DMEK procedure.

Pneumatic Dissection

Pneumatic or air dissection is a well established entity that relegates the use of microforceps or a microkeratome for dissection of the corneal stroma. An air-filled syringe is used to inject air into the stroma with the endothelial side up and is advanced under direct observation at a required depth beneath the

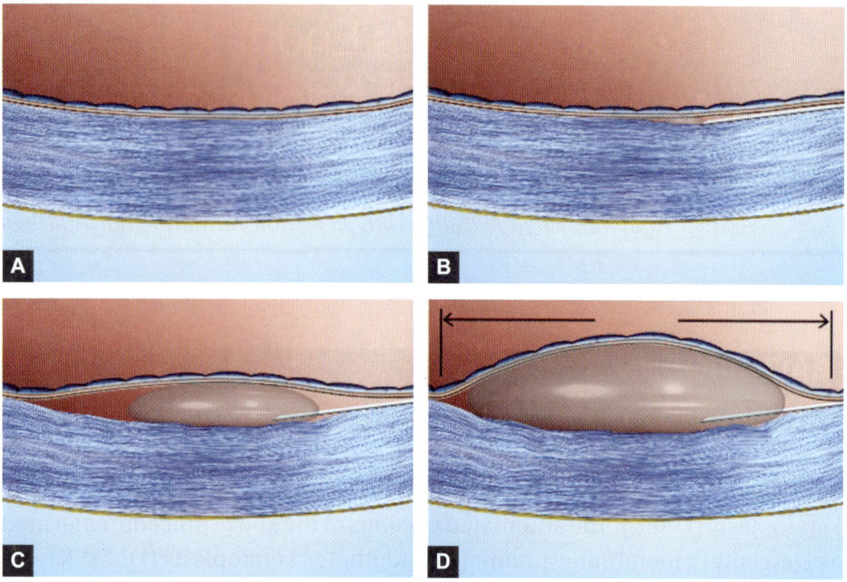

Figs. 5.1A to D: Graphical display of creation of type-1 bubble (bb). (A) The image demonstrates all the layers of cornea with graft placed with endothelial side up; (B) An air-filled 30-G needle introduced from the periphery beneath the pre-Descemet's layer (PDL). The PDL–Descemet's membrane (DM)–endothelium complex is seen lying above the bevel of the needle; (C) Further injection of air lifts the entire PDL–DM–endothelium complex that comprises Pre-Descemet's endothelial keratoplasty graft above the residual stroma; (D) Fully formed type-1 bb is formed. (*Courtesy*: Agarwal/Kim book on Endothelial Keratoplasty by Thieme, USA)

endothelium. The advantage with air dissection is that it is cost effective as it is done manually by the surgeon and the major drawback with it is that it requires a certain amount of surgical skill set on behalf of the surgeon as the needle that is employed to inject air must be introduced at the correct depth below the DM-endothelium complex.

Big Bubble Type 1

This is the kind of bb that is essential to obtain for performing a PDEK procedure. This bb typically spreads from center to periphery and is dome shaped. The diameter of the bb usually varies from 7.5 mm to 8.5 mm; this bb never extends to extreme periphery due to adhesions between the PDL and the residual stroma. Injection of air leads to separation of the PDL-DM-endothelium complex in toto from the residual stromal bed (Figs. 5.1A to D). This type-1 bb is created using a 30 G needle connected to a 5 mL syringe with bevel up (Figs. 5.2A and B).

Big Bubble Type 2

This type of bb is typically formed when the air enters the plane between the PDL and the DM-endothelium complex. Type-2 bb typically spreads from

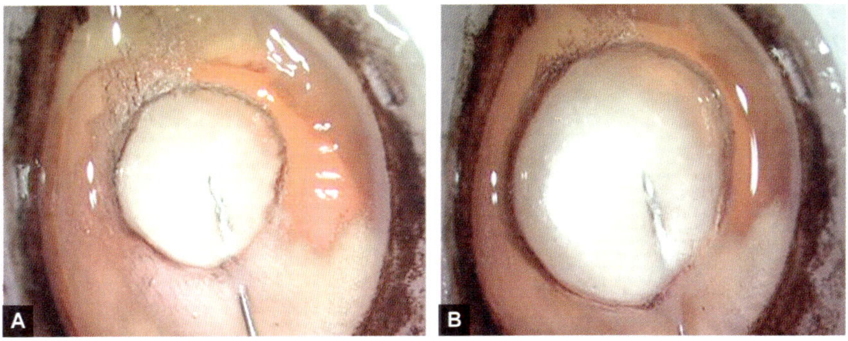

Figs. 5.2A and B: Type-1 big bubble—donor graft preparation. (A) Small type-1 bubble formed and (B) Type-1 bubble enhanced with air. The air is between the pre-Descemet's layer and the stroma. Note the bubble starts from the center and never reaches the periphery. This graft when dissected will give a pre-Descemet's endothelial keratoplasty (PDEK) graft. This is not dependent on donor age and can be produced even in an infant donor cornea. As the pre-Descemet's layer is attached to the DM and endothelium, the PDEK graft is easier to handle compared to a Descemet's membrane endothelial keratoplasty graft. (*Courtesy*: Agarwal/Kim book on Endothelial Keratoplasty by Thieme, USA)

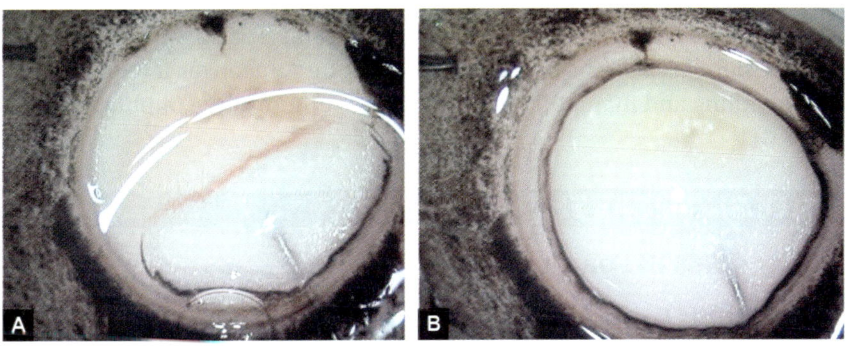

Figs. 5.3A and B: Type-2 big bubble. (A) Type-2 big bubble starts from the periphery and extends to the center; (B) The entire cornea up to the periphery is involved in the bubble formation. In a type-1 big bubble, notice it never goes up to the periphery. A type-2 big bubble means the air is between Descemet's membrane and pre-Descemet's layer. So, one can prepare a DMEK graft if this happens and the donor cornea can be used. (*Courtesy*: Agarwal/Kim book on Endothelial Keratoplasty by Thieme, USA)

periphery to center and is around 10–11 mm in diameter. It extends up to extreme periphery, as there are no adhesions between the PDL and the DM (Figs. 5.3A and B). With the formation of type 2 bb, the surgeon proceeds with a DMEK instead of a PDEK procedure. Immense care should be taken when a type-2 bb is formed as it has a thin wall and if it is subjected to excessive air push then the bb can rupture leading to perforation of graft and eventually transcending into donor tissue wastage.

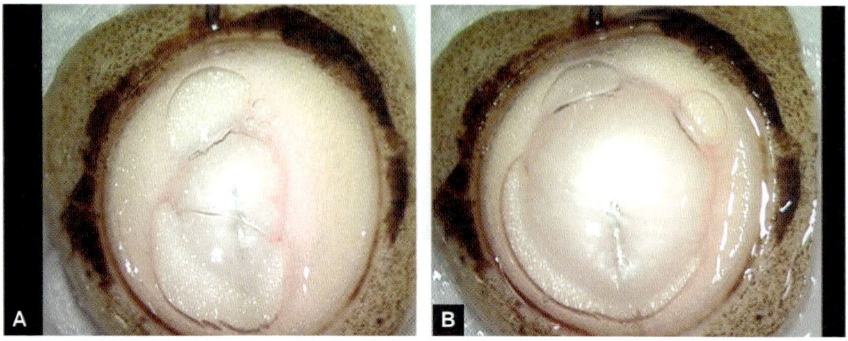

Figs. 5.4A and B: Type-3 big bubble. (A) and (B) Both type-1 and -2 bubbles are formed. Note the central type-1 big bubble and with it there is peripheral bubble forming also which is a type-2 big bubble. In such cases if the type-2 big bubble is small, we can just puncture it with a needle and dissect the type-1 big bubble and prepare the pre-Descemet's endothelial keratoplasty (PDEK) graft and use it. If the type-2 big bubble is too large, it is better to discard this donor cornea and take a new one for PDEK. (*Courtesy*: Agarwal/Kim book on Endothelial Keratoplasty by Thieme, USA)

Big Bubble Type 3

When both type-1 and -2 bb are formed and they coexist; mixed bubble is said to have been achieved. This is a type-3 big bb (Figs. 5.4A and B). These types of bubbles pose a surgical challenge to the surgeon, as it requires delicate handling and manipulation to avoid the rupture of the bubble (Figs. 5.5 and 5.6).

PDEK SURGICAL TECHNIQUE

Donor Graft Preparation

PDEK Bubble Formation

The donor button with the corneoscleral rim is placed with the endothelial side up. A 30 G needle attached to an air filled 5 mL syringe is used for bubble formation. The needle is introduced with a bevel up position from the periphery up to the mid-peripheral area at a considerable depth from the DM so as to create a plane of separation between the PDL and the residual stroma (Fig. 5.7A). If one does not get a bubble after repeated attempts (more than 10 at least) with air, one can try with fluid using the MK medium or Optisol or BSS (balanced salt solution). If still it does not come, one can use viscoelastic. Air is injected and a type-1 bb is formed that is dome shaped and is around 8 mm in diameter.

Donor Graft Staining

Staining of the graft is done with trypan blue that allows a considerable clear visualization of the graft. The bb is penetrated with a side port blade at the

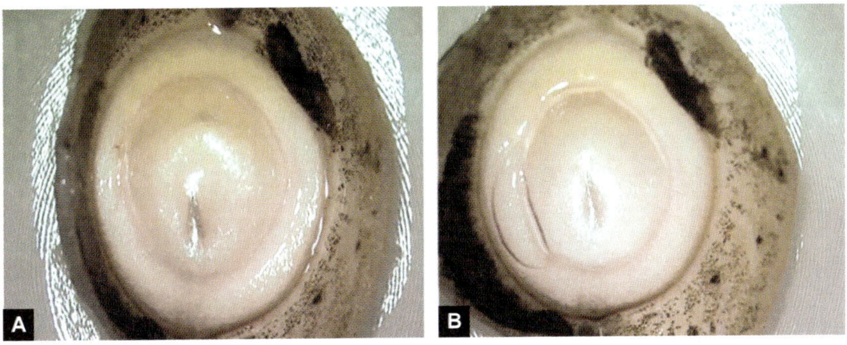

Figs. 5.5A and B: Big bubble. (A) Type-1 big bubble has been created; (B) Suddenly a small peripheral type-2 big bubble is starting. At this stage one can just puncture the type-2 big bubble with a needle and dissect the type-1 big bubble as it is large enough and complete the pre-Descemet's endothelial keratoplasty graft. (*Courtesy*: Agarwal/Kim book on Endothelial Keratoplasty by Thieme, USA)

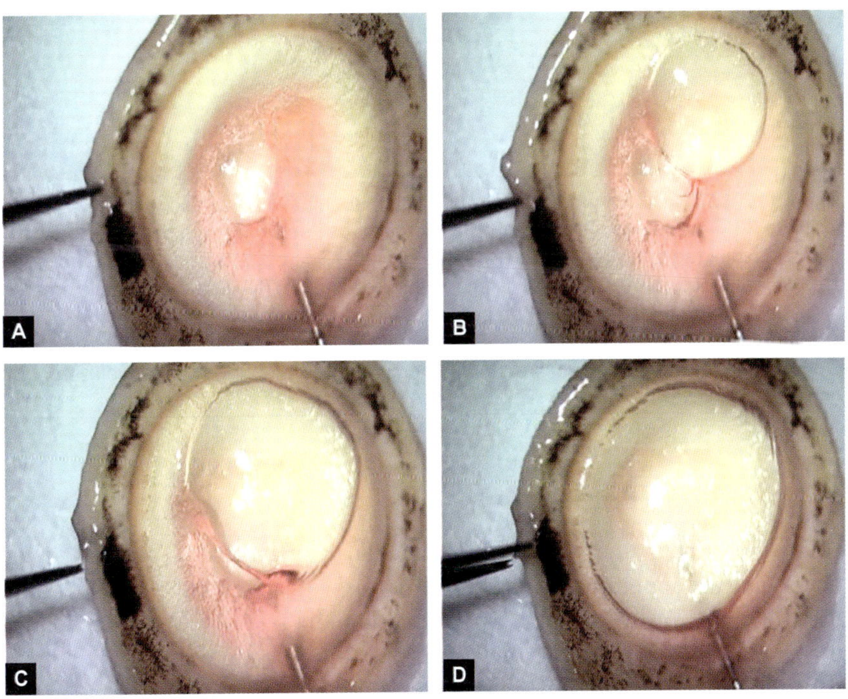

Figs. 5.6A to D: Formation of a DMEK graft. (A) Type-1 big bubble has started to form; (B) Suddenly a type-2 big bubble starts to form also; (C) The type-2 big bubble becomes larger and engulfs the type-1 big bubble; (D) The type-2 big bubble has become complete. In such a scenario prepare a DMEK graft and use the graft. (*Courtesy*: Agarwal/Kim book on Endothelial Keratoplasty by Thieme, USA)

extreme periphery (Fig. 5.7B) and trypan blue is injected inside (Fig. 5.7C). The bb is then cut all across the periphery with a corneoscleral scissors (Fig. 5.7D) and is placed in the storage media. The donor is loaded onto the injector when ready for insertion (Figs. 5.8 and 5.9).

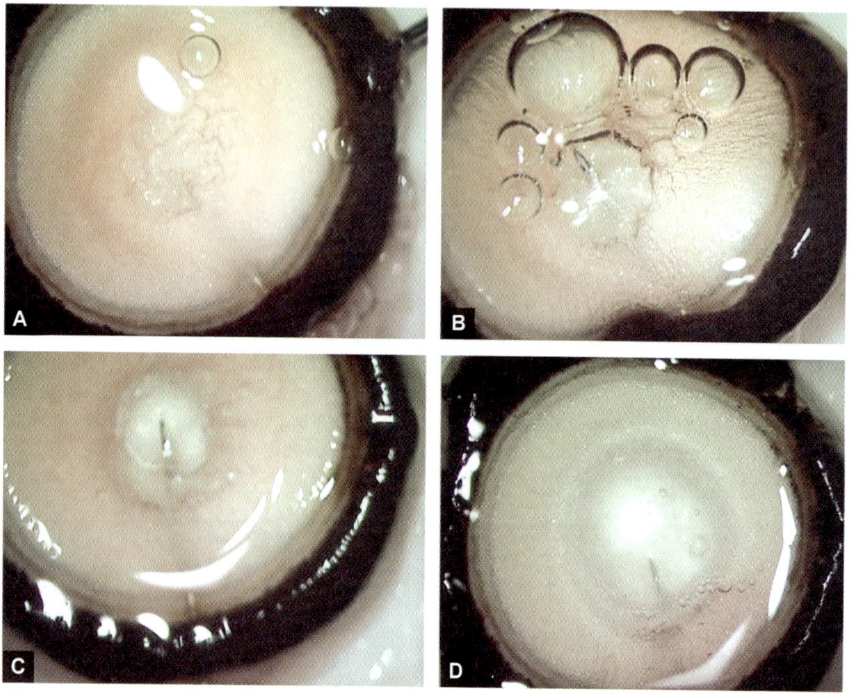

Figs. 5.7A to D: Donor graft preparation with viscoelastic or Optisol medium. (A) An air-filled 30-G needle is introduced from the corneoscleral rim up to the mid-periphery and air is injected to create a type-1 bubble (bb); (B) The bb gets punctured by mistake and air leaks out; (C) Viscoelastic is injected inside the bb; (D) The viscoelastic creates the type-1 big bubble. This can then be dissected, but before using rinse it in the Optisol medium to wash off the viscoelastic. One can also create the type-1 big bubble with the Optisol medium if the big bubble is not forming with air. (*Courtesy*: Agarwal/Kim book on Endothelial Keratoplasty by Thieme, USA)

Recipient Bed Preparation

Under peribulbar anesthesia, the epithelial debridement is performed for enhancing intraoperative visualization in eyes with an epithelial hypertrophy. An ACM or a Trocar anterior chamber maintainer (T-ACM)[6] is introduced into the eye that is connected to the air pump. This helps to maintain adequate depth of AC at all times and it also ensures appropriate shift between air and fluid infusion as and when required (Figs. 5.10A to F). A 2.8 mm corneal tunnel is made and two side port incisions are framed. With the AC completely inflated with air, DM is scored and stripped using a reverse sinskey hook. Inferior iridectomy is performed with a vitrectomy probe introduced from the corneal incision. This maneuver ensures prevention of pupillary block at a later stage.

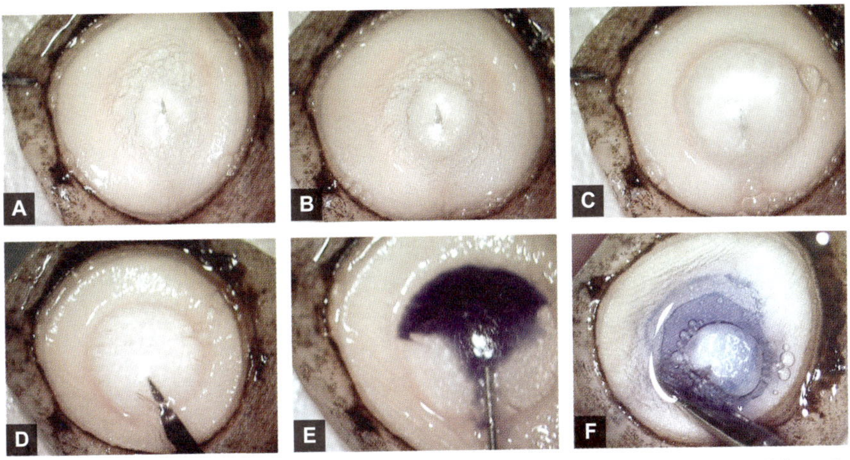

Figs. 5.8A to F: Preparing the pre-Descemet's endothelial keratoplasty (PDEK) graft. (A) 30-G needle enters the stroma and air is injected. Small bubbles are formed. One is looking at the endothelium; (B) Type-1 big bubble is forming. Note the bubble starts from the center and extends up to the mid-periphery. It does not go up to the periphery; (C) Type-1 big bubble; (D) Knife entry into the big bubble; (E) Trypan blue injected into the bubble to stain; (F) Scissor dissects the bubble creating a PDEK graft. (*Courtesy*: Agarwal/Kim book on Endothelial Keratoplasty by Thieme, USA)

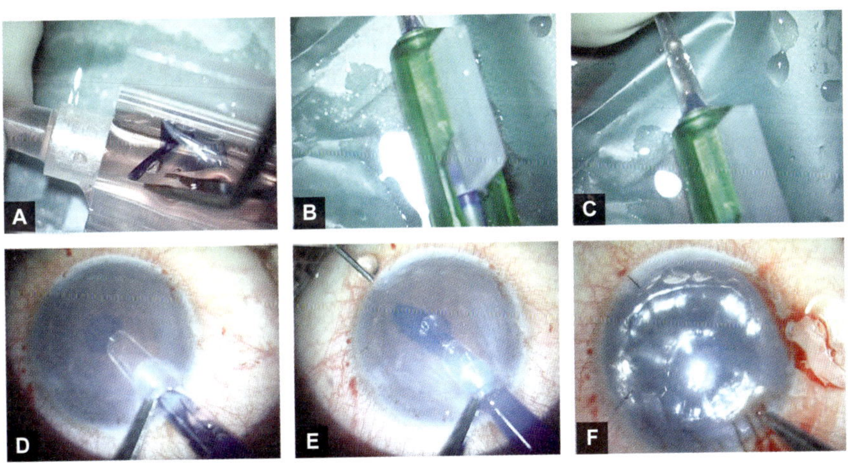

Figs. 5.9A to F: Loading and injecting the graft. (A) The sponge tip from the injector is removed; The spring of the injector is grasped and pulled out and the graft is placed on the cartridge; (B) The sponge tip is re-fixed onto the injector and the injector fixed onto the cartridge; (C) The injector pushes the PDEK graft into the nozzle of the cartridge; (D) The cartridge is loaded onto the injector and the graft is ready to be injected into the anterior chamber-AC. Cartridge nozzle passed into the AC; (E) PDEK graft injected into the AC; (F) PDEK graft unrolled and attached.

PDEK Graft Insertion

The prepared PDEK is held gently with a nontoothed forceps and is placed into the cartridge of a foldable IOL that is filled with BSS (Figs. 5.10A to F).[7]

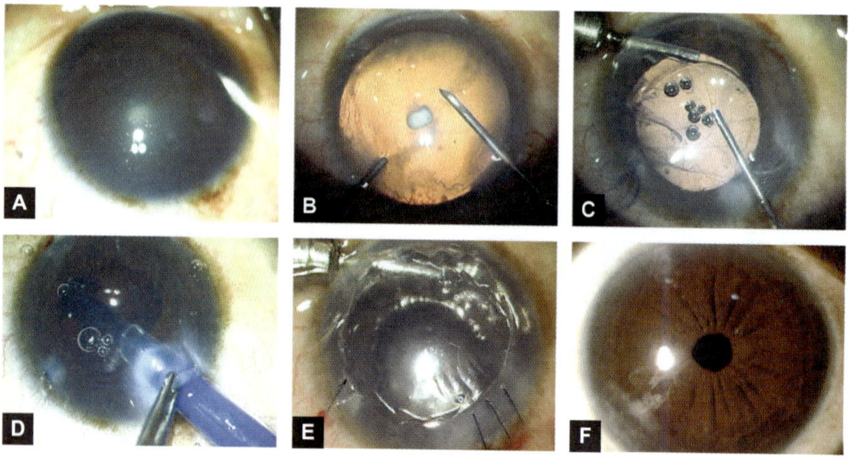

Figs. 5.10A to F: Pre-Descemet's endothelial keratoplasty with cataract. (A) Preoperative status of the recipient eye. Fuchs dystrophy with cataract; (B) Rhexis started for cataract removal; (C) Side-port incision made to introduce an anterior chamber maintainer. Notice IOL in the eye. Now descemetorhexis will be started; (D) Donor graft is inserted into the anterior chamber. Wound-assisted graft insertion is avoided; (E) Graft unrolling is attempted with air and fluidics. Endoilluminator is used to enhance the graft visualization and also to check the correct orientation; (F) Postoperative 1 month of the patient. (*Courtesy*: Agarwal/Kim book on Endothelial Keratoplasty by Thieme, USA)

Air infusion is stopped and the graft is gently injected into the AC through a clear corneal incision, avoiding wound-assisted implantation. Graft orientation is verified and the graft is gently unfolded using air and fluidics. Corneal indentation and massaging is also performed to facilitate the graft unrolling. Once the graft has partly unrolled, a small air bb is injected beneath the graft that helps it to adhere to the corneal surface. The peripheral edges of the graft can be unrolled by gently manipulating it with reverse sinskey hook. Once the graft has fully unrolled, air infusion is started. This facilitates total adherence of the graft to the recipient bed. Corneal wounds are adequately so that a well formed AC is achieved postoperatively (Figs. 5.11A and B).

POSTOPERATIVE MANAGEMENT

The patient is advised to lie in strict supine position for approximately 3 hours in the immediate postoperative period and advised to maintain supine position predominantly in the next 2 days. Slit lamp examination is done to confirm the graft centration and location. On the second postoperative day, intraocular pressure is checked and the patency of inferior iridectomy is confirmed. Topical antibiotics and steroids are prescribed that are slowly tapered over a period of 4 months.

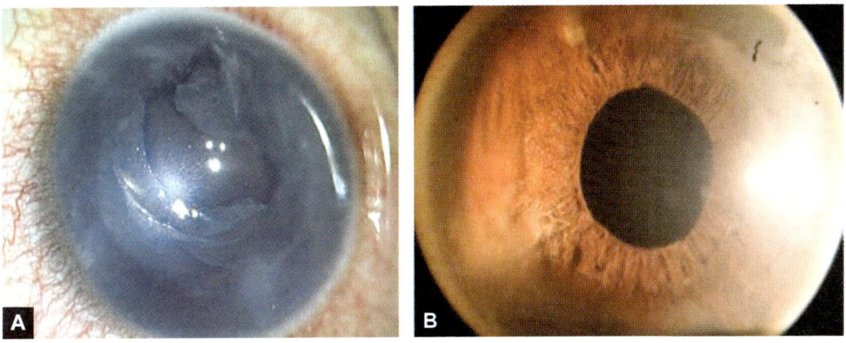

Figs. 5.11A and B: Preoperative and postoperative image of pre-Descemet's endothelial keratoplasty using a young donor. (A) Preoperative pseudophakic bullous keratopathy; (B) Three months postoperative Vision 20/20. (*Courtesy:* Agarwal/Kim book on Endothelial Keratoplasty by Thieme, USA)

PDEK VERSUS OTHER EK

Endothelial keratoplasty as a technique has evolved from deep lamellar endothelial keratoplasty (DLEK) and transitioned to DSEK/DSAEK and further to DMEK. PDEK being a latest entry into this horizon is expected to have a broad acceptance due to its similar characteristics of rapid visual recovery, predictable wound strength, and a significant greater optical predictability similar to a DMEK procedure with an added advantage of less chances of donor tissue loss due to tearing away of the DM and also of better graft maneuverability due to extra strength and splinting effect of the PDL to the DM-endothelium complex (Figs. 5.11A and B). Differences between DSEK, DMEK, and PDEK are shown in Table 5.1. Like DMEK, preparation of PDEK graft does not require large investment in addition to all the other benefits of a DMEK procedure. PDEK involves the addition of the PDL in the donor graft that increases the thickness of the graft to approximately 30–35 microns as measured with an optical coherence tomography (OCT). The graft is comparatively thicker than that of the DMEK but is thinner as compared to DSEK/DSAEK or an ultra-thin DSAEK (UT-DSAEK). Visual rehabilitation after PDEK is comparatively faster as compared to other EK techniques except DMEK that involves pure DM transplantation.

Clinically, in our series we have observed that the incidence of graft dislocation and re-bubbling rate are comparatively less in PDEK as compared to DMEK and that can probably be attributed to the addition of the PDL to the donor graft that enhances the graft sustainability. The risk of donor tissue loss can be minimized by the eye banks if they supply premade ready to use donor graft tissue.

Table 5.1: Comparison of the different endothelial keratoplasty techniques.

	DSEK	*DMEK*	*PDEK*
Surgical layers	Stroma + DM + Endo	DM + Endo	Pre-Descemet's + DM + Endo
Technical difficulty	Easy	Difficult	Moderate
Type of procedure	Tissue additive	Tissue neutral	Minimal tissue additive
Artificial anterior chamber	Required	NR	NR
Microkeratome	Required (DSAEK)	NR	NR
Induced hyperopia	Yes	NO	No
Corneal thickness	Increased	Normal	Minimal
Intrastromal interface	Yes	No	Minimal
Cost	Costly	Cost effective	Cost effective
Eye bank prepared donor tissue	Available	Available	Available
Graft unrolling	Easy	Difficult	Moderate
Tissue handling	Good	Difficult	Good
Visual recovery	Slow	Fast	Fast

(DSEK: Descemet's stripping endothelial keratoplasty; DMEK: Descemet's membrane endothelial keratoplasty; PDEK: Pre-Descemet's endothelial keratoplasty, DM: Descemet's membrane; Endo: Endothelium; DSAEK: Descemet's stripping automated endothelial keratoplasty; NR: Not required).

PDEK AND YOUNG DONOR

The feasibility of using infant donor graft for PDEK has been highlighted before and doing so potentially increase the pool of suitable donor tissue for PDEK.[5]

The upper age limit for donor tissue usage is considered to be around 75 years but there is still not a clear-cut consensus on the lower age limit of donor tissue usage. Under such circumstances, most centers accept tissue from pediatric donors over 6 months of age. Infant donor tissue has not been used in the past due to various reasons involved with the fear of implanting an immature tissue although it runs high on endothelial cell density (ECD) count along with the technical reason of implanting a tissue with greater corneal curvature and also increased antigenicity that would increase the risk of immune reaction. Increased steepness, elasticity, and flexibility of the infant donor tissue have limited its application for graft replacement especially for a penetrating keratoplasty (PK). The same criteria also applies for EK where difficulty in unrolling the graft is observed more so in a DMEK. Harvesting a donor tissue for DMEK with young donors below 40 years of age is believed and considered to be difficult and should be avoided due to presumed strong adhesions between the DM and stroma that can lead to tearing of the DM during harvesting of donor tissue.

Utilization of young donor tissue with favorable outcomes has been reported for DSEK[8] and of an infant donor tissue for DSAEK.[9] Sun et al. have reported conflicting results with neonate corneas in DSEK procedure[10] whereas in our study, we reported the feasibility of an infant donor tissue in PDEK.[5]

DONOR AGE AND ENDOTHELIAL KERATOPLASTY

Surgeons have performed DSEK with neonate corneas where they have reported achieving the maximum size of lenticule as 8 mm along with the thinner central lenticule as compared to a thicker peripheral rim of the lenticule. This can be attributed to the increased corneal curvature in newborns as compared to adults. They also observed that due to increased flexibility of the cornea, the unrolling of the graft was a bit difficult and that due to this there were increased chances of graft dislocation and lenticule contraction in the postoperative period.[10]

Other group of surgeons have performed DSEK with pediatric donor tissue and has reported good outcomes. The employment of young donor tissue for EK has a theoretical advantage of transferring a donor lenticule with high ECD that could compensate the issue of ECD loss that eventually occurs in postsurgery. In EK, a frequent concern among surgeons is potential tissue loss as a result of DM graft preparation failure, which is minimized with the PDEK procedure, as failure to get a type-1 bb may be associated with the formation of type-2 bb. Under such a scenario the surgeon can perform a DMEK instead of PDEK procedure.

SUMMARY

To summarize, a stepwise approach to donor preparation and donor insertion makes PDEK a standardized and reproducible procedure with a successful outcome in terms of usage of young donor corneas with high ECD. The procedure of PDEK also involves skill set on behalf of the surgeon to create a type-1 bb but this limitation is totally circumvented by the fact that PDEK does not require the employment of costly microkeratome as in a DSAEK, DMAEK, or UT-DSEK, thereby cutting the cost of surgical procedure and also inculcating the procedure of use of infant donor cornea with a graft thickness of around 35 microns that is eventually less as compared to DSAEK or UT-DSEK tissue.

REFERENCES

1. Melles GR, Eggink FA, Lander F, et al. A surgical technique for posterior lamellar keratoplasty. Cornea. 1998;17:618-26.
2. Melles GR, Ong TS, Ververs B, et al. Descemet membrane endothelial keratoplasty (DMEK). Cornea. 2006;25:987-90.
3. Agarwal A, Dua HS, Narang P, et al. Pre-Descemet's endothelial keratoplasty (PDEK). Br J Ophthalmol. 2014;98:1181-5.
4. Dua HS, Faraj LA, Said DG, et al. Human corneal anatomy redefined: a novel pre-Descemet's layer (Dua's layer). Ophthalmology. 2013;120:1778-85.
5. Agarwal A, Agarwal A, Narang P, et al. Pre-Descemet endothelial keratoplasty with infant donor corneas: a prospective analysis. Cornea. 2015;34:859-65.
6. Agarwal A, Narang P, Kumar DA, et al. Trocar anterior chamber maintainer (T-ACM): improvised technique of infusion. J Cataract Refract Surg. J Cataract Refract Surg. 2016;42(2):185-9.
7. Price FW Jr, Price MO. Descemet's stripping with endothelial keratoplasty in 200 eyes: early challenges and technique to enhance donor adherence. J Cataract Refract Surg. 2006;32:411-8.
8. Huang T1, Wang Y, Hu A, et al. Use of pediatric donor tissue in Descemet's stripping endothelial keratoplasty. Br J Ophthalmol. 2009;93:1625-8.
9. Kim P, Yeung SN, Lichtinger A, et al. Descemet stripping automated endothelial keratoplasty using infant donor tissue. Cornea. 2012;31:52-4.
10. Sun YX, Hao YS, Hong J. Descemet membrane stripping endothelial keratoplasty with neonate donors in two cases. Br J Ophthalmol. 2009;93:1692-3.

SECTION 2

Surgical Technique

CHAPTER 6

Surgical Technique of Pre-Descemet's Endothelial Keratoplasty: 15 Steps to Mastering PDEK

Priya Narang, Amar Agarwal

INTRODUCTION

Amongst all the subtypes of endothelial keratoplasty (EK), Descemet's membrane endothelial keratoplasty (DMEK) and pre-Descemet's endothelial keratoplasty (PDEK) are met with the technical challenge of handling the thin donor tissue and subsequently loading and unscrolling it in the eye that can be even more unpredictable and challenging at times. Donor tissue characteristics[1,2] often affect and influence the tendency of some tissues to resist unscrolling and behave in an inconsistent manner.

Pre-Descemet's endothelial keratoplasty[3,4] combines a simplified technique of stripping dysfunctional endothelium and Descemet's membrane (DM) with the pre-Descemet's layer (PDL) from the host cornea that is assisted by air dissection and creation of a type-1 bubble.[5] PDEK allows closed chamber manipulation of the donor graft, it successfully mitigates ocular surface complications and structural problems (including induced astigmatism and perpetually weak wounds) like other EK procedure subtypes and also immunologic graft reactions and secondary glaucoma from prolonged topical corticosteroid use unlike a penetrating keratoplasty (PK).

DONOR GRAFT PREPARATION

This comprises as one of the most essential and initial step of the surgery. The donor corneoscleral rim is obtained from the whole globe and is placed with the endothelial side up.

- *Bubble creation*: A 30 G needle attached to an air-filled 5 mL syringe is introduced from the periphery of the corneoscleral rim of the graft up to the center. The needle is entered at a considerable depth below the DM so as to create a plane between the PDL and the residual stroma. The needle is introduced in a bevel up position under direct supervision and air is injected. A type-1 bubble is formed that characteristically spreads from the center to periphery, is dome-shaped and is around 8 mm in diameter.
- *Staining and harvesting the graft*: Staining the graft is extremely essential for enhancing the visualization of the graft and also to identify the correct

orientation. The edge of the bubble is entered with a side port blade and trypan blue is injected inside to stain the graft. The graft is then cut with the corneoscleral scissors all around the periphery of the bubble and is placed in the storage media (Figs. 6.1A to F).

RECIPIENT BED PREPARATION AND GRAFT INSERTION

This procedure can be commemorated in short with 15 steps that need to be followed sequentially in the chronological order.

Step 1: Fix the Infusion Cannula

Trocar anterior chamber maintainer[6] (T-ACM; Fig. 6.2) or even a routine ACM can also be fixed if the surgeon is not well versed with the use of a T-ACM. Fixing up an infusion setup allows the surgeon to easily switch over between an air/fluid infusion as and when required during the surgical procedure.

Step 2: Switch on the Air Pump

Connect the T-ACM to an air pump (Fig. 6.3). This facilitates continuous air infusion into the eye and helps to perform the procedure with an anterior chamber (AC) that is always well formed.

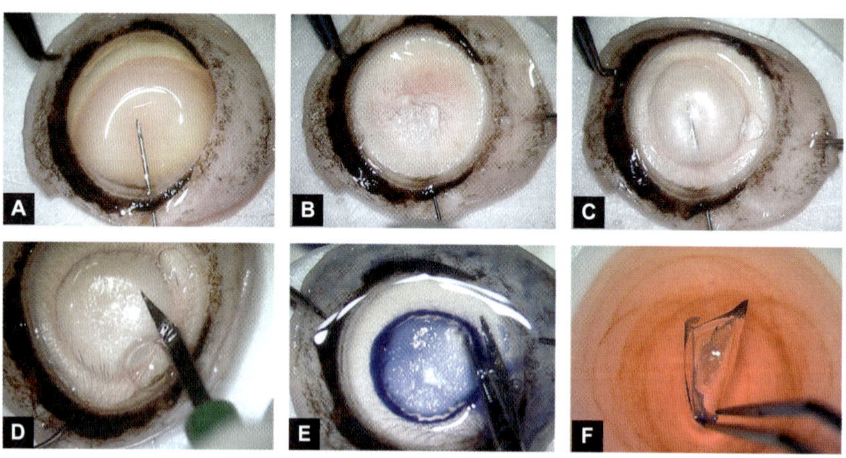

Figs. 6.1A to F: Donor graft preparation. (A) A 5 mL air-filled syringe attached to a 30 G needle is introduced from the corneoscleral edge with the endothelial side up; (B) Air being injected slowly and small bubbles start to form; (C) Air is injected and a type-1 bubble (bb) is formed; (D) The peripheral edge of the bb is ruptured with a side port blade; (E) Trypan blue is injected to stain the bubble. The edge of the bb is cut with the corneoscleral scissors; (F) The graft is placed in the storage media (*Courtesy*: Agarwal/ Kim book Endothelial Keratoplasty by Thieme, USA)

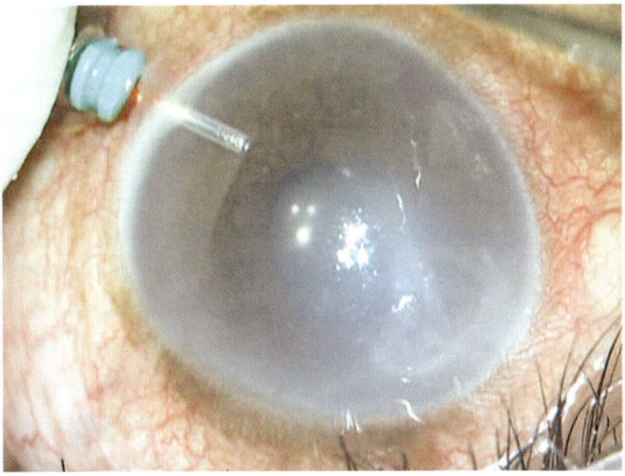

Fig. 6.2: Trocar anterior chamber maintainer (T-ACM) is introduced into the eye (*Courtesy*: Agarwal/Kim book Endothelial Keratoplasty by Thieme, USA)

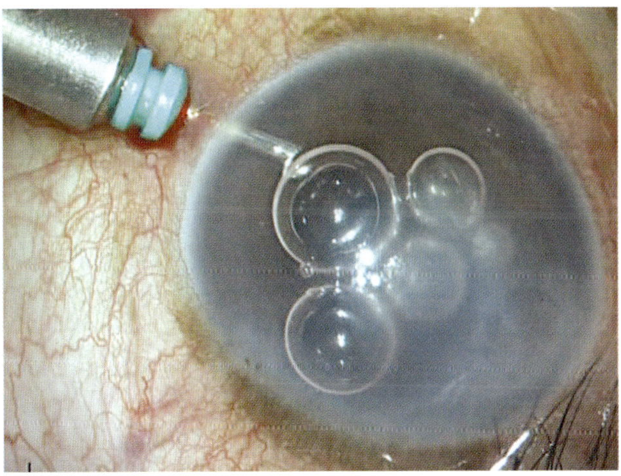

Fig. 6.3: Trocar anterior chamber maintainer (T-ACM) is connected to the air pump (*Courtesy*: Agarwal/Kim book Endothelial Keratoplasty by Thieme, USA)

Step 3: Frame Side-port Incisions

Two side-port incisions are made at superotemporal and superonasal position (Fig. 6.4). This is done so as to allow these sites to be utilized in future for further intraocular manipulation.

Step 4: Perform Descemetorhexis

Descemetorhexis is performed with a reverse Sinskey hook (Fig. 6.5). This step is essentially the same as in a DMEK procedure. Two Sinskey hooks are introduced from both the side-port incisions and the diseased DM is peeled and scrapped off the recipient bed.

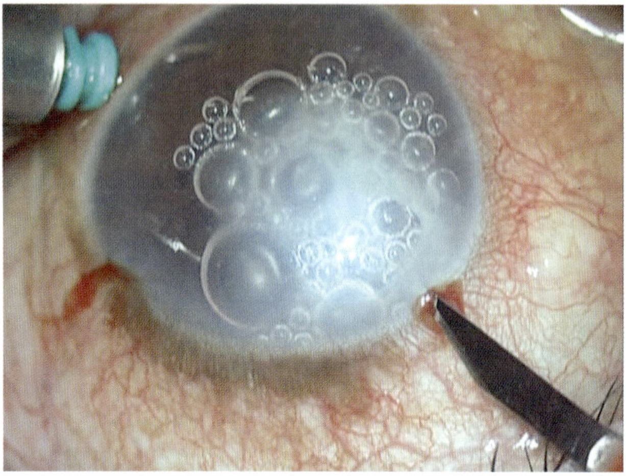

Fig. 6.4: Side-port incision being framed (*Courtesy*: Agarwal/Kim book Endothelial Keratoplasty by Thieme, USA)

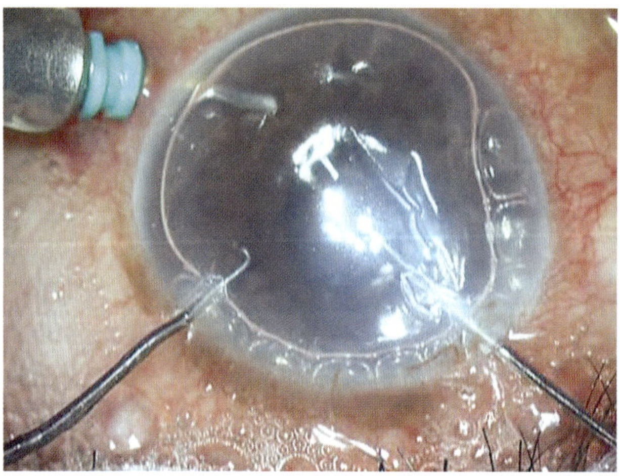

Fig. 6.5: Descemetorhexis being performed with reverse Sinskey hook (*Courtesy*: Agarwal/Kim book Endothelial Keratoplasty by Thieme, USA)

Step 5: Frame Corneal Incision Tunnel

A 2.8-mm clear corneal incision is made and the peeled DM-endothelium complex is removed (Fig. 6.6). This site is further utilized for the introduction of the graft into the eye.

Step 6: Inferior Iridectomy

Inferior iridectomy is performed with a vitrector (Fig. 6.7). This helps to prevent any incidence of pupillary blockage. The vitrectomy machine is set at

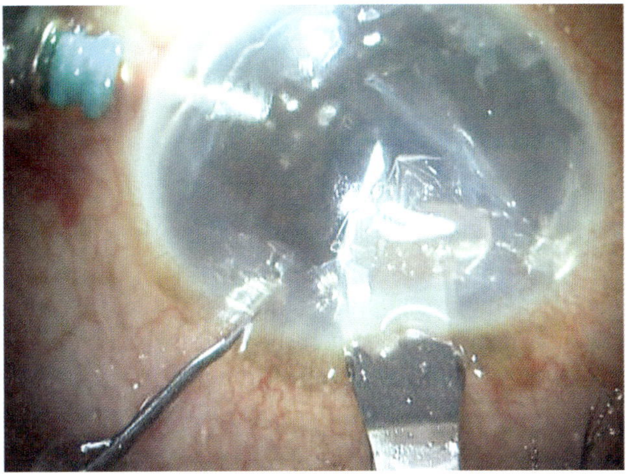

Fig. 6.6: Clear corneal incision is framed (*Courtesy*: Agarwal/Kim book Endothelial Keratoplasty by Thieme, USA)

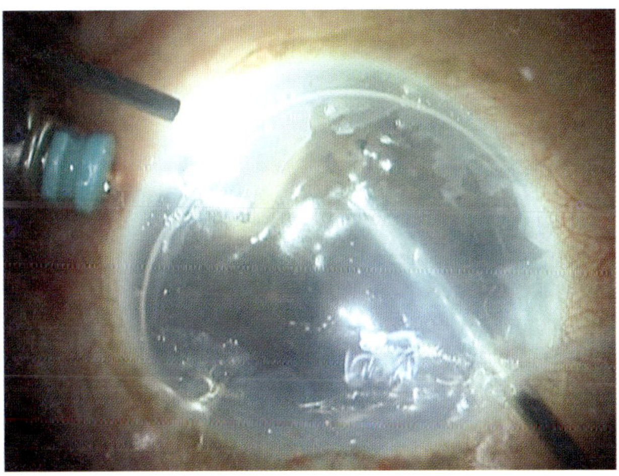

Fig. 6.7: Iridectomy being performed with a vitrectomy probe (*Courtesy*: Agarwal/Kim book Endothelial Keratoplasty by Thieme, USA)

low vacuum and at the cutter rate of around 20 cuts per minute. The cutter is then placed at the proposed iridectomy site and the iris tissue is engaged into the cutter probe initially with the aspiration mode set at low setting. Low cutting rate ensures proper aspiration of the iris tissue into the cutter followed by its cutting. The aspiration port is occluded by the iris stroma, and the iris is cut using the vitrectomy probe in a controlled manner under direct visualization, taking care not to disturb the angle structures. A customized iridectomy can thus be created in the desired quadrant, leaving the rest of the iris tissue undisturbed.

Step 7: Loading of the Graft

Load the PDEK graft in the cartridge of the foldable intraocular lens (IOL) (Fig. 6.8; originally described by Francis Price). Few drops of balanced salt solution (BSS) can be added into the cartridge to keep the graft floating and preventing it from adhering to the cartridge.

Step 8: Switch off the Air Pump

This step is performed (Fig. 6.9) before the graft is injected so that the force of the air does not displace the graft and doing so also ensures that there is enough room for the graft to enter and be properly placed into the AC.

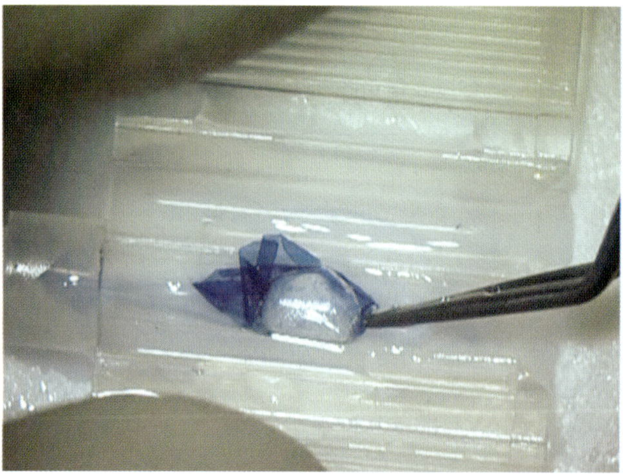

Fig. 6.8: Pre-Descemet's endothelial keratoplasty (PDEK) graft being loaded into the cartridge of the foldable intraocular lens (IOL) (*Courtesy*: Agarwal/Kim book Endothelial Keratoplasty by Thieme, USA)

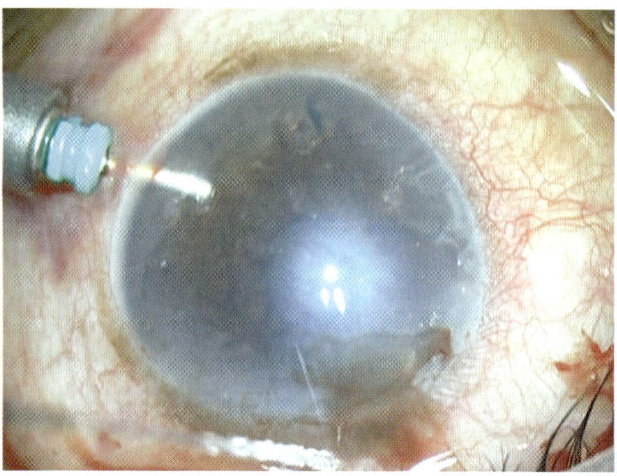

Fig. 6.9: The air pump is switched off (*Courtesy*: Agarwal/Kim book Endothelial Keratoplasty by Thieme, USA).

Step 9: Graft Injection

This is a very critical step of the surgery and the surgeon should avoid wound assisted graft injection. The PDEK graft is injected in the AC (Fig. 6.10) very slowly and carefully. Maintaining an adequate depth of AC is extremely essential at this point of surgery. If the AC is shallow then the assistant can inject a bit of fluid in AC from side-port incision. Once the graft is injected and is seen floating in the AC, the cartridge and the injector is withdrawn from the AC.

Step 10: Suture the Clear Corneal Incision

The clear corneal incision is then sutured with a 10-0 nylon (Fig. 6.11). This ensures there is no wound leakage and that the graft is placed in a well-formed AC.

Step 11: Check Graft Orientation

The correct orientation of the graft is checked (Fig. 6.12) and an endoilluminator can be used to facilitate this.[7] Obliquely directed endoilluminator light provides 3-D depth perception for the graft while allowing visualization of the entire graft. This allows proper comprehension of graft dynamics, morphology, and positioning, in turn leading to easier and faster surgery while potentially decreasing graft damage due to excessive manipulations.

Step 12: Graft Unrolling

After placing the graft in correct orientation, the donor lenticule is centered and oriented with the rolls of the scroll facing upward using short burst of BSS.

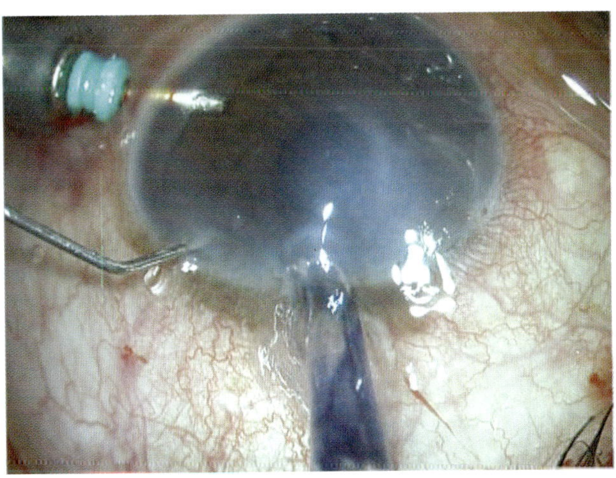

Fig. 6.10: Pre-Descemet's endothelial keratoplasty (PDEK) graft being injected into the anterior chamber (AC) (*Courtesy*: Agarwal/Kim book Endothelial Keratoplasty by Thieme, USA)

After the graft unscrolls partially, a small air bubble is injected underneath the graft to sustain the correct membrane orientation. Unroll the graft and inject a bit of air beneath the graft (Fig. 6.13).

Step 13: Switch on the Air Pump

The air pump connected to the T-ACM or an ACM is switched on. This pushes the graft up and helps it to adhere with corneal surface (Fig. 6.14) of the recipient bed.

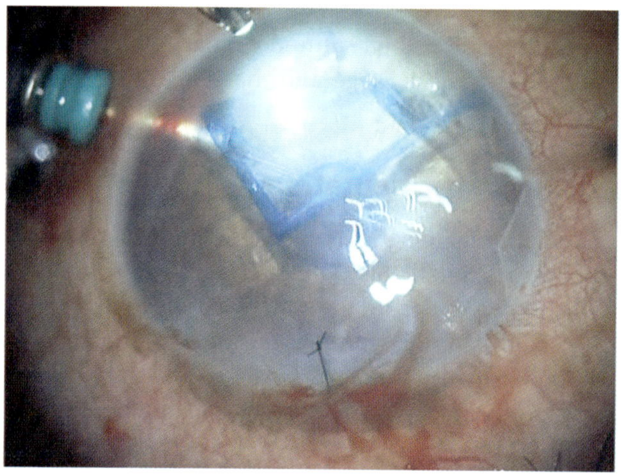

Fig. 6.11: Corneal incision is sutured to seal the anterior chamber (AC) (*Courtesy*: Agarwal/Kim book Endothelial Keratoplasty by Thieme, USA) (*Courtesy*: Agarwal/Kim book Endothelial Keratoplasty by Thieme, USA)

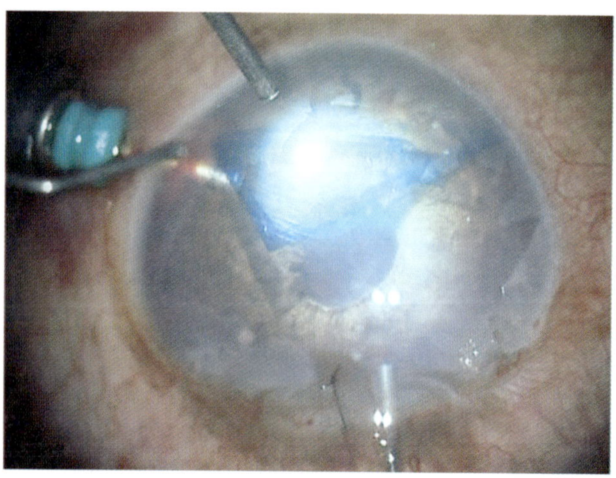

Fig. 6.12: Correct orientation of the graft is checked with an endoilluminator (*Courtesy*: Agarwal/Kim book Endothelial Keratoplasty by Thieme, USA)

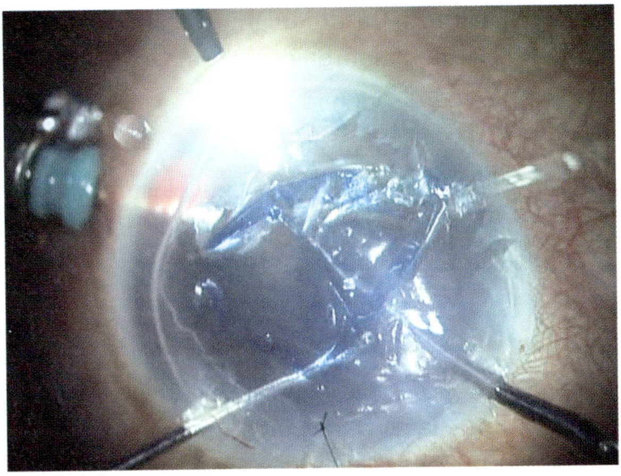

Fig. 6.13: The graft is unrolled and air is injected beneath the graft (*Courtesy*: Agarwal/Kim book Endothelial Keratoplasty by Thieme, USA)

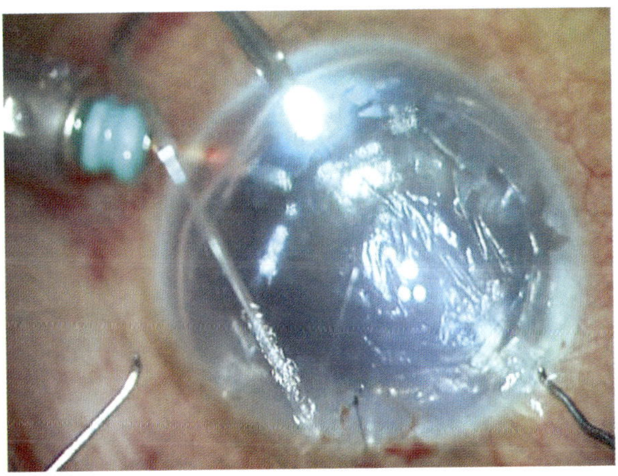

Fig. 6.14: Air pump is switched on and the anterior chamber (AC) is filled with air to facilitate further adhesion of the graft to the endothelial surface (*Courtesy*: Agarwal/Kim book Endothelial Keratoplasty by Thieme, USA)

Step 14: Unroll the Peripheral Curls of the Graft

This is an extremely important step of the surgery that helps to eliminate and curb the incidence of postoperative re-bubbling. The edges of the donor graft have a tendency to curl up and push itself away from the recipient corneal bed. These peripheral edges need to be totally unrolled or else it can lead to small peripheral separations that usually do not seal down on their own and need to be treated. A reverse Sinskey hook is used to unroll the peripheral edges of the donor graft. The entire process is done very gently taking care to minimize the endothelial touch. The graft is then centered (Fig. 6.15). Corneal massage is performed to adjust the centered position of the donor graft and to eliminate residual fluid at the donor graft-recipient interface. Residual interface fluid can also be drained through corneal venting incisions.

Step 15: Suture all the Wounds

All the corneal wounds are sutured to ensure tight closure of the globe to prevent any inadvertent air leak from the AC. The infusion is stopped and the T-ACM is removed (Figs. 6.16A and B).

DISCUSSION

The visual outcomes with PDEK procedure have been reported to be very good with good patient satisfaction. It is therefore reasonable for many surgeons to continue performing PDEK, as the overall results are satisfactory.

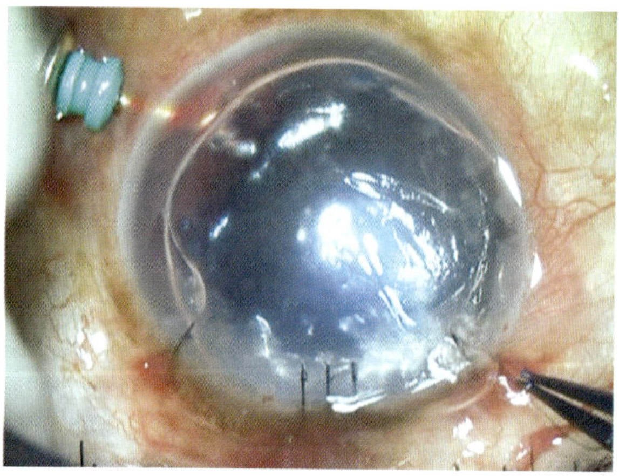

Fig. 6.15: The graft is centered (*Courtesy*: Agarwal/Kim book Endothelial Keratoplasty by Thieme, USA)

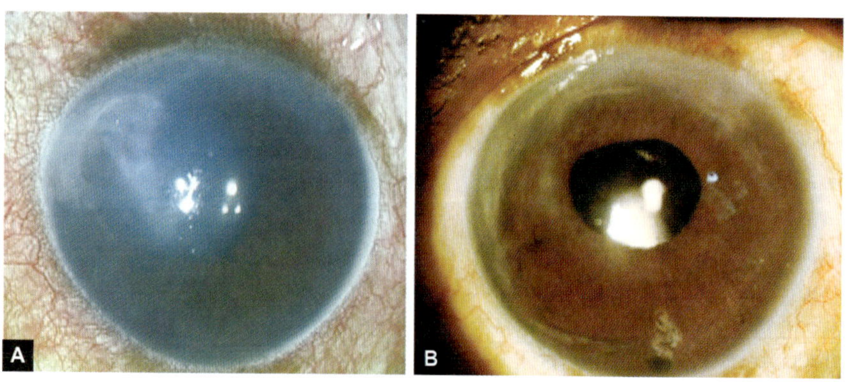

Figs. 6.16A and B: Follow-up images of the patient. (A) Preoperative image of the patient; (B) Three months postoperative image shows clearance of the corneal haze (vision 20/20) (*Courtesy*: Agarwal/Kim book Endothelial Keratoplasty by Thieme, USA)

Care should also be taken while positioning the graft, as there is a chance of graft colliding with the cannula of the ACM that is placed in the AC. The incidence is less with the use of T-ACM as the T-ACM enters the AC from the sclera and does not encroach the anterior corneal surface and is peripherally placed from the limbus. Pupilloplasty should always be performed in eyes with large iris defects as the graft may accidentally dislodge into the vitreous cavity. Pupil reconstruction also helps to maintain the depth of AC throughout the surgery.

Pre-Descemet's endothelial keratoplasty has extended itself as a lexicon amongst various EK subtypes that allows the use of adult and infant donor tissue.[3,4] The technique of PDEK scores over DMEK in this aspect as usually for DMEK older donor tissue is preferred as the thickness of DM increases with age[8] and this leads to less curling up of the donor lenticule edges. The issue of tearing of the DM due to projection of the stromal collagen fibrils in to the interfacial matrix of DM[9] during peeling from the underlying stroma is also not encountered with PDEK.

REFERENCES

1. Price MO, Giebel AW, Fairchild KM, et al. Descemet's membrane endothelial keratoplasty: prospective multi-center study of visual and refractive outcomes and endothelial survival. Ophthalmology. 2009;116:2361-68.
2. Dirisamer M, Ham L, Dapena I, et al. Efficacy of Descemet membrane endothelial keratoplasty: clinical outcome of 200 consecutive cases after a learning curve of 25 cases. Arch Ophthalmol. 2011;129:1435-43.
3. Agarwal A, Dua HS, Narang P, et al. Pre-Descemet's endothelial keratoplasty (PDEK). Br J Ophthalmol. 2014;98:1181-85.
4. Agarwal A, Agarwal A, Narang P, et al. Pre-Descemet endothelial keratoplasty with infant donor corneas: a prospective analysis. Cornea. 2015;34:859-65.
5. Dua HS, Faraj LA, Said DG, et al. Human corneal anatomy redefined: a novel pre-Descemet's layer (Dua's layer). Ophthalmology. 2013;120:1778-85.
6. Agarwal A, Narang P, Kumar DA, et al. Trocar anterior chamber maintainer: Improvised infusion technique. J Cataract Refract Surg. 2016;42:185-9.
7. Jacob S, Agarwal A, Agarwal A, et al. Endoilluminator-assisted transcorneal illumination for Descemet membrane endothelial keratoplasty: enhanced intraoperative visualization of the graft in corneal decompensation secondary to pseudophakic bullous keratopathy. J Cataract Refract Surg. 2014;40:1332-6.
8. Murphy C, Alvarado J, Juster R. Prenatal and postnatal growth of the human Descemet's membrane. Invest Ophthalmol Vis Sci. 1984;25:1402-15.
9. Schlötzer-Schrehardt U, Bachmann BO, Laaser K, et al. Characterization of the cleavage plane in Descemet's membrane endothelial keratoplasty. Ophthalmology. 2011;118:1950-7.

CHAPTER 7

Air Pump-assisted Pre-Descemet's Endothelial Keratoplasty

Soosan Jacob, Amar Agarwal

INTRODUCTION

The description of the pre-Descemet's layer (PDL) brought with it the opportunity to perform a new kind of endothelial transplantation, which included transplantation of the Dua's layer or the PDL together with the Descemet's membrane (DM), and endothelial cells. This procedure was termed as pre-Descemet's endothelial keratoplasty (PDEK).[1,2] The PDEK graft is created by creating a type 1 big bubble[3] and as opposed to DMEK graft, younger donor corneas can be used to create the graft. The PDL also gives a splinting effect to the graft and makes it a tougher tissue that is resistant to tear. The ability to use younger donor tissues with greater endothelial counts together with the tougher nature of the graft gives PDEK advantages over Descemet's membrane endothelial keratoplasty (DMEK).[4,5]

However, in contrast to a Descemet's stripping automated endothelial keratoplasty (DSAEK),[6,7] both DMEK and PDEK still have a steep learning curve as the grafts are thin, roll into scrolls and are very mobile within the anterior chamber (AC).[8-10] They may both therefore have complications ranging from difficulty in unfolding or centering the graft to complex Descemet's detachments.[11]

One of the authors (SJ) has described a technique termed as the air-pump assisted PDEK that aids in multiple key steps of PDEK surgery and makes surgery easier to learn and repeatable.[12] The technique utilizes pressurized air infusion for this purpose.

TECHNIQUE

An anterior chamber maintainer (ACM) or trocar anterior chamber maintainer[13] connected to pressurized air infusion via the fluid air exchange system present in posterior vitrectomy systems is inserted into the AC. A vitrector probe is then passed through a paracentesis to create a peripheral iridectomy (PI) in the inferior iris using 400 cuts per second with vacuum of 200 mm Hg. As this is done under continuous air infusion, any bleeding is tamponaded by the air pressure. Since this is the first step done, by the time the next step, viz. descemetorhexis is completed, the bleeding is always controlled. The DM is then scored and stripped with a reverse Sinskey hook. Any uneven tags are removed by using a microforceps or reverse Sinskey hook passed through the paracentesis. The paracentesis is enlarged with a keratome and air is then replaced with balanced salt solution (BSS). The orientation of the graft that has been loaded into a microincision lens injector is then verified using endoilluminator-assisted visualization and the graft is injected into the AC. Using E-PDEK/E-DMEK[11,14,15] technique, the graft is unrolled. A cannula connected to a syringe filled with air is passed under the graft and the graft is floated up against overlying stroma by injecting air. The ACM is then reinserted into the AC under the graft and continuous air infusion restarted. Under pressurized air infusion, the reverse Sinskey hook is used to engage the PDEK graft in the periphery and the graft is centered into position within the descemetorhexis. Under continuous air support, any graft edges that are folded inward are unfolded using a reverse Sinskey hook or a thin, blunt rod introduced between the graft and the host stroma through the side port. Wrinkles and creases in the graft are also stretched out with the reverse Sinskey hook. All incisions are closed. The ACM is finally removed and limbal paracentesis is sutured. The air fill is checked after removing speculum and if the AC is hypotonic, air is injected into the AC using a 30-G needle passed just posterior to the limbus. Intraocular pressure (IOP) and perception of light are checked and the patient asked to maintain a supine position.

ADVANTAGES OF PRE-DESCEMET'S ENDOTHELIAL KERATOPLASTY

As compared to DMEK, PDEK gives the ability to use younger grafts[2] (the authors have personally done PDEK with grafts as young as 9 months old) thus giving a higher initial count of endothelial cells to start out with. This makes the graft less susceptible to both primary and secondary graft failure. The PDEK graft also has an advantage of being more robust in nature and resistant to tear[1,3] as compared to the DMEK graft.

DISADVANTAGES OF PRE-DESCEMET'S ENDOTHELIAL KERATOPLASTY

Despite being more robust, the PDEK graft still behaves like the DMEK graft does in terms of graft handling, complete graft unfolding including edge unfolding, graft centration, graft adhesion, etc. The younger age grafts that are used in PDEK also tend to scroll more and therefore are more difficult to unroll. The learning curve is therefore more than that of a DSAEK and just as DMEK, PDEK is also difficult to perform in complex cases.

ADVANTAGES OF AIR PUMP-ASSISTED PRE-DESCEMET'S ENDOTHELIAL KERATOPLASTY

As mentioned above, PDEK still has disadvantages in terms of the surgical skill required. However, the steep learning curve can be made easier using the air pump-assisted PDEK technique. The use of air-pump has previously been described by us for phacoemulsification.[16,17] In PDEK, the air pump gives advantages of a third hand within the AC that helps maintain space within the AC and supports the graft during intraocular maneuvers, preventing its dislocation (Figs. 7.1A to F).

It has various uses during the procedure as mentioned below:

- *Descemetorhexis*: Descemetorhexis under an air bubble[18] as well as under continuous low pressure air infusion[19] have been described previously in DMEK. Having the pressurized air inflow into the chamber during descemetorhexis prevents AC collapse while at the same time giving better visualization and control. A descemetorhexis can be made following the desired size marked on the cornea. The tearing edge is always seen can be controlled under pressure of air. An appropriately sized and centered descemetorhexis is therefore possible.

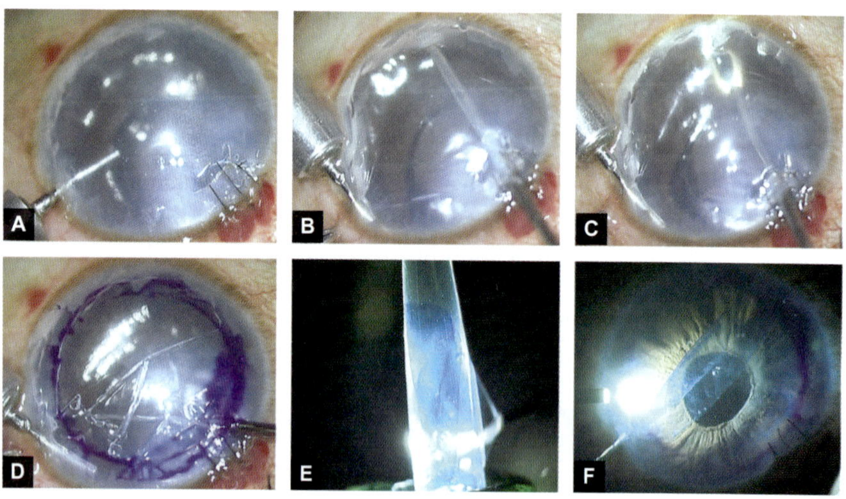

Figs. 7.1A to F: Air pump-assisted pre-Descemet's endothelial keratoplasty (PDEK): (A) Anterior chamber maintainer is inserted into anterior chamber (AC); (B) Inferior peripheral iridectomy is performed with a vitrector under pressurized air infusion; (C) Peripheral iridectomy seen clearly using the endoilluminator from the endoilluminator-assisted PDEK (E-PDEK) technique; Notice no bleeding because of air tamponade; (D) Descemetorhexis is performed under pressurized air infusion; (E) The PDEK graft is loaded into the injector and orientation identified with the E-PDEK technique; (F) Air is replaced with balanced salt solution (BSS) and the PDEK graft is injected into the AC. The E-PDEK technique is used to enhance visualization of the PDEK graft.

- *Preventing blood in anterior chamber*: Iris stroma may bleed while creating the inferior PI. Bleeding into the AC may also occur from synechiolysis or secondary to blood seeping into the AC from any peripheral corneal neovascularization. The continuous pressure head tamponades any intraocular bleeding as well as prevents blood from seeping into the AC from external bleeding sources.
- *Graft floatation*: In a DMEK, the graft needs to be completely unfolded and centered before floating it up. Complete unfolding of young grafts may be difficult in PDEK and trying to unfold extreme edge folds often takes time and more graft manipulation. With air pump-assisted PDEK, because of the tough nature of the graft, complete unfolding and centration can be done even after floatation unlike DMEK where the graft may tear if these are attempted after floatation. Therefore, once the PDEK graft is largely unfolded, it can be floated up despite the presence of small edge folds.
- *Graft centration*: Under the continuous pressurized air infusion, a reverse Sinskey is used to pull the graft into centered position. The entire graft slides en toto while the pressurized air prevents dislocation during this maneuver.
- *Graft edge unfolding*: Once centered, extreme edge folds can be unfolded using a reverse Sinskey. Unfolding is successful when started at one edge of the fold and continued through to the other side of the fold. The graft is held against the corneal stroma by the pressurized air while the reverse Sinskey or a thin, blunt rod introduced between the stroma and the graft is used to unfold inward rolled graft edges. The infusion pressure into the eye is adjusted depending on the amount of leak from the incisions (Figs. 7.2A to D).
- *Graft unwrinkling*: Wrinkles in the graft are stretched out using the reverse Sinskey hook by pulling the graft outward at its extreme edges.
- *Graft adhesion*: The pressurized air promotes earlier and better graft adherence by continuously holding the graft tightly against the overlying stroma.

Thus, we see that continuous pressurized air infusion helps in multiple steps of PDEK, making the transition to PDEK from DSAEK and DMEK easier. It makes surgery easier to adopt and repeatable.

TIPS AND TRICKS

Repeated graft touch should be decreased by minimal touching of the graft and only at peripheral edge points. Only minimally required manipulations should be performed and rough handling of the graft should be avoided. Infusion pressure of air should be titrated subjectively against the amount of leakage from the incisions in order to maintain a normotensive or slightly

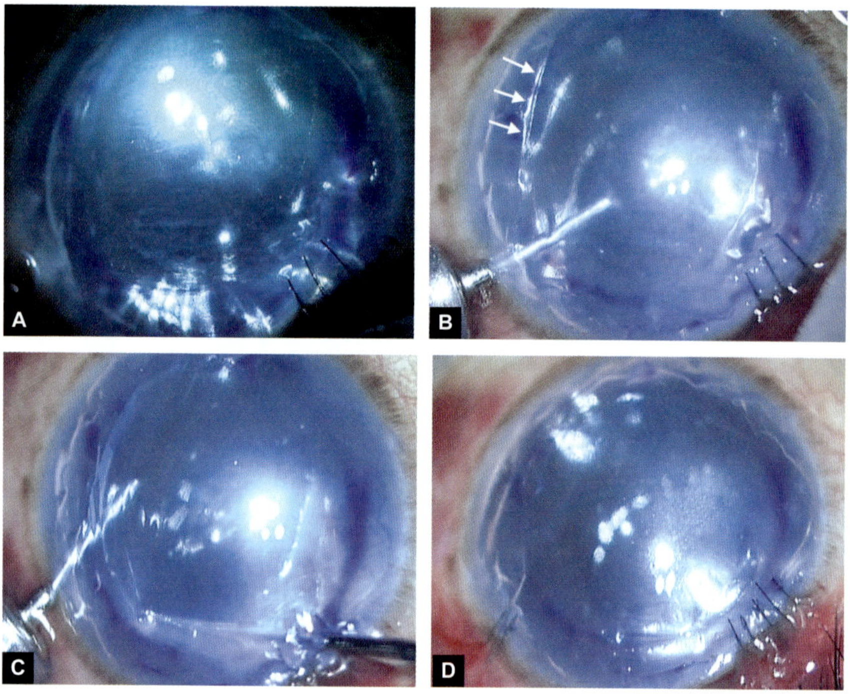

Figs. 7.2A to D: Air pump-assisted pre-Descemet's endothelial keratoplasty (PDEK): (A) Graft is unfolded and air injected to float it up; (B) The anterior chamber maintainer (ACM) is reinserted and air pump turned on, after making sure that the tip is below the PDEK graft; Notice small edge folds on the graft (arrows); (C) The graft is centered into position and graft edge is unfolded using a reverse Sinskey hook while the air acts as a third hand preventing the graft from dislocating; (D) Graft wrinkles cleared. The continuing air infusion allows incisions to be sutured without air escaping while also allowing early graft adherence.

hypertensive pressure level within the AC. The pressure level can be judged by checking the indentation of cornea with a cannula. With this technique, graft centration, edge unfolding and unwrinkling is possible in all cases when performed with adequate air support to the graft. It avoids endothelial loss secondary to repeated attempts at trying to manipulate a free-floating graft within the AC (Figs. 7.3A and B). DMEK grafts may also be centered similarly using lower infusion pressure, however, in our experience, DMEK grafts, being thinner and more fragile had a higher rate of graft wrinkling and graft edge tearing.

To conclude, air pump-assisted PDEK increases the ease, speed and success of surgery while decreasing complications. It also helps decrease the learning curve.

Disclosure: The author has no financial interests in the product or procedure mentioned. No funding has been received.

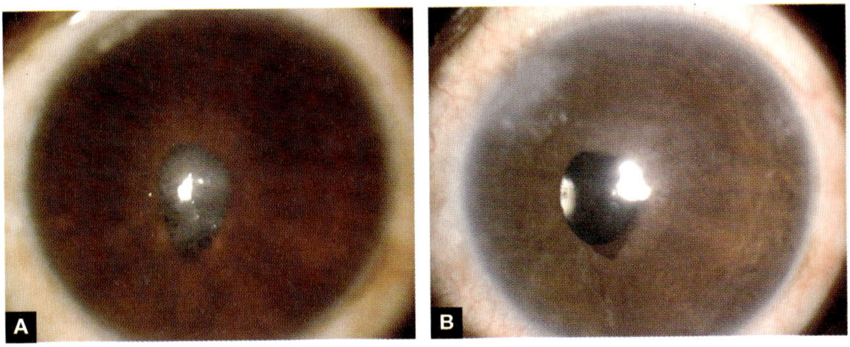

Figs. 7.3A and B: Air pump-assisted pre-Descemet's endothelial keratoplasty (PDEK): (A) Preoperative picture of patient with iridocorneal endothelial (ICE) syndrome; (B) Postoperative picture after phaco and air pump-assisted PDEK showing a well attached graft and a clear cornea.

REFERENCES

1. Agarwal A, Dua HS, Narang P, et al. Pre-Descemet's endothelial keratoplasty (PDEK). Br J Ophthalmol. 2014;98(9):1181-5.
2. Agarwal A, Agarwal A, Narang P, et al. Pre-Descemet endothelial keratoplasty with infant donor corneas: a prospective analysis. Cornea. 2015;34(8):859-65.
3. Dua HS, Faraj LA, Said DG, et al. Human corneal anatomy redefined: a novel pre-Descemet's layer (Dua's layer). Ophthalmology. 2013;120(9):1778-85.
4. Dapena I, Moutsouris K, Droutsas K, et al. Standardized "no-touch" technique for descemet membrane endothelial keratoplasty. Arch Ophthalmol. 2011;129(1): 88-94.
5. Dapena I, Ham L, Melles GR. Endothelial keratoplasty: DSEK/DSAEK or DMEK—the thinner the better? Curr Opin Ophthalmol. 2009;20:299-307.
6. Gorovoy MS, Descemet-stripping automated endothelial keratoplasty. Cornea. 2006;25(8):886-9.
7. Busin M, Albé E, Does thickness matter: ultrathin Descemet stripping automated endothelial keratoplasty. Curr Opin Ophthalmol. 2014;25(4):312-8.
8. Coster DJ, Lowe MT, Keane MC, et al. A comparison of lamellar and penetrating keratoplasty outcomes: a registry study. Ophthalmology. 2014;121(5):979-87.
9. Monnereau C, Quilendrino R, Dapena I, et al. Multicenter study of descemet membrane endothelial keratoplasty: first case series of 18 surgeons. JAMA Ophthalmol. 2014;132(10):1192-8.
10. Satué M, Rodríguez-Calvo-de-Mora M, Naveiras M, et al. Standardization of the Descemet membrane endothelial keratoplasty technique: Outcomes of the first 450 consecutive cases. Arch Soc Esp Oftalmol. 2015;90(8):356-64.
11. Jacob S, Narasimhan S, Agarwal A, et al. Air pump-assisted graft centration, graft edge unfolding, and graft uncreasing in young donor graft pre-descemet endothelial keratoplasty. Cornea. 2017;36(8):1009-13.
12. Agarwal A, Narang P, Kumar DA, et al. Trocar anterior chamber maintainer: improvised infusion technique. J Cataract Refract Surg. 2016;42(2):185-9.
13. Jacob S, Agarwal A, Chaudhry P, et al. A new clinico-tomographic classification and management algorithm for Descemet's membrane detachment. Cont Lens Anterior Eye. 2015;38(5):327-33.

14. Jacob S, Agarwal A, Agarwal A, et al. Endoilluminator-assisted transcorneal illumination for Descemet membrane endothelial keratoplasty: enhanced intra-operative visualization of the graft in corneal decompensation secondary to pseudophakic bullous keratopathy. J Cataract Refract Surg. 2014;40(8):1332-6.
15. Jacob S, Agarwal A, Kumar DA. Endoilluminator-assisted Descemet membrane endothelial keratoplasty and endoilluminator-assisted pre-Descemet endothelial keratoplasty. Clin Ophthalmol. 2015;9:2123-5.
16. Chaudhry P, Prakash G, Jacob S, et al. Safety and efficacy of gas-forced infusion (air pump) in coaxial phacoemulsification. J Cataract Refract Surg. 2010;36(12):2139-45.
17. Agarwal A, Kumar DA, Agarwal A. Gas-forced infusion prevents endothelial cell loss in phacoemulsification. J Cataract Refract Surg. 2013;39(3):481.
18. Mehta JS, Hantera MM, Tan DT. Modified air-assisted descemetorhexis for Descemet-stripping automated endothelial keratoplasty. J Cataract Refract Surg. 2008;34(6):889-91.
19. Güell JL, Morral M, Gris O, et al. Bimanual technique for insertion and positioning of endothelium-Descemet membrane graft in Descemet membrane endothelial keratoplasty. Cornea. 2013;32(12):1521-6.

CHAPTER 8

Trocar Anterior Chamber Maintainer

Amar Agarwal, Priya Narang

BACKGROUND

Postoperative self sealing wounds are the most desirable and hallmark of the advanced intraocular procedures. Controlled access to the intraocular segment structures without running risk of hypotony is the prime concern of all the surgeons. Anterior chamber (AC) maintainer[1-3] and trocar cannula are the most common methods employed for infusion by the anterior segment and posterior segment surgeons, respectively.

THE NEW TROCAR ANTERIOR CHAMBER MAINTAINER (TACM)

Continuous infusion into the eye is often imperative for performing an intraocular surgery; anterior chamber maintainer (ACM) and trocar cannula system form an essential component of it and are most commonly employed. Trocar anterior chamber maintainer (TACM)[1] is a new technique where a trocar cannula system is used for infusion into the eye at the level of limbus and it essentially works as an ACM. The basis for the wound construction is similar to the modern vitrectomy surgery, which creates a biplanar angle-based incision with the trocar system. Self-sealing wounds are the most desirable and are the hallmark of any intraocular surgery. Controlled access to the intraocular segment structures without running risk of hypotony is the prime concern of all the surgeons. ACM[2-4] and trocar cannula are the most common methods employed for infusion by the anterior segment and posterior segment surgeons, respectively.

Introduction of trocar cannula was a monumental advance in ophthalmology as it allowed, for the first time, controlled access to the posterior segment of the eye and currently it is an integral part of modern pars plana vitrectomy for maintaining infusion in the eye.[5-9] A 23-gauge (0.6 mm), 25-gauge (0.5 mm), or 27-gauge (0.4 mm) entry does not require incision of the conjunctiva and tenon's layer to expose the sclera. Instead, trocars are placed through the conjunctiva and sclera to afford access to the vitreous and also to maintain an infusion in the eye.

Taking into consideration the advantages of a trocar system, we employed a method of introduction of trocar cannula for the maintenance of AC that would be applicable and the advantages of which would be availed by the anterior segment surgeons too with equal ease and élan. Encompassing the advantages of a trocar cannula into the AC maintainer, a new device has been designed called as TACM (Figs. 8.1 to 8.3). This has been made by Mastel (USA). As compared to the conventional trocars, the overall length of the newly designed TACM has been decreased to 6 mm, so that it can be conveniently used by the anterior segment surgeons without the fear of damaging the intraocular structures (Figs. 8.4 to 8.6).

SURGICAL TECHNIQUE USING TACM

The conjunctiva is displaced with a cotton tip to keep the conjunctival puncture away from the scleral-limbal wound (Figs. 8.7 and 8.8). The cannula

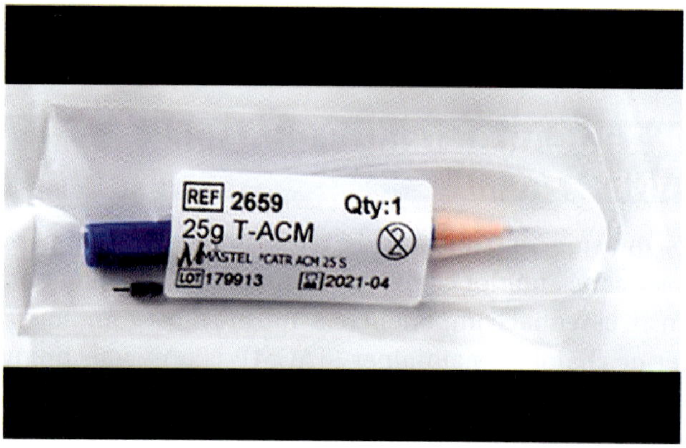

Fig. 8.1: 25-gauge trocar anterior chamber (AC) maintainer (Mastel USA).

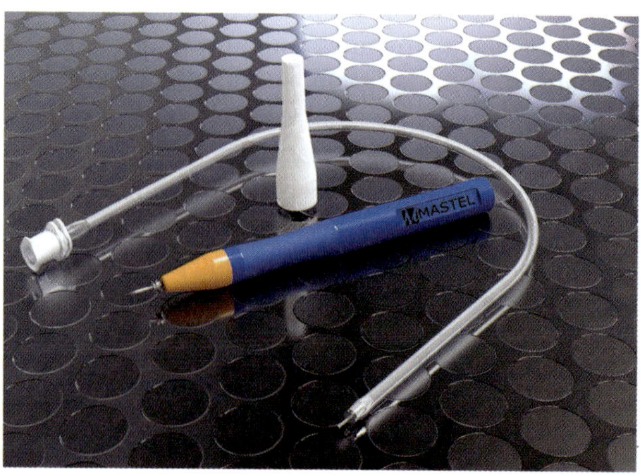

Fig. 8.2: Trocar with the cannula opened.

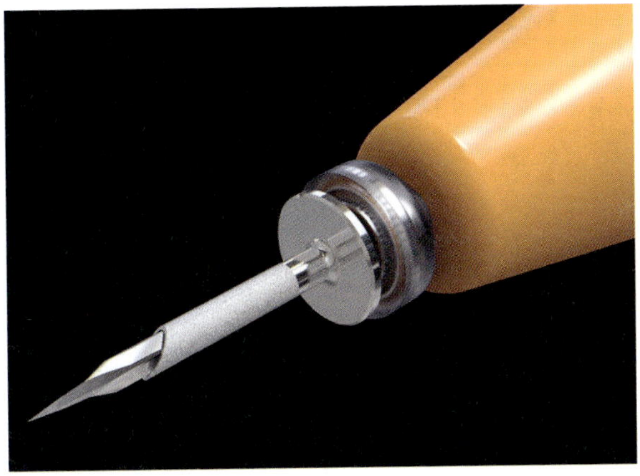

Fig. 8.3: Magnified view of the trocar.

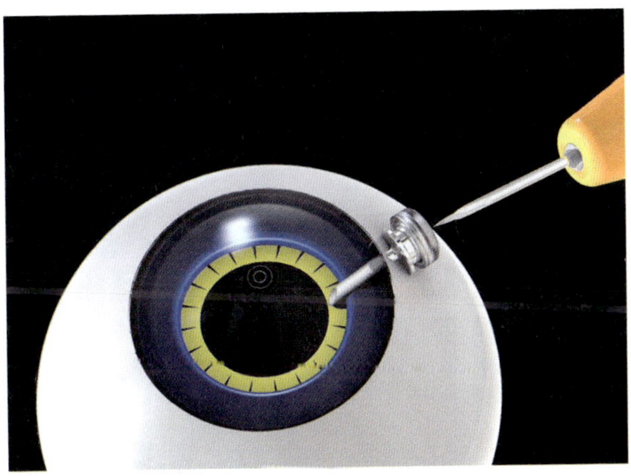

Fig. 8.4: Animation of the trocar anterior chamber maintainer (TACM) fixed in the eye.

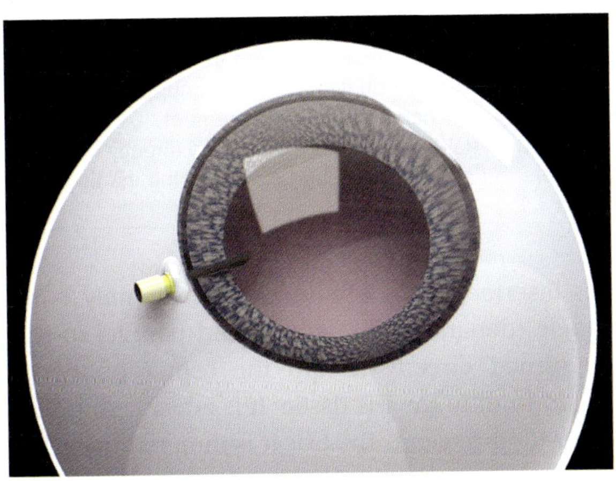

Fig. 8.5: Cannula fixed in the anterior chamber (AC).

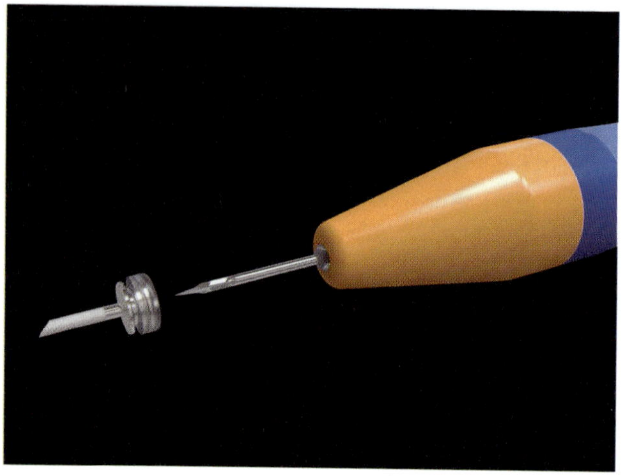

Fig. 8.6: Animation showing trocar being disconnected from the cannula.

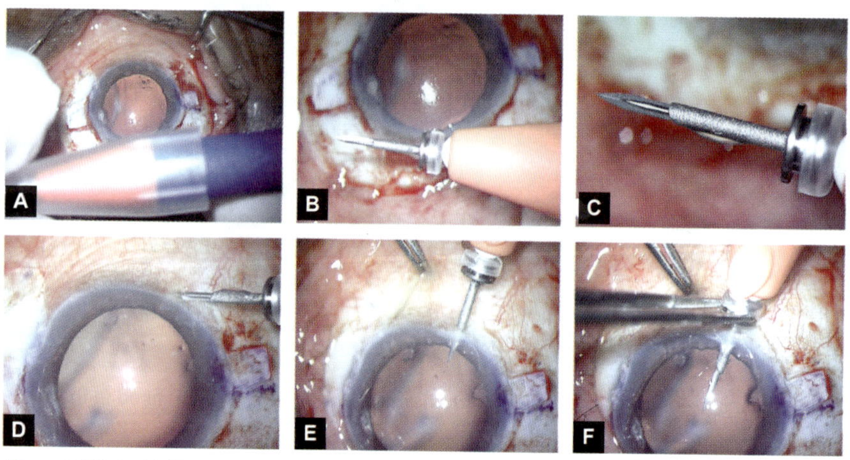

Figs. 8.7A to F: Trocar anterior chamber maintainer (TACM); surgical technique: (A) TACM in the protection cover; (B) TACM removed from the protection cover; (C) Magnified view of the TACM. Note the dusting of the cannula, which helps locking of the TACM to the sclera; (D) After conjunctival displacement, TACM being introduced 0.5 mm away from the limbus; (E) The trocar is then turned directly toward the center of the globe, so that it enters the anterior chamber in front of the iris tissue; (F) The trocar is now to be removed.

(on a trocar) is inserted into the limbus approximately 1 mm away, usually at a 45° angle (depending on gauge) and parallel to the limbus. The trocar is then turned directly toward the center of the globe, so that it enters the AC in front of the iris tissue. It is advanced until the hub of the cannula is flush with the sclera. The trocar is then removed, leaving the cannula in place. This maneuver allows a longer scleral wound and carries a lower risk of wound leakage. The infusion line is attached to the stent of the

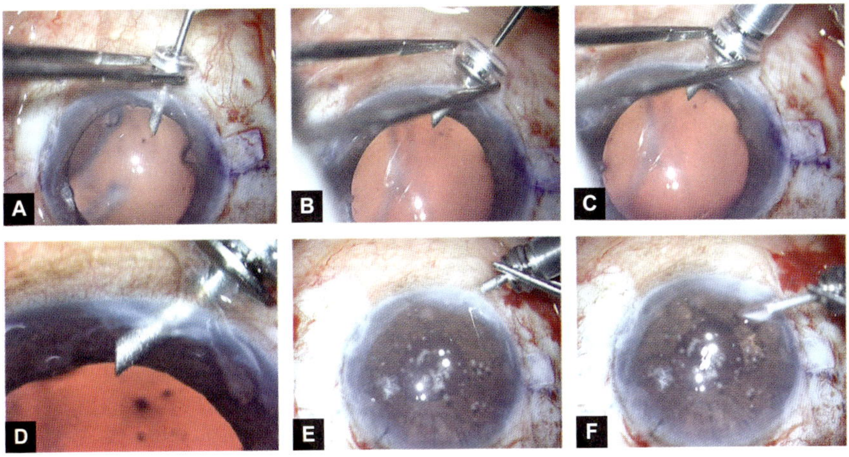

Figs. 8.8A to F: Trocar anterior chamber maintainer (TACM); surgical technique continued: (A) Trocar removed; (B) Cannula is getting fixed; (C) Cannula fixed; (D) Magnified view of the cannula. The infusion line is attached to the stent of the cannula. The infusion is turned on; (E) After surgery TACM is going to be removed; (F) TACM removed.

cannula, and the infusion is turned on. At the end of the surgical procedure, the surgeon just withdraws the TACM and as the wound is self-sealing, no leakage is observed.

ADVANTAGES OF TACM

Trocar anterior chamber maintainer allows an easy and atraumatic transconjunctival entry into the anterior segment. It also allows better endurance and ability to create auto sealing ports. Utilization of valved trocars can offer a better control of the intraocular pressure and eye outflow during the surgery, although we have not yet exploited this option in our patients.

Trocar-ACM can also be employed for maintaining continuous air/fluid infusion in the eye in cases of corneal endothelial keratoplasty. This can prevent repeated shallowing and reforming of the AC and minimize the risk of iris damage, miosis, and lens damage in phakic eye procedures. Some surgeons even prefer using vitrectomy air exchange pumps for the same.[10]

The additional advantage of TACM is the induction of less astigmatism. Moreover, the same TACM can be used in both anterior and posterior segment surgeries.

TACM IN ANTERIOR SEGMENT SURGERY

The maintenance of a deep AC is a prerequisite for a safe anterior segment surgery. An AC maintainer helps to prevent AC collapse apart from serving as an important tool during intraocular lens (IOL) insertion, post-IOL insertion maneuvers, during vitrectomy or secondary IOL implantation, obviating

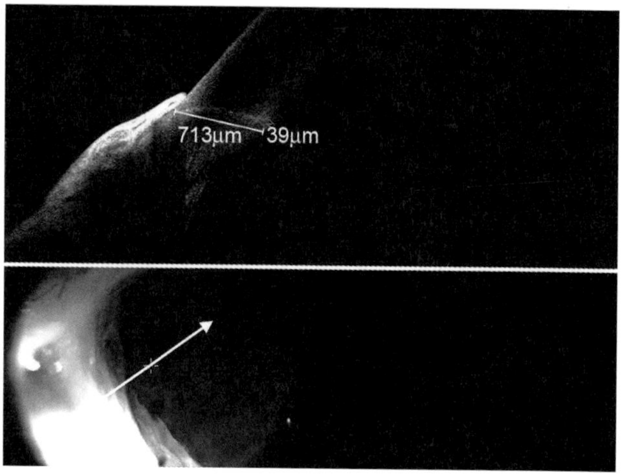

Fig. 8.9: Anterior segment optical coherence tomography (OCT) showing the track of the trocar anterior chamber maintainer (TACM). Good apposition is seen.

the need for use of an ophthalmic viscosurgical device (OVD). Fluid is the natural milieu of the anterior segment and its use during surgery does not disturb any of the anatomical relationships in the eye.[4]

The surgical wound creation for introduction of ACM necessitates the use of paracentesis wound with a side-port incision in the peripheral cornea. The ACM must be exactly the right size and the knife must be withdrawn along the tract of entry as any sideway movement during entry or withdrawal will produce an incision that is too large and the ACM wound will leak. Suturing an incision is often required to prevent postoperative hypotony and also to minimize the continuous leak and the induced postoperative astigmatism.[11] All these shortcomings are outweighed by the use of TACM.

Optical coherence tomography (OCT) study on these incisions demonstrated proper wound apposition and stability that completely healed at the period of one month (Fig. 8.9). To conclude, TACM is effective in obtaining better wound closure and results in a significantly lower incidence of postoperative hypotony. Although, it is necessary to state that a certain level of skill is necessary to make these tunnel-based incisions. The sclerotomy wound should be checked thoroughly and in case of any persistent leakage noted from the sclerotomy site, the scleral wound should be sutured to prevent any overt hypotony.

Another disadvantage that can be associated is the occurrence of subconjunctival hemorrhage that can occur due to disruption of the conjunctival blood vessels either during the insertion or removal of the TACM. Withholding the intake of aspirin or anticoagulants taken by patients as a medication before the operation along with gentle maneuvering of tissues might help to decrease the risk of this complication.

CONCLUSION

In TACM, oblique incision parallel to the limbus displaces the circumferentially oriented scleral fibers laterally, rather than cutting it. Creation of a biplanar incision seals the wound perfectly. The use of TACM has applications, which in our opinion may facilitate some complex ophthalmic surgeries. A word of caution is to choose an appropriate distance from the limbus while introducing a TACM in a phakic eye, so as to curtail the possibility of hitting the transparent lens.

REFERENCES

1. Agarwal A, Narang P, Kumar DA, et al. Trocar anterior chamber maintainer: improvised infusion technique. J Cataract Refract Surg. 2016;42:185-9.
2. Thrasher B. Maintaining an anterior chamber with the Cavitron unit. Am Intra-Ocular Implant Soc J. 1978;4:220-1.
3. Lewicky AO, Lopez OI, Petkus RW, et al. The chamber maintainer system (CMS). Ophthalmic Surg. 1982;13:921-7.
4. Blumenthal M, Moisseiev J. Anterior chamber maintainer for extracapsular cataract extraction and intraocular lens implantation. J Cataract Refract Surg. 1987;13:204-6.
5. Chen JC. Sutureless pars plana vitrectomy through self-sealing sclerotomies. Arch Ophthalmol. 1996;10:1273-5.
6. Kwok KK, Tham CC, Lam DS, et al. Modified sclerotomies in pars plana vitrectomy. Am J Ophthalmol. 1999;6:731-3.
7. De Juan E, Hickingbotham D. Refinements in micro-instrumentation for vitreous surgery. Am J Ophthalmol. 1990;2:218-20.
8. Fujii GY, De Juan E, Humayun MS, et al. A new 25-gauge instrument system for transconjunctival sutureless vitrectomy surgery. Ophthalmology. 2002;10: 1807-12; discussion 1813.
9. Eckardt C. Transconjunctival sutureless 23-gauge vitrectomy. Retina. 2005;2: 208-11.
10. Leyland M. Anterior chamber maintenance during Descemet stripping [letter]. Cornea. 2007;26:1292-3.
11. Ashkenazi, Avni I, Blumenthal M. Maintaining nearly physiologic intraocular pressure levels prior to tying the sutures during cataract surgery reduces surgically induced astigmatism. Ophthalmic Surg. 1991;22:284-6.

CHAPTER 9

Endoilluminator-assisted Pre-Descemet's Endothelial Keratoplasty

Soosan Jacob, Amar Agarwal

INTRODUCTION

Though Descemet's Stripping Automated Endothelial Keratoplasty (DSAEK) is widely practiced, this is not the case with Descemet Membrane Endothelial Keratoplasty (DMEK) and Pre-Descemet's Endothelial Keratoplasty (PDEK), partly because of the difficult learning curve associated with these two surgeries. Poor visibility and a thin, flimsy graft make surgery more difficult. Though staining of the graft with trypan blue is performed in an attempt to increase visibility, visualization is still difficult, especially through edematous and hazy corneas. Prolonged surgery also results in the trypan blue dye washing off, thereby increasing the difficulty in visualization again. One of us (SJ) has described a technique called the E-DMEK/E-PDEK (endoilluminator-assisted DMEK/PDEK) to allow good visualization of the graft and to make surgery easier and faster. This technique utilizes oblique illumination from an endoilluminator.[1-4]

TECHNIQUE

It is important to determine the descemetic side of the graft in PDEK as it must be ascertained that this side faces the stroma and the endothelium downwards. Because of the intrinsic elastic nature of the Descemet's membrane, the graft always tends to scroll toward the Descemet's membrane. Therefore a graft that has the edges curled upwards is in the correct orientation and can be unscrolled and floated up. However, the thin, flimsy and transparent nature of the graft makes identification of side difficult. This is more so when perpendicular light from the operating microscope is used as this decreases three dimensional perception. In the E-DMEK/E-PDEK technique, once the graft is injected into the AC, the microscope light is turned off. Light from a vitreoretinal light probe (20G, 23G or 25G) is then shone obliquely onto the graft and thus used to determine graft orientation. The light probe is held obliquely near the limbus and moved in order to see the direction of the curls. The oblique focused light beam highlights details of the graft and thus allows good visualization and three-dimensional perception. The light reflexes created at the edges of the graft on tapping the corneal surface gently allows verification of the direction of the graft in a non-touch manner without even having to enter the anterior chamber. Once the surgeon has verified orientation, the light probe is handed over to the assistant while the surgeon proceeds with unscrolling the graft and then floating it up (Figs. 9.1 to 9.3). Once this is done, the microscope light is turned back on and further surgery continued with using the air pump assisted PDEK technique also been described by one of us (SJ).[5]

ADVANTAGES OF ENDOILLUMINATOR-ASSISTED PDEK

Though chandelier illumination has been described for DSAEK in 2011 by using a chandelier illumination fiber inserted through a paracentesis to provide sclerotic scattering-like illumination from the sclerocorneal margin and endoillumination from the anterior chamber to increase visibility in DSAEK, endoilluminator use has not been described for either DMEK or PDEK to determine graft orientation. This technique has advantages over other techniques that have been described in being able to determine graft orientation in a non-touch manner, thus decreasing unnecessary manipulation within the anterior chamber. This helps decrease uncontrolled movements of the graft secondary to manipulations as well as decreases cell loss. The entire graft can be visualized at the same time and the graft orientation can be determined definitively before floatation unlike those that utilize a mark. No preoperative marking are required and therefore graft manipulation is minimized. It thus makes surgery easier, faster and decreases endothelial loss secondary to intraocular maneuvering/graft marking.

To conclude, the E-DMEK/E-PDEK technique allows better three-dimensional visualization and depth perception, thus providing better understan-

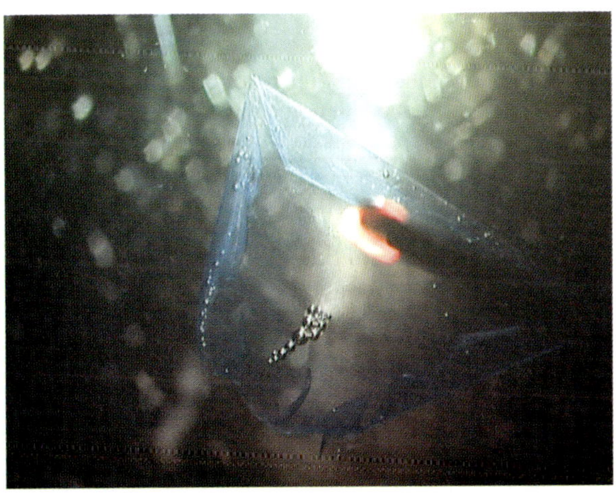

Fig. 9.1: The E-PDEK technique allows easy identification of orientation of the graft in a non-touch manner and without the need for any markings on the graft. It allows visualization of the entire extent of the graft.

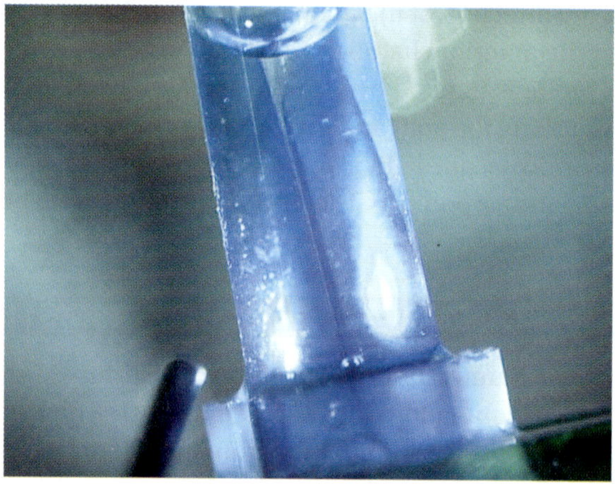

Fig. 9.2: The direction of the graft can be verified easily before injection as well by shining the endoilluminator light on to the graft within the injector.

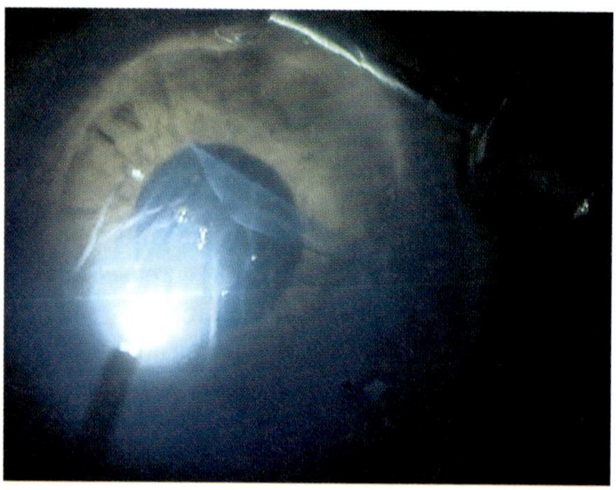

Fig. 9.3: The oblique light from the endoilluminator bouncing off the edges of the graft gives very good three-dimensional depth perception and helps in determining graft orientation. It also helps in other steps of surgery by improving visualization.

ding of graft morphology, position, orientation, and dynamics. It enhances surgical ease, speed, and success of the endothelial keratoplasty (EK) surgery. Potential graft damage caused by excessive handling and maneuvering within the eye is decreased.

REFERENCES

1. Jacob S, Agarwal A, Agarwal A, et al. Endoilluminator-assisted transcorneal illumination for Descemet membrane endothelial keratoplasty: enhanced intraoperative visualization of the graft in corneal decompensation secondary to pseudophakic bullous keratopathy. J Cataract Refract Surg. 2014;40(8):1332-6.

2. Jacob S, Agarwal A, Kumar DA. Endoilluminator-assisted Descemet membrane endothelial keratoplasty and endoilluminator-assisted pre-Descemet endothelial keratoplasty. Clin Ophthalmol. 2015;9:2123-5.
3. Agarwal A, Dua HS, Narang P, et al. Pre-Descemet's endothelial keratoplasty (PDEK). Br J Ophthalmol. 2014;98(9):1181-5.
4. Dua HS, Faraj LA, Said DG, et al. A novel pre-Descemet's layer (Dua's layer). Ophthalmology. 2013;120:1778-85.4.
5. Jacob S, Narasimhan S, Agarwal A, et al. Air pump-assisted graft centration, graft edge unfolding, and graft uncreasing in young donor graft pre-descemet endothelial keratoplasty. Cornea. 2017;36(8):1009-13.

Chapter 10

Infant and Young Donor Pre-Descemet's Endothelial Keratoplasty

Priya Narang, Amar Agarwal

INTRODUCTION

Good visual outcomes have been reported with the utilization of pediatric donor tissue for Descemet's stripping endothelial keratoplasty (DSEK) and infant donor tissue for Descemet's stripping automated endothelial keratoplasty (DSAEK) procedure. We have used infant donor cornea for transplantation in pre-Descemet's endothelial keratoplasty (PDEK)[1-4] and also young donor tissues.

DESCEMET'S MEMBRANE ENDOTHELIAL KERATOPLASTY AND YOUNG DONOR

Donor tissue characteristics have been assumed to be associated as a possible reason for long-term donor graft survival. The Descemet's membrane endothelial keratoplasty (DMEK) graft from young donors is more difficult to harvest and is also difficult to unfold inside the eye because younger donor tissue tends to curl up tightly. For this reason, surgeons now prefer to use tissue from donors older than 40 years for DMEK cases to facilitate uncurling and positioning the tissue after it is inside the eye.

PRE-DESCEMET'S ENDOTHELIAL KERATOPLASTY BUBBLE CREATION AND YOUNG DONOR

The ease of air injection and bubble creation was essentially the same as compared to adult donor tissues, and no specific difficulty was encountered during bubble creation. In an infant/young donor tissue, the presence of strong adhesions between Descemet's membrane (DM) and the pre-Descemet's layer (PDL) obviates any chances of accidental creation of a type-2 bubble. It is for this reason that infant donor tissue is not ideal for a DMEK procedure as it is difficult to peel the DM layer off the residual cornea. These adhesions help in PDEK surgery as this decrease the chances of creating a type-2 bubble and its subsequent conversion to DMEK (Figs. 10.1 and 10.2).

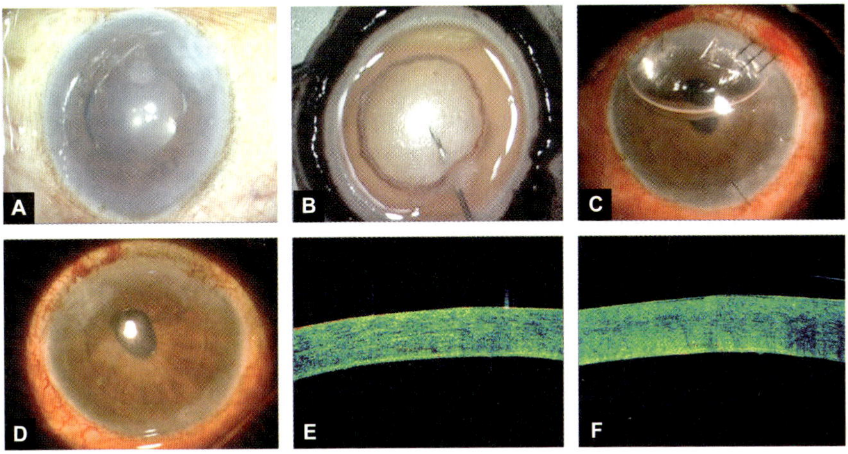

Figs. 10.1A to F: PDEK done using a 1 year old donor (Part 1). (A) Pseudophakic bullous keratopathy; (B) Type 1 big bubble prepared for PDEK graft; (C) Postoperative day 1 after PDEK; (D) Postoperative 1 week after PDEK (Vision 6/9); (E) Anterior segment OCT postoperative day 1; (F) Anterior segment OCT postoperative 1 week.
(PDEK: Pre-Descemet's endothelial keratoplasty; OCT: Optical coherence tomography)

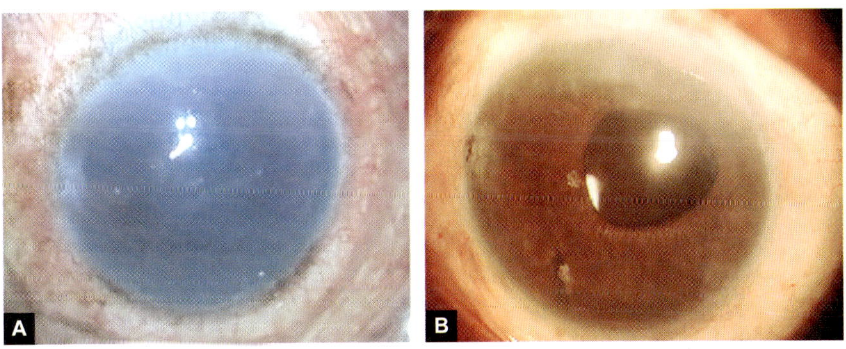

Figs. 10.2A and B: Pre-Descemet's endothelial keratoplasty (PDEK) using a young donor; (A) Pseudophakic bullous keratopathy. See severe corneal haze; (B) 1 month postoperative after PDEK Vision 6/9.

DISCUSSION

The use of infant donor corneas has an inherent advantage of abundant endothelial cells that should theoretically translate into faster resolution of corneal edema and greater longevity of the graft. The donor graft size achieved in PDEK is comparatively small irrespective of the use of adult or infant donor tissue because of adhesions present in the periphery in between the collagenous layers. Transplantation of a larger graft has an inherent advantage of better covering the visual axis and transferring a greater amount of endothelial cells as compared with a smaller graft. But in the PDEK procedure, the applicability and feasibility of using an infant donor cornea seems to override this advantage by providing donor tissue with a high endothelial cell count. Moreover, a smaller graft undergoes less compression during lenticule insertion resulting in lesser damage to the endothelial cells. In addition to this with a smaller graft, unfolding is better, and the presence of PDL to the DM-endothelium complex provides an extra splinting effect to the tissue leading to better maneuverability inside the anterior chamber. With the presence of a thin donor lenticule, although the surgical challenges increase, no specific difficulty was encountered in handling the infant donor lenticule. The ease of insertion can be attributed to the extra splinting effect provided by the presence of minimal stroma present in the PDL. No incidence of tissue wrinkling with a thinner lenticule was seen that could have theoretically resulted in a lower best corrected visual acuity (BCVA). It has been reported that thinner lenticules with minimal posterior stromal lamellae have better visual outcomes (Figs. 10.3 to 10.5). Thus, PDEK, a procedure in which the replacement of the posterior corneal lamella is limited to the PDL with a DM-endothelium complex, is expected to result in better functional rehabilitation.

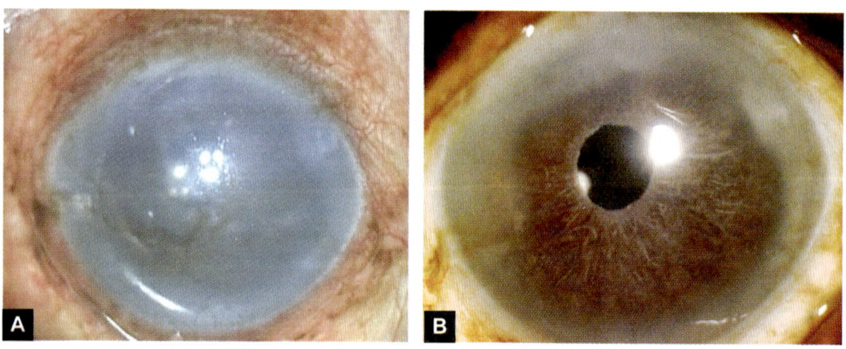

Figs. 10.3A and B: Pre-Descemet's endothelial keratoplasty (PDEK) pre- and postoperative with a young donor. *Note:* The severe corneal haze has cleared postoperative vision 20/20.

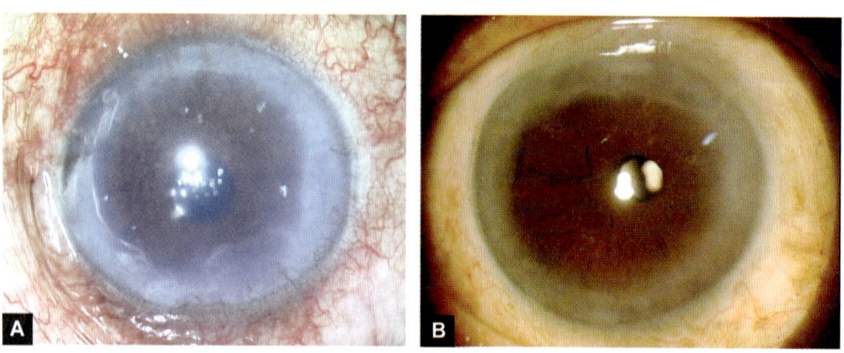

Figs. 10.4A and B: Pre-Descemet's endothelial keratoplasty (PDEK) pre- and postoperative with a young donor postoperative vision 20/20.

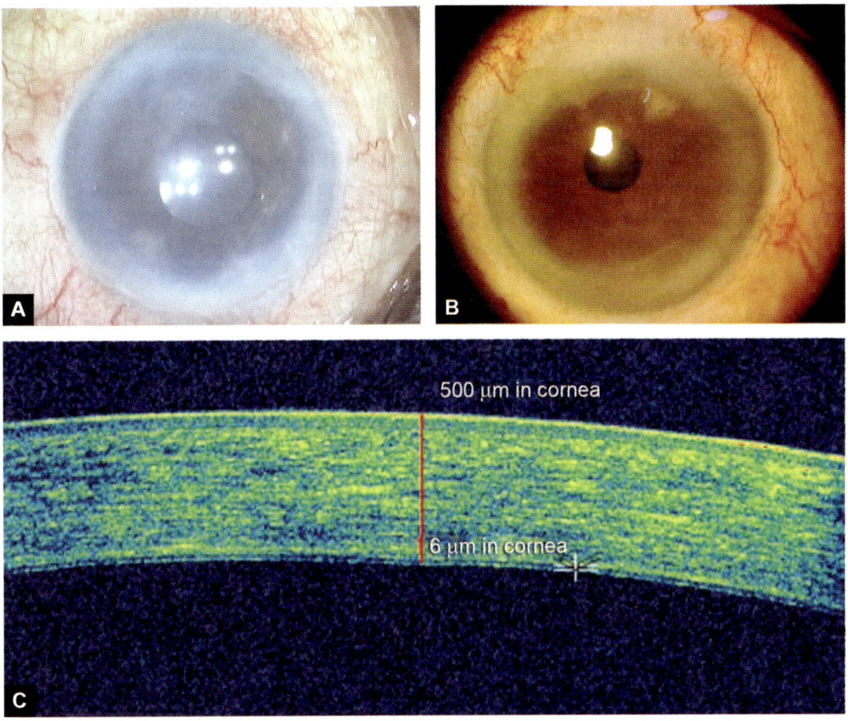

Figs. 10.5A to C: PDEK pre- and postoperative with a young donor. Anterior segment OCT shows an attached graft postoperative vision 20/20.
(PDEK: Pre-Descemet's endothelial keratoplasty; OCT: Optical coherence tomography).

At this juncture, an advantage of DMEK is that it allows selective transplantation of the DM-endothelium complex. But the use of infant donor tissue is not an ideal proposition for the DMEK procedure because it does not allow its usage. It has been observed that it is surgically possible to dissect an approximately 35 mm graft from the donor corneas of both adults and infants with the help of air dissection.

CONCLUSION

Although optimal donor tissue selection remains controversial and in some areas, is dependent on the availability of corneal grafts, the limited availability of infant donor tissue adds to the limitation. However, the potential advantage of using an infant donor cornea is that it represents a new source of tissue that was previously unusable.

REFERENCES

1. Agarwal A, Dua HS, Narang P, et al. Pre-Descemet's endothelial keratoplasty (PDEK). Br J Ophthalmol. 2014;98(9):1181-5.

2. Dua HS, Faraj LA, Said DG, et al. Human corneal anatomy redefined: a novel pre-Descemet's layer (Dua's layer). Ophthalmology. 2013;120(9):1778-85.
3. Agarwal A, Kumar DA, Jacob S, et al. Fibrin glue-assisted sutureless posterior chamber intraocular lens implantation in eyes with deficient posterior capsules. J Cataract Refract Surg. 2008;34(9):1433-8.
4. Jacob S, Agarwal A, Agarwal A, et al. Endoilluminator-assisted transcorneal illumination for Descemet membrane endothelial keratoplasty: enhanced intraoperative visualization of the graft in corneal decompensation secondary to pseudophakic bullous keratopathy. J Cataract Refract Surg. 2014;40(8):1332-6.

SECTION 3

Special Situations

CHAPTER 11

Glued Intraocular Lens

Athiya Agarwal, Amar Agarwal

INTRODUCTION

Posterior capsular rupture (PCR)[1,2] can occur in the early learning curve in phacoemulsification.[1-15] Intraoperative dialysis or a large PCR will prevent intraocular lens (IOL) implantation in the capsular bag. Implantation of an IOL in the sulcus will be possible in cases of adequate anterior capsular support. The first glued posterior chamber IOL (PCIOL) implantation in an eye with a deficient capsule was done on 14th December, 2007. In eyes with inadequate anterior capsular rim and deficient posterior capsule, the new technique of IOL implantation is the fibrin glue (FG)-assisted (Figs. 11.1A to C) sutureless IOL implantation with scleral tuck.[3-7] Since 2007, a large number of cases have been done with this technique. The technique has also evolved since then and extended its application to many different scenarios and as part of combined surgeries. The scleral tuck and intrascleral haptic fixation of a PCIOL was first started by Gabor Scharioth from Germany.[8] Maggi had done previously a sutureless scleral fixation of a special IOL.[9]

WHITE-TO-WHITE MEASUREMENT

One should always measure the corneal white-to-white (WTW) diameter. If the horizontal WTW is about 11 mm then one can do a horizontal glued IOL. This means the flaps can be made at 3 and 9 o'clock positions. If the WTW

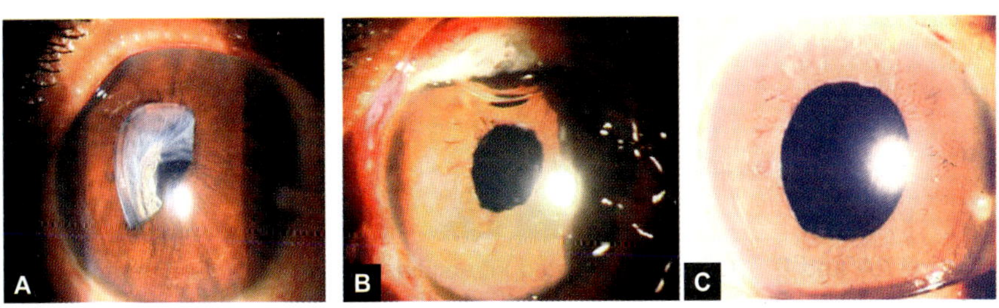

Figs. 11.1A to C: (A) Preoperative slit lamp image showing anterior subluxated intraocular lens (IOL); (B) Day 1 postoperative period; (C) 3 months after surgery.

is more then it would be better to do a vertical glued IOL, which means the sclera flaps are made at 12 and 6 o'clock positions. The vertical WTW is sometimes shorter than the horizontal WTW so one will have more haptic to tuck (Figs. 11.2A and B). This idea was suggested by Jeevan Ladi from India.

CONJUNCTIVAL PERITOMY

If one is performing a manual nonphaco technique or a nonfoldable glued IOL implantation, then it is better to have the superior rectus secured as exposure is better. In such cases, one should prepare the conjunctival peritomy in the areas where the scleral flaps are to be made. Adequate but not over excessive cautery should be done to stop any bleeding vessels.

SCLERAL MARKING

It is imperative that the scleral flaps are 180° apart, if not the IOL will be decentered. For this reason, it is better to use a scleral marker which creates marks on the cornea to see that the sclera flaps created are diagonally opposite (Figs. 11.3A to D). One of the sclera markers is designed by Ashvin Agarwal (Fig. 11.4).

SCLERAL FLAP PREPARATION

The size of the flaps should be 2.5 mm by 2.5 mm with the base at the limbus. Too large a flap is not ideal as the haptic has to traverse a longer distance to get tucked. There are many ways by which the scleral flap can be prepared just like one prepares a trabeculectomy flap. Sometimes it is cumbersome to create these flaps as one might have to use the nondominant hand. A simple

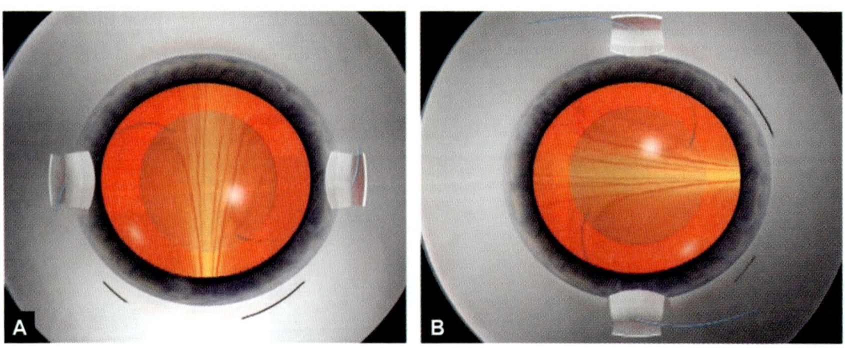

Figs. 11.2A and B: (A) Horizontal glued intraocular lens (IOL). *Note:* The amount of haptic available to tuck and glue is less; (B) Vertical glued IOL. *Note:* The amount of haptic available to tuck and glue is more.

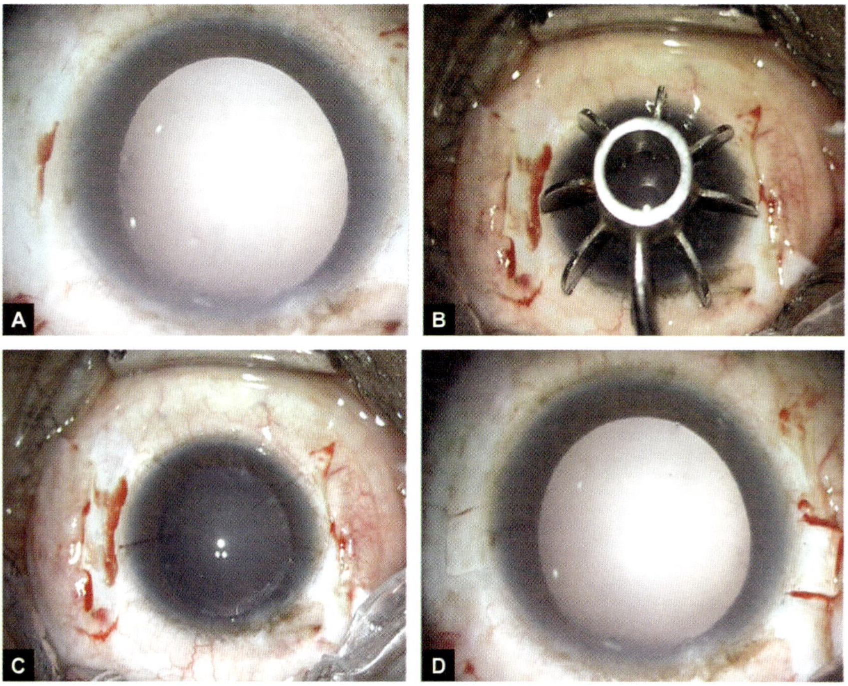

Figs. 11.3A to D: Scleral marker creating marks on the cornea and sclera. (A) Aphakic eye; (B) Scleral marker; (C) Scleral and corneal marks made; (D) Scleral flaps made.

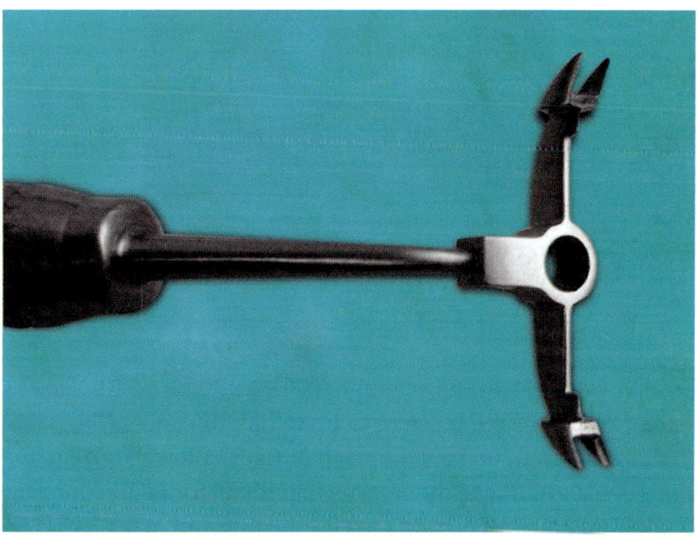

Fig. 11.4: Ashvin Agarwal's scleral marker (Epsilon, India). The special feature of this is that it makes marks for the scleral flaps. It also measures 11 mm so one can know immediately if the white-to-white (WTW) is too large.

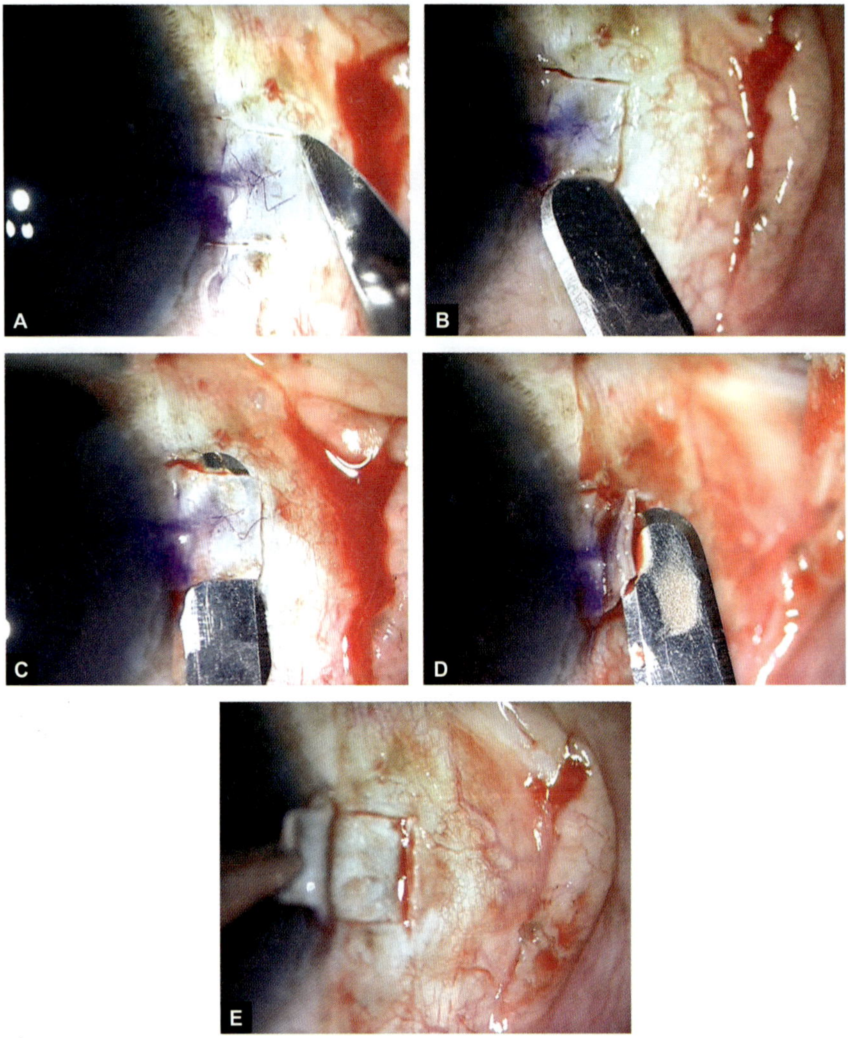

Figs. 11.5A to E: Scleral flap creation. (A) Knife first makes half thickness marks; (B) The dissector passes from one end of the flap; (C) Dissector comes out from the other end; (D) The dissector is moved outward to complete the flap; (E) Flap is lifted and checked.

way by which we perform the scleral flaps (Figs. 11.5A to E) is to first use a knife to create a mark on the sclera to up to half thickness (Fig. 11.5A). One should be careful not to make it too deep or too shallow. Once the marks are made, then one should take the hockey flap dissector (same one which one uses to make a scleral tunnel) and pass it from one end of the flap (Fig. 11.5B) till it comes out from the other end (Fig. 11.5C). Then move the dissector outwards so that the flap is created (Fig. 11.5D). The flap is then lifted (Fig. 11.5E) and any bleeding vessels can be cauterized.

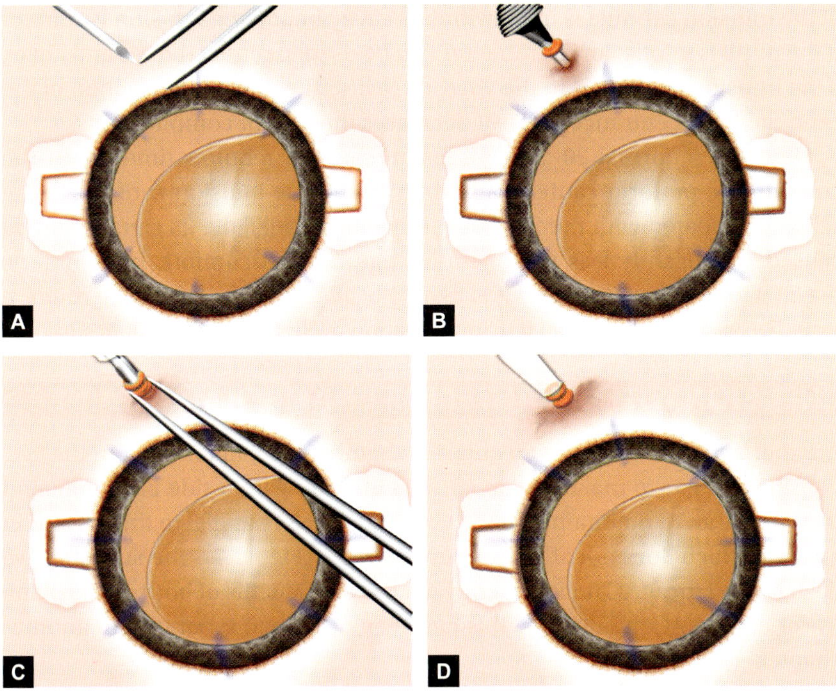

Figs. 11.6A to D: Insertion of 23 gauge trocar and cannula for glued intraocular lens (IOL) surgery. (A) A 23 gauge trocar is placed 3.0 mm from the limbus. The distance is measured using a caliper; (B) The trocar is inserted into the pars plana; (C and D) The inserter is removed and an infusion cannula connected to the infusion bottle is inserted.

INFUSION WITH A TROCAR CANNULA

One should get infusion of fluid into the eye. This can be done using a sutureless 23G/25G trocar cannula (Figs. 11.6A to D). The advantage is that there is no disruption of conjunctival integrity, no need for suturing the sclerotomy, and a reduction in surgical time. Insertion and removal of the cannula is faster than with a conventional 20 gauge infusion cannula. The trocar infusion kit is available separately and can be used by anterior segment surgeons in special situations. It contains a scleral guide, an inserter, and an infusion cannula. The scleral guide is inserted into the pars plana about 3.0 mm from the limbus with the help of the inserter (Figs. 11.6A and B), the inserter is removed, and the infusion cannula connected to the infusion bottle is then inserted (Figs. 11.6C and D). During removal of the cannula, the infusion is switched off and the scleral guide is removed. No suture is applied in the sclerotomy site. We noted that the surgical time needed to fixate the infusion cannula was reduced when 23 gauge infusion was used. It was also safe and easy in the hands of the anterior segment surgeons as one had to insert only the trocar and fixate the infusion cannula. One should always ensure the tip of the infusion cannula is in the vitreous cavity before the infusion is started. If the pupil is miotic, an iris retractor can be used to retract the iris and check if the infusion cannula is in the vitreous cavity. The direct visualization of the cannula during entrance and exit decreases the risk for complications.

Fixating a normal 20 gauge infusion cannula requires time to cut the conjunctiva, perform cautery, and then suture the infusion cannula to the sclera. Compared with the 20 gauge infusion cannula, the 23 gauge cannula caused significantly less postoperative pain and discomfort. In summary, if a 23 gauge trocar cannula kit is readily available in the operating room, it would be easy to use in glued IOL implantation by the anterior segment surgeon.

INFUSION WITH AN ANTERIOR CHAMBER MAINTAINER

Another alternative is to fix an anterior chamber (AC) maintainer in the eye. For this one has to make a clear corneal incision with a side port knife and then pass the AC maintainer in the eye. It should be parallel to the iris and in an area, which does not affect the surgical view (Fig. 11.7). The authors have designed a Trocar AC maintainer which has the benefits of both a pars plana trocar and an AC maintainer. This has been described separately in another chapter.

TROCAR CANNULA VERSUS ANTERIOR CHAMBER MAINTAINER

Infusion of fluid can be done with either a trocar cannula or an AC maintainer. The advantage of a trocar cannula is that it is in the vitreous cavity so does not hamper the surgical view. It also does not push back the iris or touch

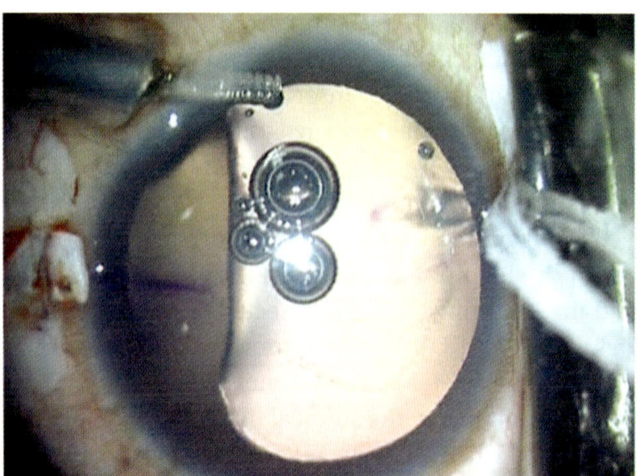

Fig. 11.7: Anterior chamber (AC) maintainer.

the iris. The disadvantage is that an anterior segment surgeon might not have easy access to a trocar cannula compared to a posterior segment surgeon. Another problem is that one should check the trocar cannula is in the vitreous cavity before turning on the infusion so that the fluid does not go into the subretinal space. Sometimes this may be difficult to visualize in small pupils, etc.

The advantage of an AC maintainer is that it is easily available for an anterior segment surgeon, can be reautoclavable and also there is no issue of one having to be careful that the tip is in the subretinal space. The disadvantage of the AC maintainer is that the clear corneal incision does not always match the size of the AC maintainer accurately. This can lead to the AC maintainer coming out in the middle of the surgery and would then have to be refixed. Another issue with the AC maintainer is that when the AC maintainer fluid is turned on it pushes the iris back creating a deep AC. When one has to make the 22 G needle sclerotomy under the scleral flaps one can hit the iris root as the iris is pushed back by the fluid. A solution to this is to fix the AC maintainer, create the 22 G sclerotomies, and then turn on the infusion.

Scleral Flaps or Infusion—Which Comes First?

One has to decide whether to create the scleral flaps first or fix the infusion for fluid. If one is operating a fresh case, for example a patient posted for secondary IOL in aphakia or a fresh ectopia lentis, it is better to create the scleral flaps first. The reason is that the globe is firm and it is easy to create the scleral flaps. In a case of a posterior capsular rupture (PCR) where the corneal or scleral tunnel is open and one is preparing for a glued IOL surgery, it is better to first fix the infusion. This way fluid is flowing inside the eye. One can suture the open wound (either clear corneal or scleral tunnel) then fix the infusion for fluid. This way the globe becomes firm. Then it is easy to create the scleral flaps. Creating the scleral flaps in eyes which are open is tricky as the eyeball is soft.

SCLEROTOMIES UNDER THE FLAP

Two straight sclerotomies with a 22 G needle are made about 1.0 mm from the limbus under the existing scleral flaps (Fig. 11.8). The sclerotomies are to be directed obliquely into the mid-vitreous cavity so that one does not hit the iris which can happen if the sclerotomies are made in a horizontal direction.

VITRECTOMY

Vitrectomy is performed using a 23/25 G vitrectomy probe. A good vitrectomy is crucial so that there is no vitreous traction and chances of retinal breaks and retinal detachments. If one is using a 23/25 G vitrectomy probe, which are available with posterior vitrectomy machines, one can pass the probe through the sclerotomy under the scleral flap (Fig. 11.9). If one is

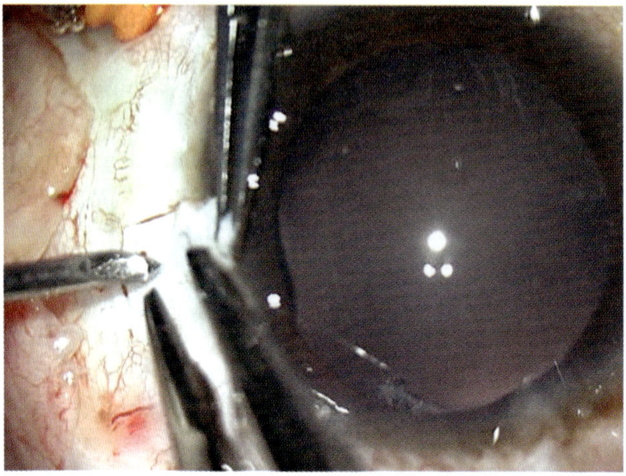

Fig. 11.8: Sclerotomy made 1 mm from the limbus under the sclera flap using a 22 G needle.

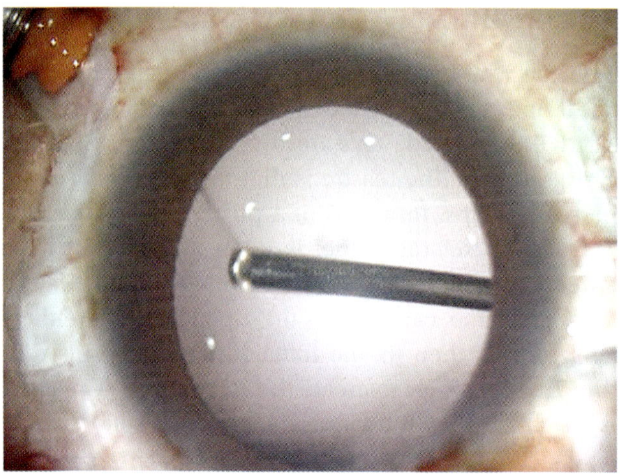

Fig. 11.9: 23 G vitrectomy to remove anterior and mid-vitreous.

using the vitrectomy setup of a phaco machine one should remember that those vitrectomy probes are 20 G and will not pass through the 22 G needle sclerotomies made. In such a case, one should make a clear corneal incision (Fig. 11.10) and do the vitrectomy through the clear corneal incision.

INTRAOCULAR LENS TYPES

Glued IOL can be performed well with rigid polymethylmethacrylate (PMMA) IOL, three-piece PCIOL, or IOLs with modified PMMA haptics. One, therefore, does not need to have an entire inventory of special sutured scleral fixated

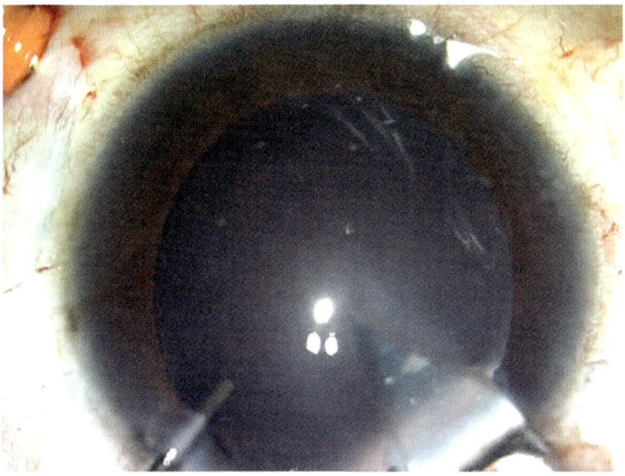

Fig. 11.10: Clear corneal incision.

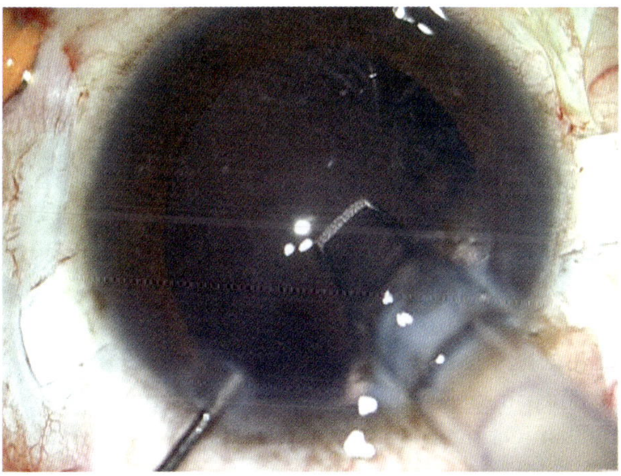

Fig. 11.11: Foldable three-piece intraocular lens (IOL) being injected slowly. *Note:* The cartridge is inside the eye. One should not do wound assisted injection. This can either break the IOL or push it so fast that it might go into the vitreous cavity.

IOLs (SFIOLs) with eyelets. In dislocated PC PMMA IOL or three-piece IOLs, the same IOL can be repositioned thereby reducing the need for further manipulation. The one IOL that cannot be glued is the single-piece foldable IOL as one needs a firm haptic to tuck and glue.

The best IOL to use is a three-piece IOL as the haptics do not break compared to a single-piece nonfoldable IOL (Fig. 11.11). A foldable three piece IOL is even better for the simple reason the incision has not to be enlarged. The length of a normal foldable three-piece IOL is 13 mm. The three-piece nonfoldable IOLs are also 13.5 mm.

FOLDABLE INTRAOCULAR LENS INJECTORS

It is preferable to have a plunger-type injector for better coordination although a screwing mechanism type injector may also be used. In the latter case, the assistant gently maneuvers the IOL forward as the surgeon holds the injector with one hand and the glued IOL forceps with the other hand. While introducing the injector, it is advisable to have the injector tip within the mouth of the incision and not use wound-assisted injection of the IOL that can lead to a sudden, uncontrolled entry of the IOL into the eye, and a consequent IOL drop into the vitreous cavity.

LEADING HAPTIC EXTERNALIZATION

When we are using a foldable IOL one has to take a three-piece foldable IOL. Once the lens is loaded, see that the haptic is slightly out of the cartridge (Figs. 11.12A to E). The cartridge is passed into the AC (Figs. 11.13A to D). The glued IOL forceps is passed through the sclerotomy and grasps the tip of the haptic. The IOL is then gradually injected into the eye. If the injector is a screwing mechanism one then the assistant screws the injector. One should not externalize the haptic till the optic totally unfolds inside the eye, otherwise the optic can break. Once the optic is unfolded the glued IOL forceps pulls the haptic out and externalizes it. The haptic can then be caught by an assistant.

At this stage, George Beiko from Canada, Roger Steinert from USA and Steve Safran from USA have suggested to put the silicone plugs of an iris hook onto the haptic which has been externalized to prevent the haptic from slipping back. Priya Narang from India has suggested a no assistant technique where the trailing haptic is passed into the eye near the inferior portion so that due to physic principles the leading haptic cannot slip back.

When one is injecting the IOL one hand is holding the tip of the haptic. Fear of the IOL falling into the vitreous cavity is not there as:

- The tip of the haptic is caught with the forceps so the IOL cannot go down and
- The trailing haptic is still outside the eye. If the forceps slips and the haptic is missed the trailing haptic can still be caught and the IOL would not fall into the vitreous cavity.

TRAILING HAPTIC EXTERNALIZATION

The trailing haptic is caught with the first glued IOL forceps and flexed into the AC (Figs. 11.14A to G). The haptic is transferred from the first forceps to the second using the handshake technique. The second forceps is passed through the side port. The first forceps is then passed through the sclerotomy under the scleral flap. The haptic is transferred from the second forceps back to the first using the handshake technique once again. The haptic tip is

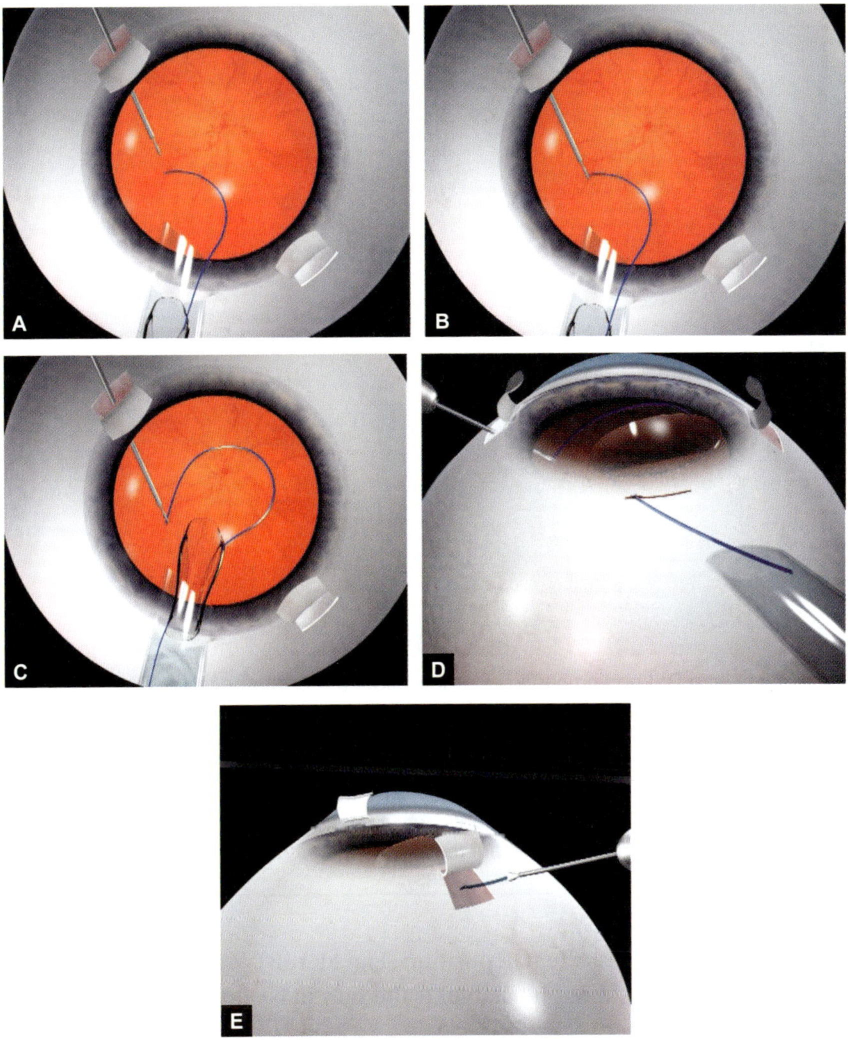

Figs. 11.12A to E: Illustration showing leading haptic externalization. (A) Haptic outside the cartridge. Glued IOL forceps ready to grasp the haptic tip; (B) Haptic tip caught with the forceps; (C) Injection of the IOL is continued till the optic unfolds inside the AC. One should not externalize the haptic till entire optic has unfolded otherwise the optic can break; (D) Haptic externalization started; (E) Haptic externalized.
(AC: Anterior chamber; IOL: Intraocular lens)

grasped with the first forceps and pulled towards the sclerotomy and externalized (Figs. 11.15A and B).

VITRECTOMY AROUND THE SCLEROTOMY

While all these maneuvers are being done, some vitreous might be in the sclerotomy site. Vitrectomy should be done around the sclerotomy (Fig. 11.16A).

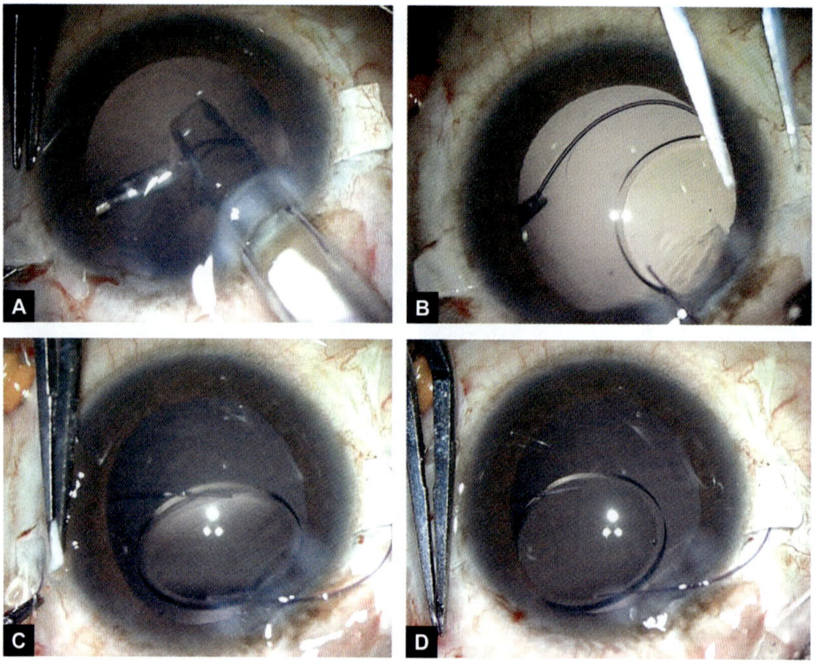

Figs. 11.13A to D: Leading haptic externalization. (A) Cartridge inside the AC with the haptic slightly outside. The glued IOL forceps is passed through the sclerotomy and is ready to grasp the haptic tip; (B) Haptic tip grasped with the glued IOL forceps. Foldable IOL injection continued with one hand. This injector has a pushing mechanism so one hand can be used. If the injector has a screwing mechanism, the assistant continues the injection; (C) Forceps pulls the haptic while injection of the foldable IOL is continued; (D) Haptic externalized. Assistant then holds the haptic which is externalized.
(AC: Anterior chamber; IOL: Intraocular lens)

Then one should assess the IOL position (Fig. 11.16B). Without anyone holding the IOL the lens must be stable. If the haptic is slipping back then it is possible:

- The eye is large and has a large WTW in which case a vertical glued IOL would have to be done.
- The sclerotomy made is too far back so very little haptic has been externalized.

If the haptics are slipping back then a fresh sclerotomy should be made more anterior to the previous one, the haptic pushed back into the vitreous cavity and using the handshake technique again grasped and re-externalized through the fresh anterior sclerotomy. When one comes anterior to create the sclerotomy about 0.5 mm from the limbus the iris can get hit and damaged so in such cases it is better to do a small peripheral iridectomy in the area of the scleral flaps. The 22 G needle then passes through the iridectomy and inadvertent iris damage does not occur.

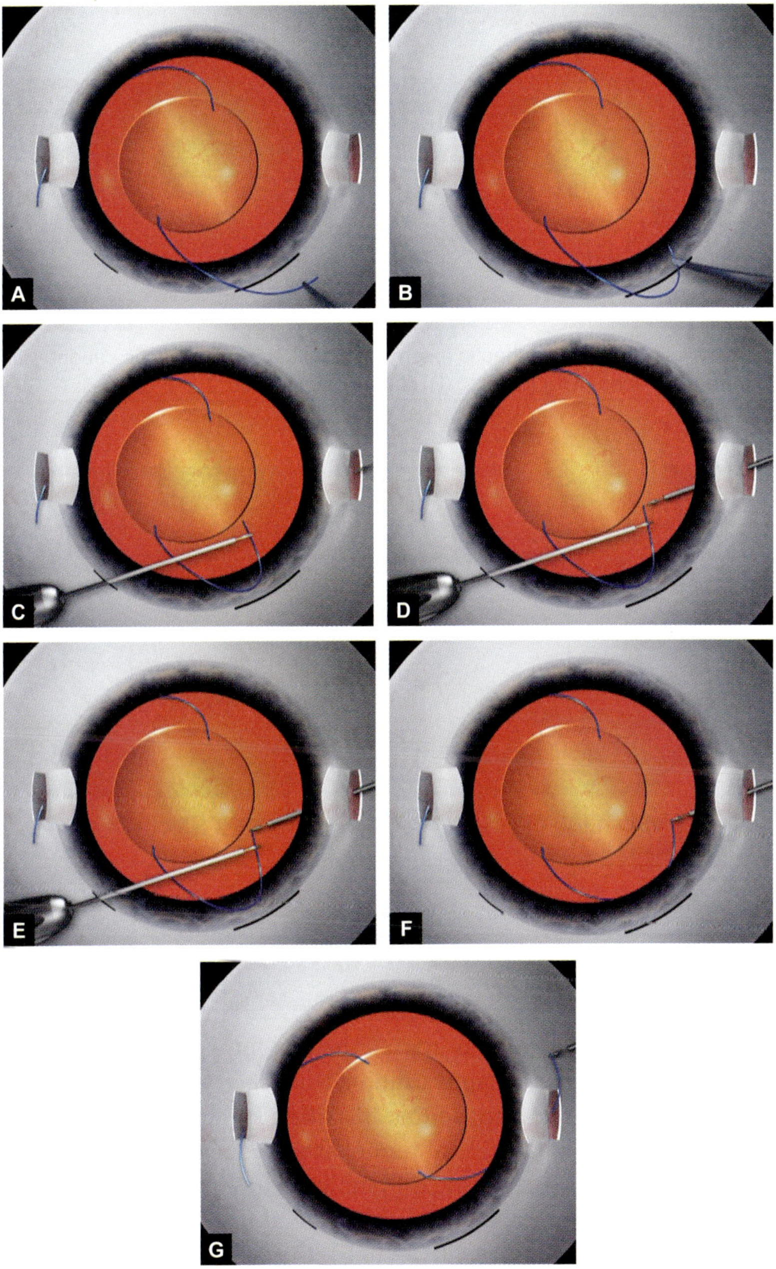

Figs. 11.14A to G: Handshake technique—illustration of trailing haptic externalization. (A) The trailing haptic is caught with the first glued IOL forceps; (B) Haptic flexed into the AC; (C) Haptic is transferred from first forceps to the second using the handshake technique. The second forceps is passed through the side port; (D) First forceps is passed through the sclerotomy under the scleral flap; (E) Haptic is transferred from second forceps back to the first using the handshake technique; (F) Haptic tip grasped with the first forceps; (G) Haptic is pulled towards the sclerotomy. Haptic externalized.
(AC: Anterior chamber; IOL: Intraocular lens)

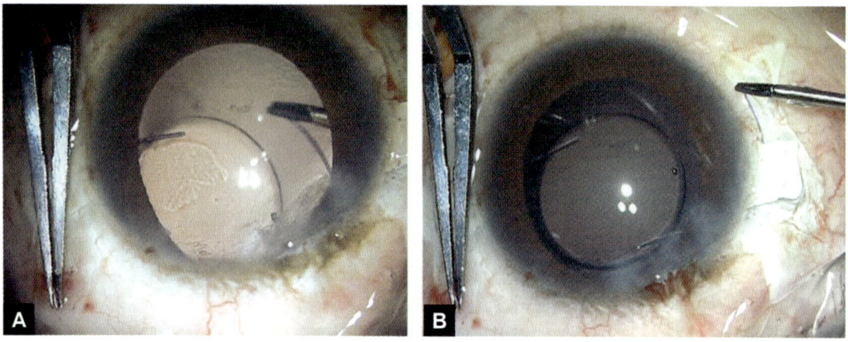

Figs. 11.15A and B: Trailing haptic externalization. (A) Trailing haptic caught with the glued intraocular lens (IOL) forceps; (B) Haptic externalized.

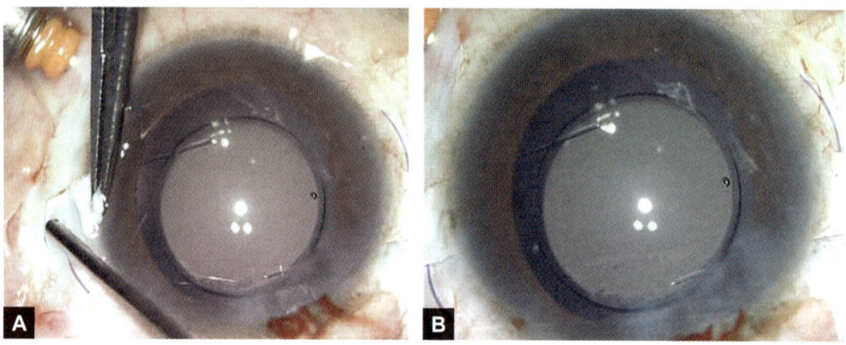

Figs. 11.16A and B: (A) Vitrectomy around the sclerotomy site; (B) Intraocular lens (IOL) stable without the tuck.

SCHARIOTH SCLERAL POCKET AND INTRASCLERAL HAPTIC TUCK

Gabor Scharioth from Germany started the first intrascleral haptic fixation in 2006. It is the intrascleral haptic fixation, which gives stability to the IOL. A 26 G needle is taken and bent so that it is like a keratome (Fig. 11.17). The 26 G needle then creates a scleral tunnel at the edge of the flap where the haptic is externalized. The haptic is then flexed and tucked into the scleral pocket. One can also mark the Scharioth scleral pocket and create it even before the eye is opened (Figs. 11.18A to E). The 26 G needle is marked with the marker pen to leave a mark in the sclera where the scleral pocket is created. This can be done adjacent to the area where the sclerotomy will be made. It is now easy to know where the scleral pocket is located. Another way is to pass a rod in the area of the scleral pocket to check its location (Figs. 11.19A to C).

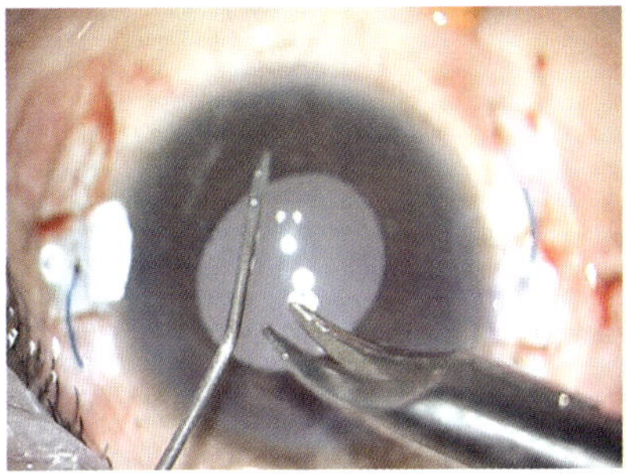

Fig. 11.17: 26 G needle bent like a keratome.

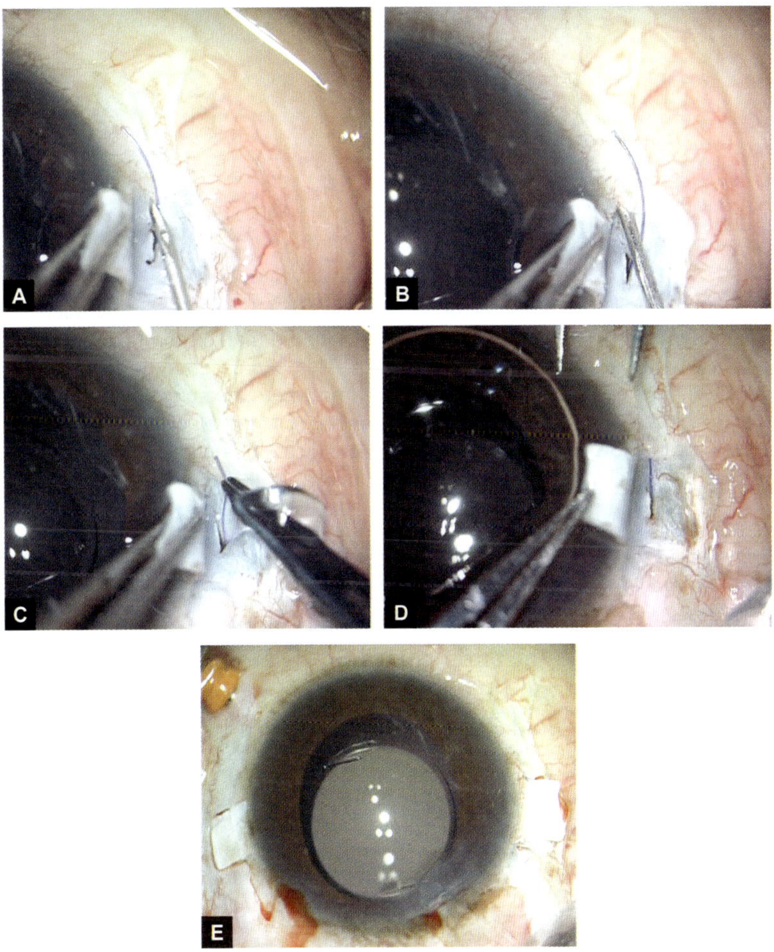

Figs. 11.18A to E: Scharioth scleral pocket creation with intrascleral haptic tuck. (A) 26 G needle creating a scleral tunnel at the edge of the flap where the haptic is externalized; (B) Scharioth scleral pocket; (C) Haptic flexed to be tucked into the scleral pocket; (D) Haptic tucked in the scleral pocket; (E) Intraocular lens (IOL) centered and stable with haptics tucked.

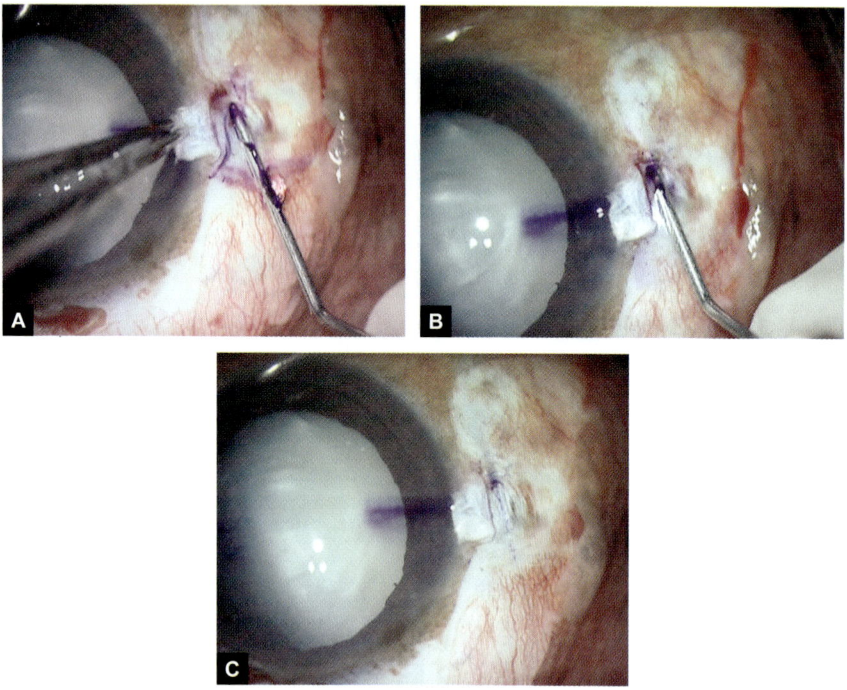

Figs. 11.19A to C: Marked Scharioth scleral pocket creation before intraocular lens (IOL) implantation. (A) 26 G needle is marked with the marker pen to leave a mark in the sclera where the scleral pocket is created. This can be done before opening the eye as it will have to be done adjacent to the area where the sclerotomy will be made; (B) Marked scleral pocket created by 26 G needle; (C) Marked scleral pocket created. It is now easy to know where the scleral pocket is located. Another way is to pass a rod in the area of the scleral pocket to check its location.

AIR IN THE ANTERIOR CHAMBER

Air is now injected into the AC and the fluid from the infusion cannula is turned off (Fig. 11.20). The fibrin glue (FG) has to work in a dry area so the fluid has to be turned off. Otherwise, fluid might keep on coming from the sclerotomy site. Once fluid is turned off there could be intraoperative hypotony and also postoperative hypotony. To prevent this we inject air in the AC to have a firm globe intra- and postoperatively.

FIBRIN GLUE

The fibrin kit we use is Tisseel (Baxter, USA). The fibrinogen and thrombin are first reconstituted according to the manufacturer's instructions. The commercially available FG is virus inactivated and is checked for viral antigen and antibodies with polymerase chain reaction; hence, the chances of transmission of infection are very low. The glue is applied over the flaps and after

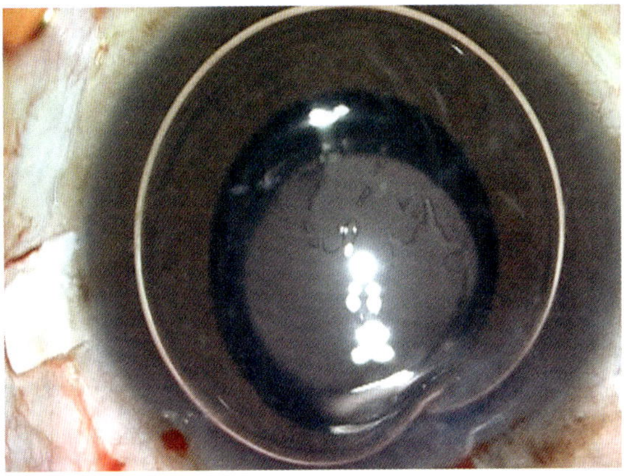

Fig. 11.20: Air in the anterior chamber (AC).

sealing them it can be used over the conjunctiva and clear corneal incisions to seal them too (Figs. 11.21A to D).

Role of Fibrin Glue

The FG plays a multifactorial role in glued IOL surgery that is as follows:

- The glue seals the flaps so that there is no opening from inside the eye to the outside. This prevents any chances of endophthalmitis even some years later where one could get conjunctivitis leading to endophthalmitis as there is an opening from inside to the outside of the eye.
- The glue prevents any trabeculectomy opening as the flaps are now firmly stuck.
- The glue helps seal the cut conjunctiva.
- The glue helps seal the clear corneal incisions.

POSTOPERATIVE REGIMEN

One should keep a watch on the patients postoperatively as these are worst case scenarios being operated upon (Figs. 11.22A and B). They need post-operative antibiotic steroids for 6 weeks. If there is temporary elevation of IOP antiglaucoma medications can be given. If there is a reaction if necessary subconjunctival antibiotic-steroids can also be given.

STABILITY OF THE INTRAOCULAR LENS HAPTIC

As the flaps are manually created, the rough apposing surfaces of the flap and bed heal rapidly and firmly around the haptic, being helped by the FG early on. Because postoperative fibrosis starts early, the flaps become stuck secondary to fibrosis even prior to full degradation of the glue (Fig. 11.23A). To further

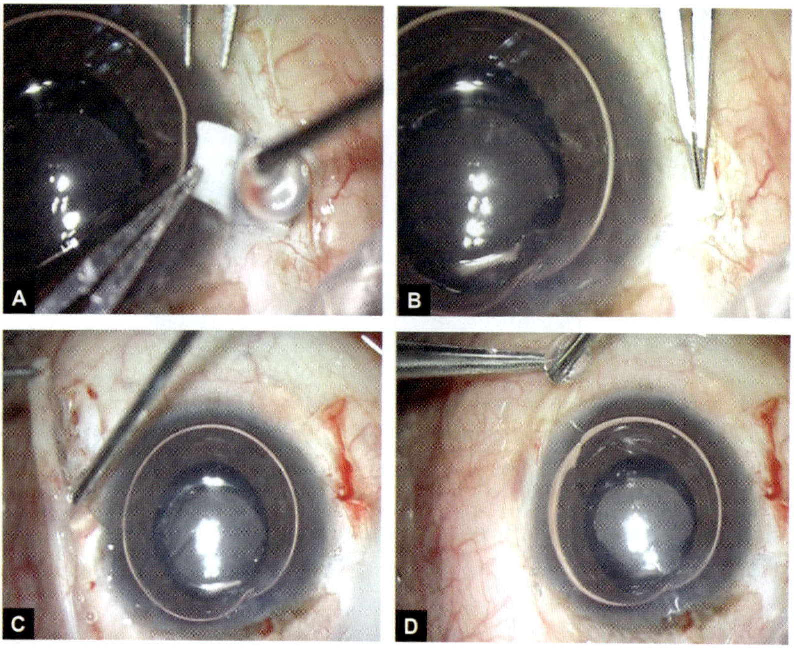

Figs. 11.21A to D: Fibrin glue application. (A) Fibrin glue applied under the flaps; (B) Scleral flaps stuck; (C) Fibrin glue applied to seal the conjunctiva; (D) Conjunctiva sealed with the glue.

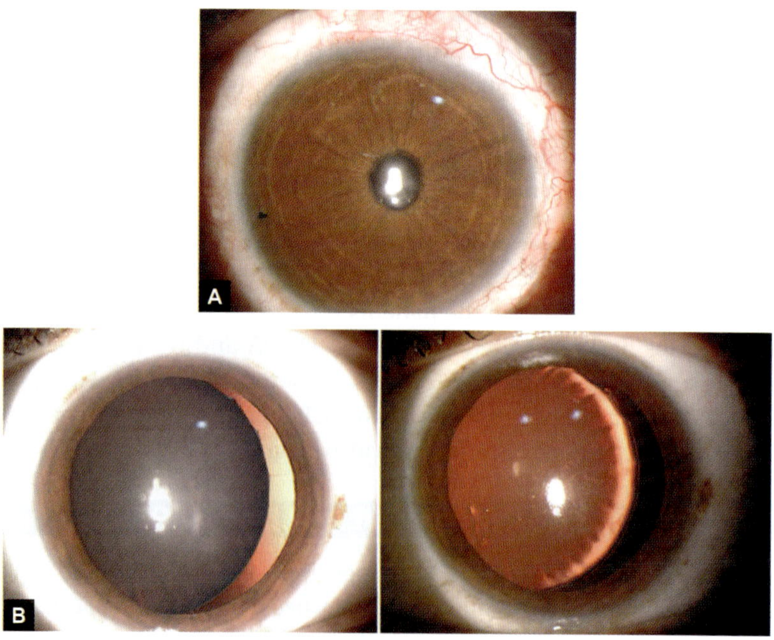

Figs. 11.22A and B: Glued intraocular lens (IOL). (A) Glued IOL done in right eye 1.5 years postoperative; (B) Subluxated cataract in left eye.

make the IOL rock stable, we tuck the haptic tip into the scleral wall through a tunnel. This prevents all movement of the haptic along the transverse axis as well (Fig. 11.23B). The stability of the lens first comes through the tucking of the haptics in the scleral pocket created. Externalization of the greater parts of the haptics along its curvature stabilizes the axial positioning of the IOL and thereby prevents any IOL tilt.

ADVANTAGES

This FG-assisted sutureless PCIOL implantation technique would be useful in a myriad of clinical situations where SFIOLs are indicated, such as luxated IOL, dislocated IOL, zonulopathy, or secondary IOL implantation.

- *No special intraocular lenses*: It can be performed well with rigid PMMA IOL, three-piece PCIOL or IOLs with modified PMMA haptics. One therefore, does not need to have an entire inventory of special SFIOLs with eyelets, unlike in sutured SFIOLs. In dislocated PC PMMA IOL, the same IOL can be repositioned thereby reducing the need for further manipulation.
- *No tilt*: Since the overall diameter of the routine IOL is about 12–13 mm, with the haptic being placed in its normal curved configuration and without any traction, there is no distortion or change in shape of the IOL optic (Figs. 11.24A to D). Externalization of the greater part of the haptics along its curvature stabilizes the axial positioning of the IOL and thereby prevents any IOL tilt.
- *Less pseudophacodonesis*: When the eye moves, it acquires kinetic energy from its muscles and attachments and the energy is dissipated to the internal fluids as it stops. Thus, pseudophacodonesis is the result of oscillations of the fluids in the anterior and posterior segment of the eye. Since the IOL haptic is stuck beneath the flap, it would prevent the further movement of the haptic and thereby reducing the pseudophacodonesis.

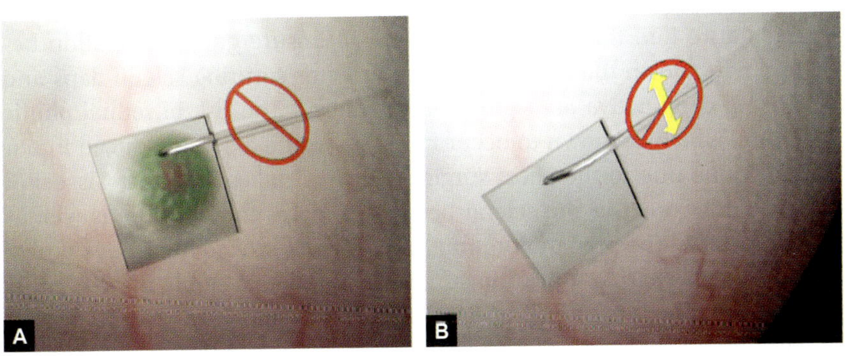

Figs. 11.23A and B: Stability of the intraocular lens (IOL). (A) Long axis movement is not possible in the scleral Scharioth pocket; (B) Transverse axis movement is prevented by the scleral tuck.

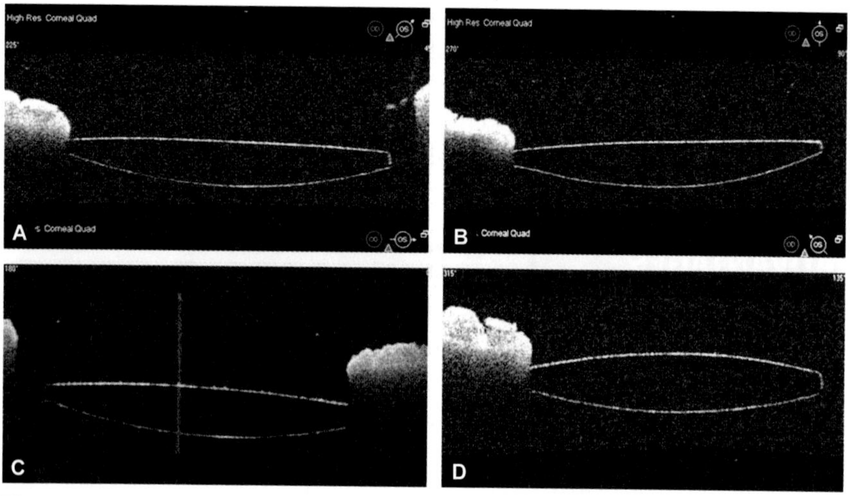

Figs. 11.24A to D: Anterior segment OCT showing 360° good centration of the IOL. (IOL: Intraocular lens; OCT: Optical coherence tomography)

- *Less uveitis-glaucoma-hyphema syndrome*: We expect less incidence of uveitis-glaucoma-hyphema (UGH) syndrome in FG-assisted IOL implantation as compared to sutured SFIOL. This is because; in the former, the IOL is well stabilized and stuck onto the scleral bed and thereby, has decreased intraocular mobility whereas in the latter, there is increased possibility of IOL movement or persistent rub over the ciliary body.
- *No suture-related complications*: Visually significant complications due to late subluxation, which has been known to occur in sutured SFIOL, may also be prevented as sutures are totally avoided in this technique. Another important advantage of this technique is the prevention of suture-related complications like suture erosion, suture knot exposure or dislocation of IOL after suture disintegration, or broken suture.
- *Rapidity and ease of surgery*: Since all the time taken in SFIOL for passing suture into the IOL haptic eyelets, to ensure good centeration before tying down the knots as well as time for suturing scleral flaps and closing conjunctiva are significantly reduced. The risk of retinal photic injury, which is known to occur in SFIOL would also be reduced in our technique due to the short surgical time. FG takes less time Tisseel (3 seconds)] to act in the scleral bed and it helps in adhesion as well as hemostasis. The preparation time can also be reduced in elective procedures by preparing it prior to surgery as it remains stable up to 4 hours from the time of reconstitution. FG has been shown to provide airtight closure and by the time the fibrin starts degrading, surgical adhesions would have already occurred in the scleral bed. This is well shown in the follow-up anterior segment optical coherence tomography (OCT) (Figs. 11.25A and B) where postoperative perfect scleral flap adhesion is observed.

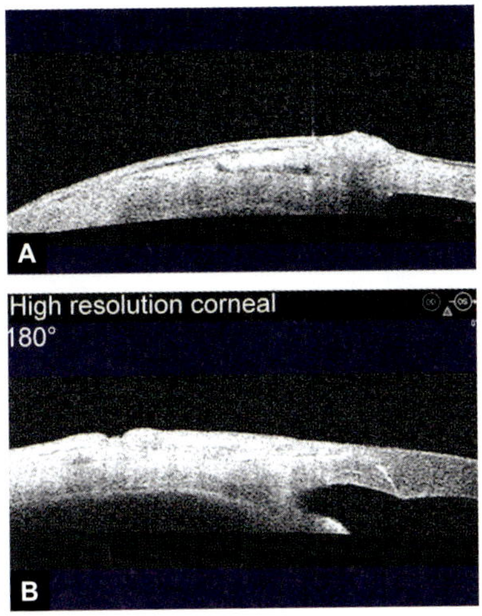

Figs. 11.25A and B: (A) Anterior segment optical coherence tomography (OCT) showing the scleral flap placement on day 1; (B) Adhesion well maintained till 6 weeks.

SURGICAL STEPS OF GLUED INTRAOCULAR LENS

Figures 11.26A to P show the steps of glued IOL with animated figures.

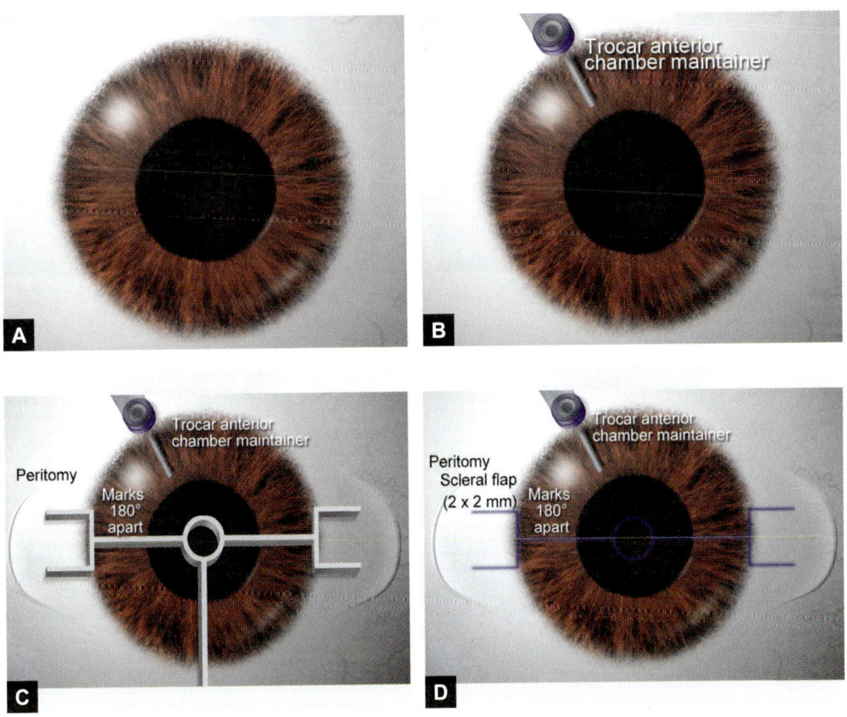

Figs. 11.26A to D

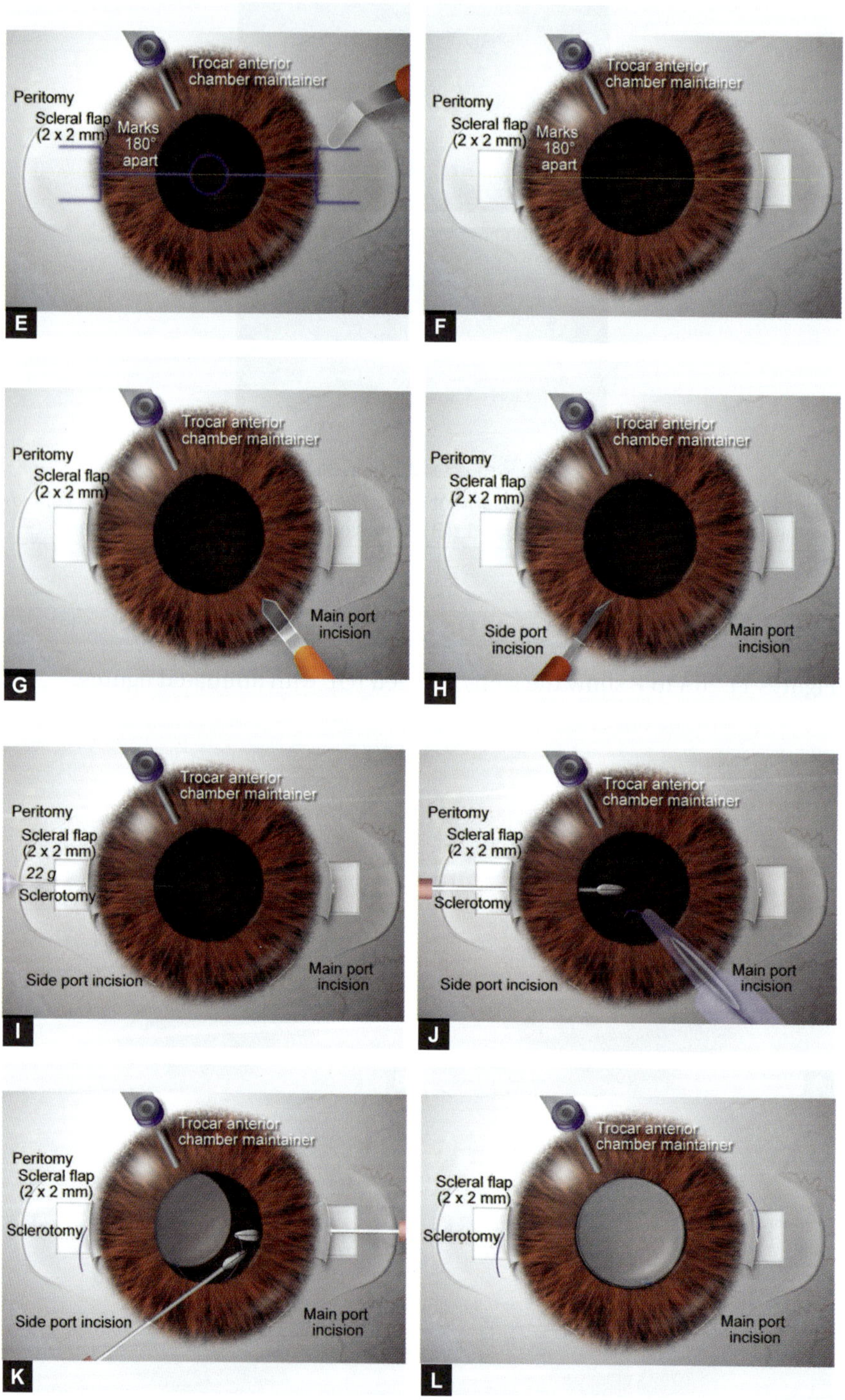

Figs. 11.26E to L

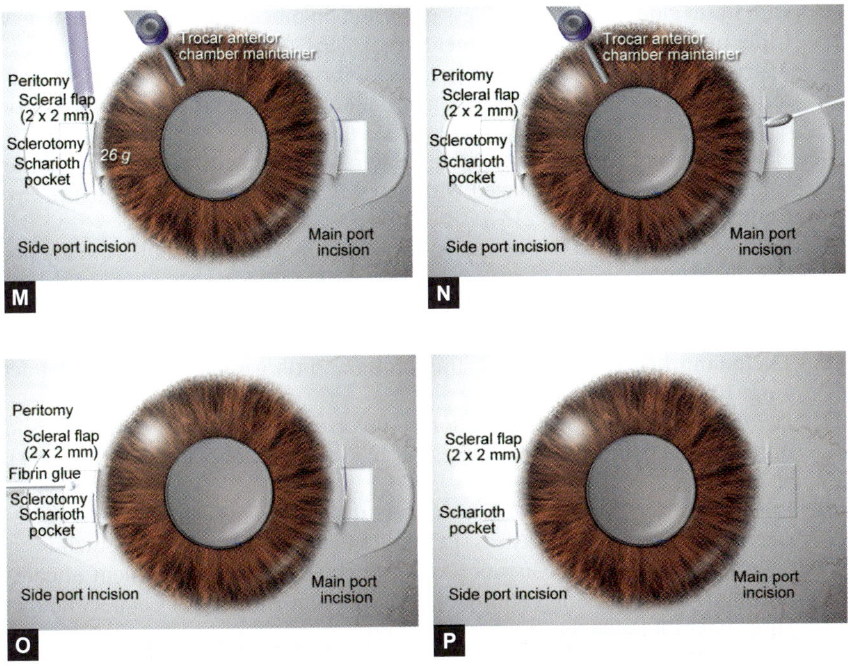

Figs. 11.26A to P: Surgical steps of glued IOL explained through animated figures (A) Aphakic eye without any capsule; (B) Trocar AC maintainer fixed. One can fix an AC maintainer or a retina trocar cannula instead; (C) Conjunctival peritomy done. Scleral marks created for scleral flaps; (D) Scleral marks created; (E) Dissector dissects the scleral flap; (F) Scleral flap dissection completed; (G) Main port incision; (H) Side port incision; (I) 22 G needle creates sclerotomy under the scleral flaps 1 mm behind the limbus; (J) Three-piece IOL with cartridge passed into the AC. *Note:* The haptic slightly out of the cartridge. Glued IOL forceps passed through the sclerotomy ready to grasp the tip of the haptic; (K) Handshake technique for trailing haptic; (L) Both haptics externalized; (M) 26 G needle creates Scharioth pocket; (N) Haptic tucked in Scharioth pocket; (O) Fibrin glue applied once trocar AC maintainer is removed; (P) Glued IOL completed. (AC: Anterior chamber; IOL: Intraocular lens)
(*Courtesy:* Dr Agarwal's eye hospital, India).

REFERENCES

1. Vajpayee RB, Sharma N, Dada T, et al. Management of posterior capsule tears. Surv Ophthalmol. 2001;45(6):473-88.
2. Wu MC, Bhandari A. Managing the broken capsule. Curr Opin Ophthalmol. 2008;19(1):36-40.
3. Agarwal A, Kumar DA, Jacob S, et al. Fibrin glue-assisted sutureless posterior chamber intraocular lens implantation in eyes with deficient posterior capsules. J Cataract Refract Surg. 2008;34(9):1433-8.
4. Prakash G, Ashokumar D, Jacob S, et al. Anterior segment optical coherence tomography-aided diagnosis and primary posterior chamber intraocular lens implantation with fibrin glue in traumatic phacocele with scleral perforation. J Cataract Refract Surg. 2009;35(4):782-4.

5. Prakash G, Jacob S, Ashok Kumar D, et al. Femtosecond-assisted keratoplasty with fibrin glue-assisted sutureless posterior chamber lens implantation: a new triple procedure. J Cataract Refract Surg. 2009;35(6):973-9.
6. Agarwal A, Kumar DA, Prakash G, et al. Fibrin glue-assisted sutureless posterior chamber intraocular lens implantation in eyes with deficient posterior capsules. J Cataract Refract Surg. 2009;35:795-6.
7. Nair V, Kumar DA, Prakash G, et al. Bilateral spontaneous in-the-bag anterior subluxation of PCIOL managed with glued IOL technique: A case report. Eye Contact Lens. 2009;35(4):215-7.
8. Gabor SG, Pavlidis MM. Sutureless intrascleral posterior chamber intraocular lens fixation. J Cataract Refract Surg. 2007;33(11):1851-4.
9. Maggi R, Maggi C. Sutureless scleral fixation of intraocular lenses. J Cataract Refract Surg. 1997;23(9):1289-94.
10. Teichmann KD, Teichmann IA. The torque and tilt gamble. J Cataract Refract Surg. 1997;23(3):413-8.
11. Jacobi KW, Jagger WS. Physical forces involved in pseudophacodonesis and iridodonesis. Albrecht Von Graefes Arch Klin Exp Ophthalmol. 1981;216(1):49-53.
12. Price MO, Price FW, Werner L, et al. Late dislocation of scleral-sutured posterior chamber intraocular lenses. J Cataract Refract Surg. 2005;31(7):1320-6.
13. Solomon K, Gussler JR, Gussler C, et al. Incidence and management of complications of transsclerally sutured posterior chamber lenses. J Cataract Refract Surg. 1993;19(4):488-93.
14. Asadi R, Kheirkhah A. Long-term results of scleral fixation of posterior chamber intraocular lenses in children. Ophthalmology. 2008;115(1):67-72.
15. Lanzetta P, Menchini U, Virgili G, et al. Scleral fixated intraocular lenses: an angiographic study. Retina. 1998;18:515-20.

CHAPTER 12

Single-Pass Four-Throw Technique for Pupilloplasty

Priya Narang, Amar Agarwal

INTRODUCTION

The single-pass four-throw (SFT) pupilloplasty[1,2] is a simple technique of repositioning the iris structure and pupil reconstruction with a single-pass four-throw technique, which entails intertwining of thread around itself that acts as a lock mechanism and ensures nonloosening of the loop.

Among various techniques that have been described for pupil reconstruction, SFT is one of the newer techniques that can be employed for pupilloplasty. As the name suggests, a single pass of the 10-0 prolene suture on a long-arm needle is passed through the iris tissue followed by creation of a loop with four throws around it that slide inside the eye. This creates a helical configuration that prevents the suture from opening up. This is a modification of the Siepser sliding knot technique.

A knot essentially consists of an initial approximating loop followed by a second throw of sutures that creates a securing loop. SFT technique employs the creation of only the initial approximating loop but it comprises four throws thereby creating an intertwining of sutures that has a self-locking mechanism and prevents loosening of the suture loop (Figs. 12.1 to 12.3).

CONNECTION TO PDEK OR EK

The reason why pupilloplasty is connected to pre-Descemet's endothelial keratoplasty (PDEK) or for that matter any endothelial keratoplasty (EK) technique is that in eyes without a capsule and endothelial damage, one performs a glued IOL procedure. Now in such cases the pupil might be distorted and mydriatic. The air when infused in the anterior chamber (AC) for the PDEK graft fixation goes into the vitreous cavity postoperatively. This creates absence of air in the AC in the immediate postoperative period. The air isessential to be in the AC to keep the PDEK graft attached.

The main purpose of the SFT pupilloplasty is that once the pupil is made miotic the air remains in the AC and does not migrate to the vitreous cavity. This then helps the graft remaining attached with a good air fill in the AC.

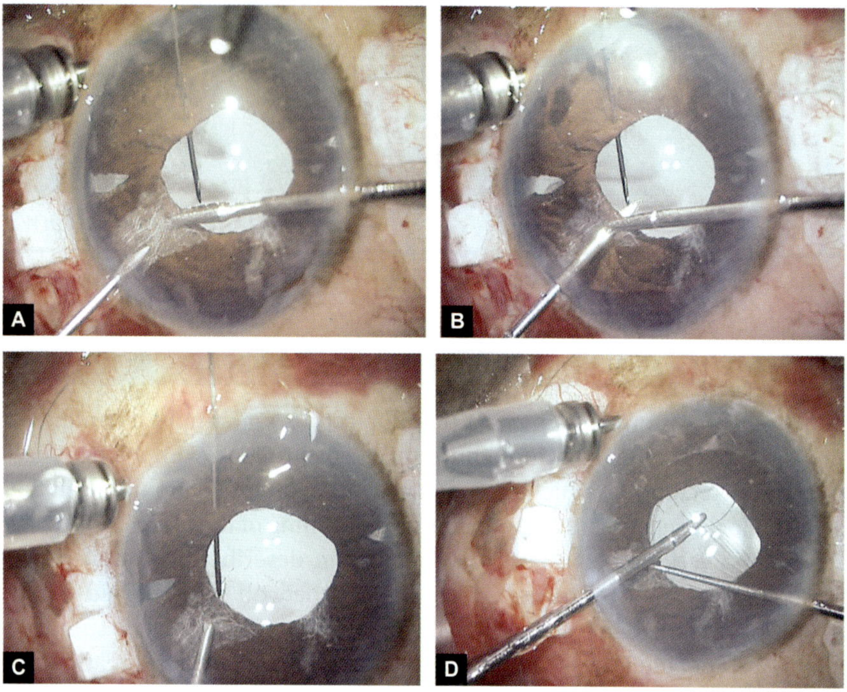

Figs. 12.1A to D: Steps in the pupilloplasty procedure to prevent a captive iris in a normal pupil with glued IOL procedure (Part 1). (A) Two side-port incisions are created parallel to each other along the same longitudinal plane. A 10-0 prolene suture long needle is passed from 1 edge of pupil, and a 26 G needle is introduced from the other side-port incision; (B) The other end of the pupil edge along the proposed tract of passage of needle is held with a glued IOL forceps that helps to provide countertraction and eases the passage of a 26 G needle; (C) The needle is docked into the barrel of 26 G needle that is then withdrawn from the anterior chamber (AC); (D) A sinskey hook is passed into the AC and suture is hooked onto and a loop is created in the AC. The loop is pulled out of the AC with the glued IOL forceps.

SINGLE-PASS FOUR-THROW PUPILLOPLASTY

In this procedure, two stab incisions are created on either side in the limbal area along the axis of the area of iris defect. A 10-0 polypropylene single-arm suture on the long arm of the needle is introduced and the needle is passed from the proximal iris defect after grasping the iris leaflet with an end-opening forceps (Figs. 12.4 and 12.5). A 26 G needle is then passed through the opposite stab incision and the distal end of the iris defect is grasped with end opening forceps and the 26 G needle is passed through it. The suture needle end is anchored on to the barrel of 26 G needle that is then withdrawn along with the suture needle end. A sinskey hook is introduced and a loop is formed into the AC by hooking along the suture as it emerges out of the opposite paracentesis incision. The loop is pulled out of the AC and is positioned on the conjunctiva. The suture end is then passed through the

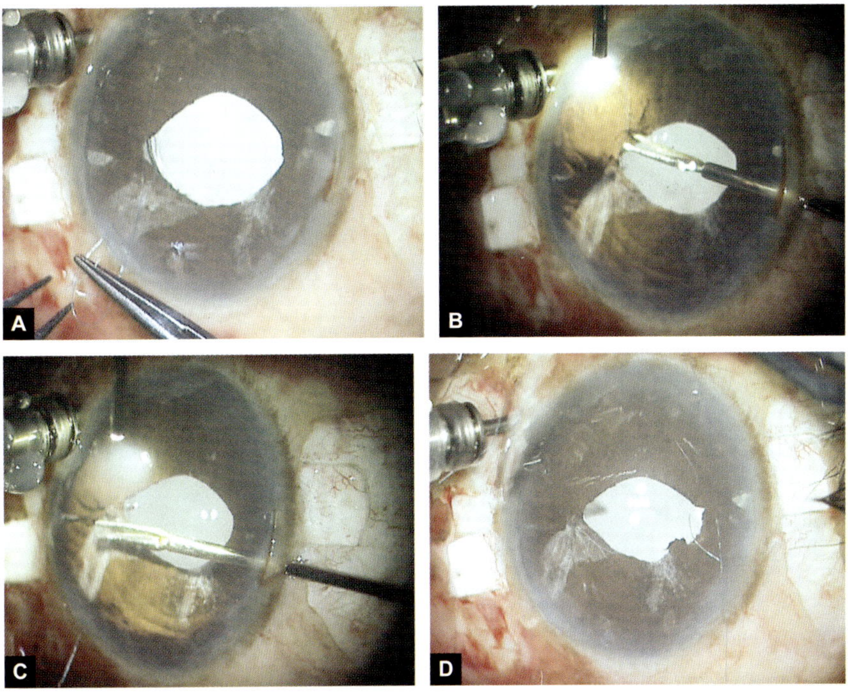

Figs. 12.2A to D: Steps in pupilloplasty procedure to prevent captive iris in normal pupil with glued IOL procedure (Part 2). (A) The free end of the suture is passed four times through the loop, and both ends of the suture are pulled so a knot is created and slides automatically into the eye; (B) A microscissors is introduced, and one end of the knot is cut; (C) The other end of the knot is also cut with the microscissors; (D) Pupilloplasty is performed at the opposite end across the same plane.

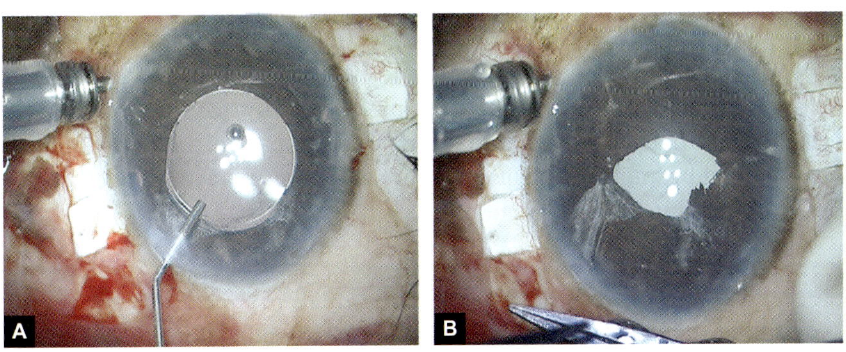

Figs. 12.3A and B: Steps in the pupilloplasty procedure to prevent a captive iris in a normal pupil with glued IOL procedure (Part 3). Intraoperative and immediate intraoperative image after single pass 4 throw pupilloplasty. (A) Intraoperative image showing the pupil size to be same as that of the IOL optic; (B) Immediate intraoperative image of the pupil following pupilloplasty.

loop until four throws are taken, with each throw passing through the loop. Both the suture ends are pulled and the approximating loop slips inside the eye. The suture ends are then cut with microscissors in a way that 1 mm of

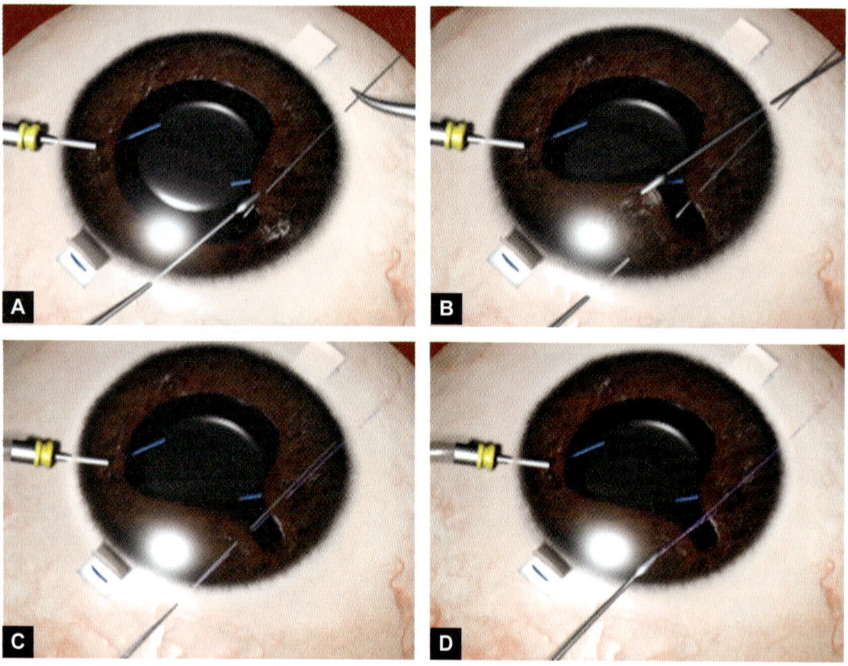

Figs. 12.4A to D: Animation showing single pass 4 throw pupilloplasty for PDEK cases (Part 1): (A) 10/0 straight needle prolene suture passed through the clear cornea and iris. A glued IOL forceps holds the iris for counter traction. Note infusion in the eye through a trocar AC maintainer and a glued IOL has also been done; (B) 26 G needle passes through a paracentesis and then iris. A glued IOL forceps gives counter traction so that no accidental iridodialysis is created when passing the needle through the iris; (C) Railroad technique. The prolene suture with needle is passed through the 26 G needle and brought out through the paracentesis; (D) A loop with a single pass is created of the suture and brought out through the paracentesis.

cut ends are left in situ at the terminal end. The helical configuration created helps to approximate the edges of the pupil followed by securing them closely to each other. The helical structure prevents the slippage of the suture into the helix created by intertwining of the suture and in turn prevents loosening or opening up of the suture configuration.

TECHNIQUE

Two side-port incisions are created on the opposite sides along the line of iris defect that is to be repaired. A single arm 10-0 polypropylene suture threaded on the long-arm needle is introduced from the incision in a way that it engages the proximal part of the iris defect (Fig. 12.6) that needs to be corrected. A 26 G needle is introduced from the opposite end and is passed so that it engages the distal part of the iris defect (Fig. 12.7) that needs to be approximated. An end opening forceps is introduced and is used to grab the edge of iris defect so that 26-G needle can pass through it easily (Figs. 12.6 and 12.7).

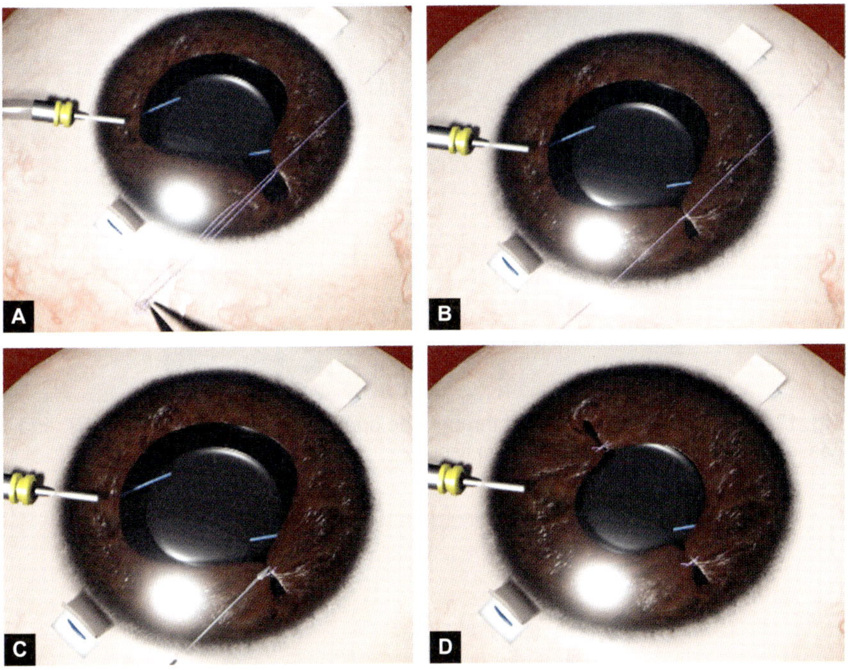

Figs. 12.5A to D: Animation showing single pass 4 throw pupilloplasty for PDEK cases (Part 2): (A) Single pass loop created and 4 throws done; (B) The two sends of the suture are pulled like in a Siepser sliding knot technique; (C) Microscissor cuts the ends of the suture; (D) Pupilloplasty completed.

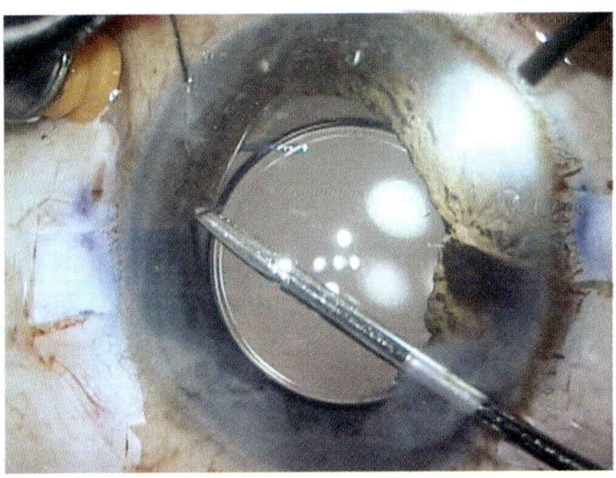

Fig. 12.6: The proximal end of the iris leaflet is held with an end-opening forceps, and a 10-0 long-arm needle with prolene suture is passed through it.

The tip of the long-arm needle is then passed into the barrel of the 26 G needle that is then withdrawn from the eye thereby pulling the needle and the suture along with it (Fig. 12.8). A sinskey's hook is introduced from the side-port incision and a loop is created (Fig. 12.9) and is pulled out and the cut end of the suture is passed four times through the loop (Fig. 12.10). Both the ends of the suture are pulled and as it is done so, the loops slip inside the

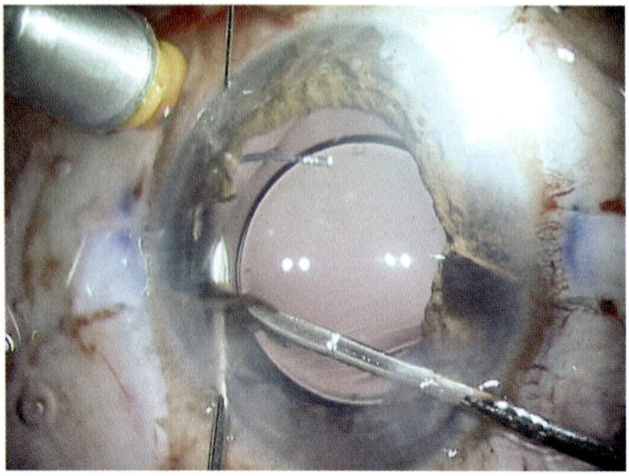

Fig. 12.7: A 26 G needle is passed through the opposite side via a paracentesis, and it passes from the distal edge of the iris tissue.

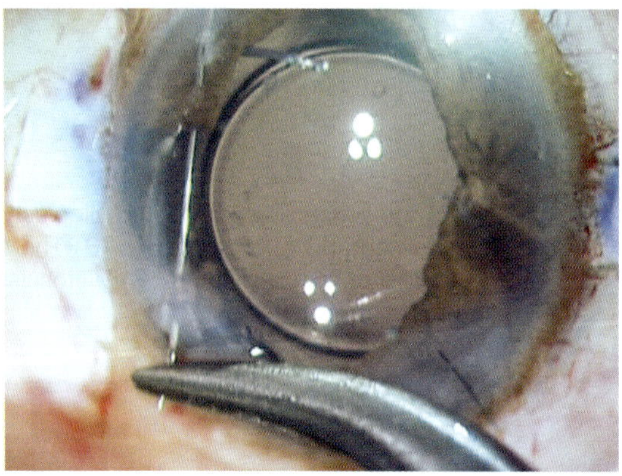

Fig. 12.8: The long-arm needle is passed into the barrel of the 26 G needle and is pulled out of the eye.

eye as in a modified Siepser's technique. This creates an intertwining and interlocking mechanism that secures the loop and prevents it from opening. A microscissors is then introduced into the AC and the sutures are cut (Fig. 12.11).

ENDOILLUMINATOR

We use the endoilluminator in most cases especially if the cornea is hazy when performing SFT. This helps in visualization. This gives the extra light source and one can see the suture clearly.

TROCAR ANTERIOR CHAMBER MAINTAINER

Always have fluid in the eye when performing pupilloplasty. This helps in maintain the AC very well rather than doing the same with viscoelastic. One

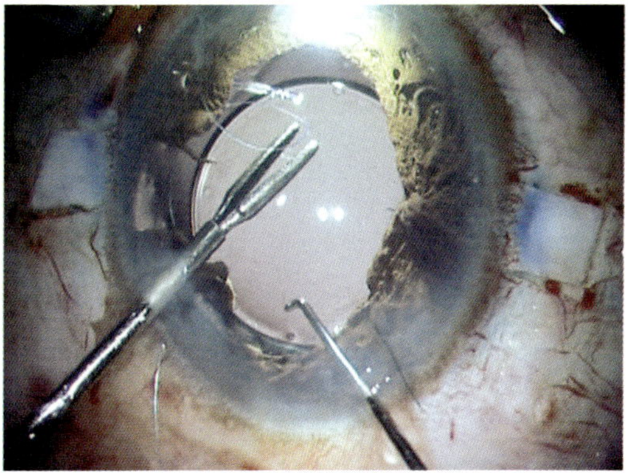

Fig. 12.9: A sinskey's hook is passed and it engages the suture that is pulled inside the AC creating a loop. This is a single pass.

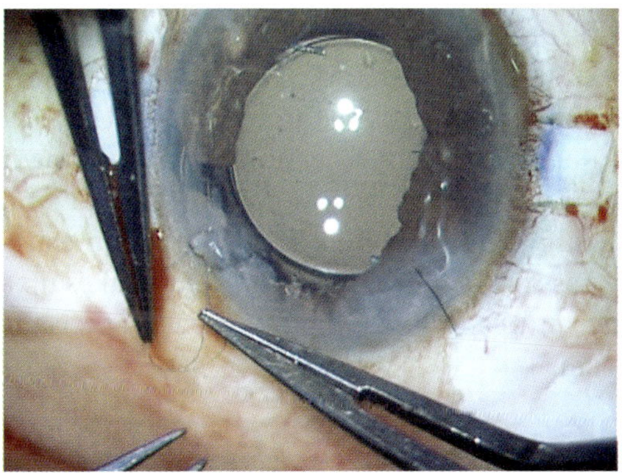

Fig. 12.10: The loop is pulled out and the suture end is passed four times through the loop.

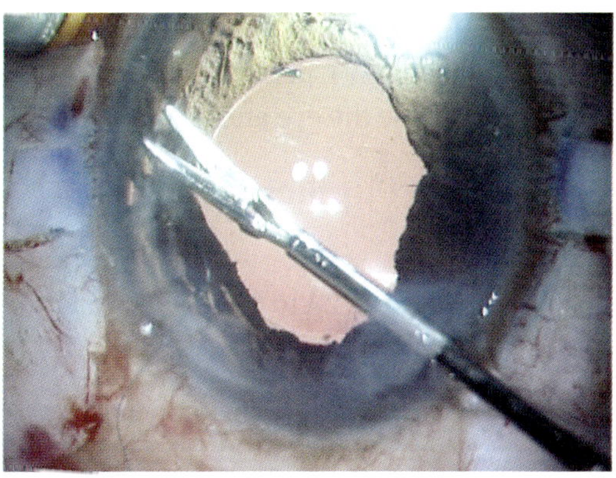

Fig. 12.11: Microscissor cuts the ends of the suture.

can use for this a trocar AC maintainer, an AC maintainer, or a retina trocar. But the principle is simple that if fluid is in the eye all the time, the AC does not collapse and one can perform the SFT easily.

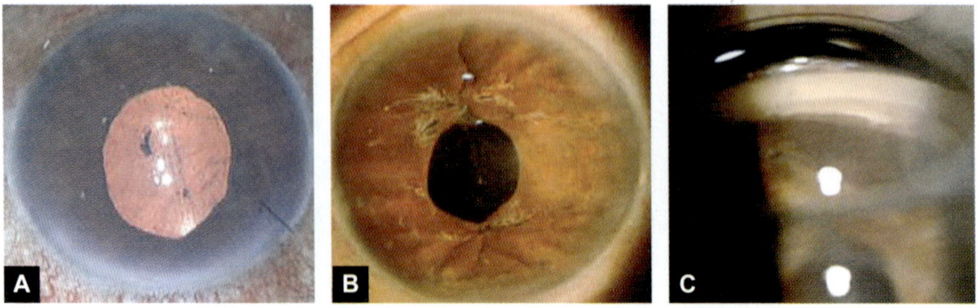

Figs. 12.12A to C: Single pass 4 throw pupilloplasty for closed angle glaucoma. (A) Iris bombe with peripheral anterior synechiae and closed angle glaucoma; (B) After single pass 4 throw pupilloplasty angles are opened; (C) Gonioscopy shows angles open after pupilloplasty.

DISCUSSION

The knot is the most important part of the suture closure in vivo, and essentially comprises the initial approximation loop followed by a second pass that helps to secure a knot with the securing loop. Ideally, an initial approximating loop is taken with either two or three throws followed by a securing loop that helps to tie the knot. In our technique, only the approximating loop is taken with four throws that creates a helical configuration. Extra throws are not recommended as they only add bulk and do not add extra strength to the knot. Due to the passage of four throws, the suture takes up a helical pattern that prevents the sutures from slipping past each other and creates a self-locking mechanism.

ADVANTAGES OF SFT OVER OTHER TECHNIQUES

The advantage of SFT is that one just does one pass. The main issue in pupilloplasty is the pass. Every time a pass is made one has to enter the eye and there are chances of endothelium damage or iris damage or tapping the IOL producing a tilt or dislocation. In SFT, just once we create the pass to form the loop. The four throws are outside the eye and are easy to perform.

Single-Pass Four-Throw Pupilloplasty for Closed Angle Glaucoma

In closed angle glaucoma (Figs. 12.12A to C), the SFT helps to pull the iris and open the angles.

REFERENCES

1. Narang P, Agarwal A. Single-pass four-throw technique for pupilloplasty. Eur J Ophthalmol. 2017;27(4):387-512.
2. Narang P, Agarwal A. Pupilloplasty for pupil size attenuation to prevent pupillary capture: theory of quintet in glued IOL. J Cataract Refract Surg. 2017;43(1):3-7.

CHAPTER 13

Pre-Descemet's Endothelial Keratoplasty with Glued Intraocular Lens

Priya Narang, Amar Agarwal

INTRODUCTION

Glued intraocular lens (IOL) was introduced in 2007 as a technique for sutureless scleral fixation of the IOL via transscleral haptic tuck in patients with absent or deficient capsular support.[1-13] This may be done as a primary procedure during cataract extraction in case of posterior capsular rupture and deficient capsule or as a secondary procedure in an aphakic patient. It may also be used for closed chamber translocation of a malpositioned or subluxated three-piece IOL. However, many of these patients who need primary or secondary glued IOL implantation have already undergone complicated cataract surgery with inability to implant an IOL in the bag during the cataract extraction. Therefore, the chances of endothelial damage and the consequent need for a keratoplasty are also higher in these patients. Depending on the severity of endothelial damage and corneal scarring the patient may require either a penetrating keratoplasty (PK) or an endothelial keratoplasty (EK).

GLUED INTRAOCULAR LENS WITH ENDOTHELIAL KERATOPLASTY

In patients with predominantly endothelial damage, an EK may be performed instead of a PK. This has advantages over PK of being a closed chamber technique with faster visual recovery, better quality of vision, lesser induction of irregular astigmatism, lesser chances of rejection, and less surface- and suture-related problems. There is also likely to be less postoperative refractive surprise with EK as compared with PK. Glued IOL can be combined with DSAEK (Descemet's stripping automated endothelial keratoplasty), DMEK (Descemet's membrane endothelial keratoplasty), or PDEK (Pre-Descemet's endothelial keratoplasty). It may also be done as a staged procedure performing the glued IOL first and the EK in a second sitting.[1-13]

PRINCIPLES OF COMBINING GLUED IOL WITH PDEK

In aphakic eyes, a loss of bicamerality of the eye occurs that leads to posterior migration of the air bubble used for attaching the PDEK graft.

This increases the risk for a consequent postoperative partial or total graft detachment, forward bowing of the iris, iris-graft touch, graft dislocation into the vitreous and so on, all of which can necessitate secondary procedures such as refloating, rebubbling, vitrectomy, AC formation and so on, in turn increasing graft endothelial cell loss. An effective compartmentaliztion of the eye can be obtained through the glued IOL technique. The glued IOL offers advantages of posterior chamber IOL placement, ease of centration, scleral fixation as well as stable and sturdy fixation without pseudophakodonesis. It is therefore our preferred technique when combining with PDEK unlike AC IOL, which has disadvantages of decreased AC space, iris fixated IOLs which require intact iris all around as well as sutured scleral fixated IOL which has disadvantages of greater pseudophakodonesis and greater difficulty in centration (Figs. 13.1 to 13.3).

The procedure is started as a conventional glued IOL. An anterior chamber (AC) maintainer or a trocar AC maintainer is inserted. Conjunctival flaps and lamellar scleral flaps are made 180° apart as explained earlier. Twenty-two gauge sclerotomies are made under the scleral flap about 1 mm from the limbus. This is followed by limited 23 G vitrectomy through the sclerotomies followed by glued IOL implantation. The haptics are tucked in the Scharioth pockets and the flaps may be glued down. As the posterior capsule is unlikely

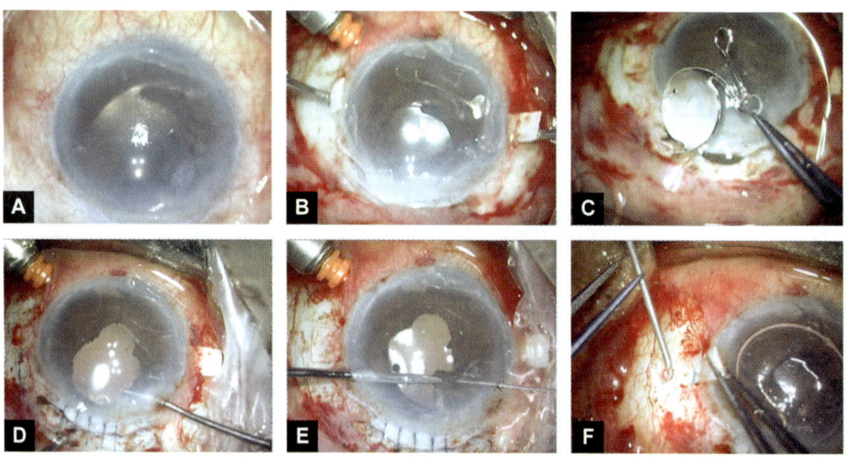

Figs. 13.1A to F: Pre-Descemet's endothelial keratoplasty (PDEK) with glued IOL (Part 1). (A) Pseudophakic bullous keratopathy. Note the corneal haze and an AC IOL in the eye; (B) Trocar cannula fixed. Two scleral flaps created 180° apart and a 22 G sclerotomy created with a needle 1 mm from the limbus; (C) After vitrectomy, the haptics are grasped with glued IOL forceps and AC IOL explanted; (D) Glued IOL in place. Note the haptics externalized under the scleral flaps. Suturing of the scleral tunnel done; (E) Single-pass four-throw pupilloplasty (SFT) is done to make the pupil smaller so that air remains in the AC and does not go into the vitreous cavity when PDEK will be done; (F) Fibrin glue applied.
(IOL: Intraocular lens; AC: Anterior chamber).

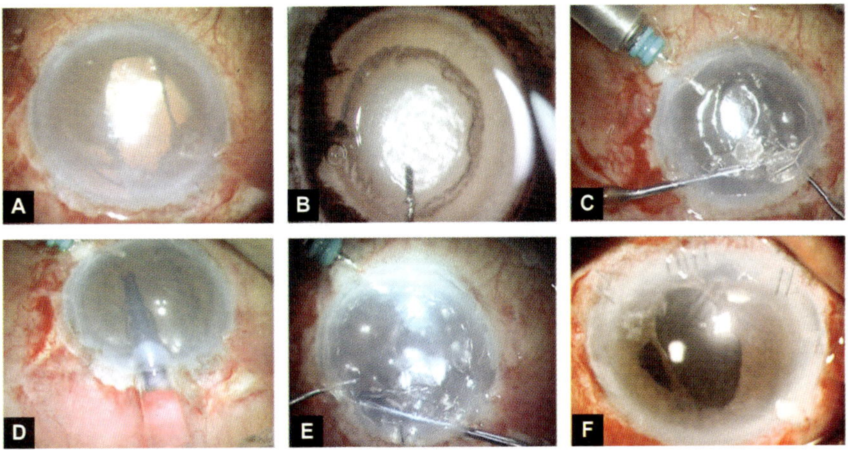

Figs. 13.2A to F: Pre-Descemet's endothelial keratoplasty (PDEK) with glued IOL (Part 2). (A) One month after glued IOL. Note the corneal haze; (B) Type 1 big bubble created. One can do the PDEK in one sitting with the glued IOL. It is better to do in two steps so that the glued IOL heals well and a month later PDEK is done. Another advantage is that donor corneas are not readily available and one can do the glued IOL and wait for a good donor cornea to do the PDEK; (C) Descemetorhexis is being performed. Air pump-assisted PDEK. In this the air pump is connected to the trocar AC maintainer or AC maintainer so that air is continuously flowing inside the AC. If one is doing PDEK with glued IOL in one sitting, it is better to have a trocar cannula in the pars plana with fluid being passed inside and an AC maintainer or a trocar AC maintainer in the AC passing air. This way there will not be any hypotony and one can control the amount of fluid being passed inside the eye; (D) PDEK graft is injected inside the AC; (E) PDEK graft is unrolled with the help of endoilluminator-assisted PDEK; (F) One week postoperative.
(IOL: Intraocular lens; AC: Anterior chamber)

to be intact, there is still a chance of posterior migration of air that is injected into the AC for graft support. Migration of air behind the IOL leads to insufficient support for the graft with consequent graft detachment. It is therefore imperative to have a good iris-IOL diaphragm separating the AC from the vitreous cavity. Therefore, when combining a glued IOL with PDEK, the sclerotomy should be made slightly closer to the limbus than usual in order to decrease the potential gap between the iris and the IOL. At the same time, a single pass 4 throw pupilloplasty should be done to obtain a round pupil that overlaps the IOL optic all around. Once this is done the adequacy of air fill is checked by turning off the infusion and checking for the air fill. If inadequate, the pupil may need to become smaller or the IOL may need to come closer to the iris. A well-formed iris-IOL diaphragm prevents air from going back into the vitreous cavity and allows good postoperative support for the graft. Once the air fill is found to be adequate, air is attached to the ACM through an air-pump and host descemetorhexis is performed. The PDEK graft is then injected into the AC, unfolded and floated up using air. In cases with subluxated or

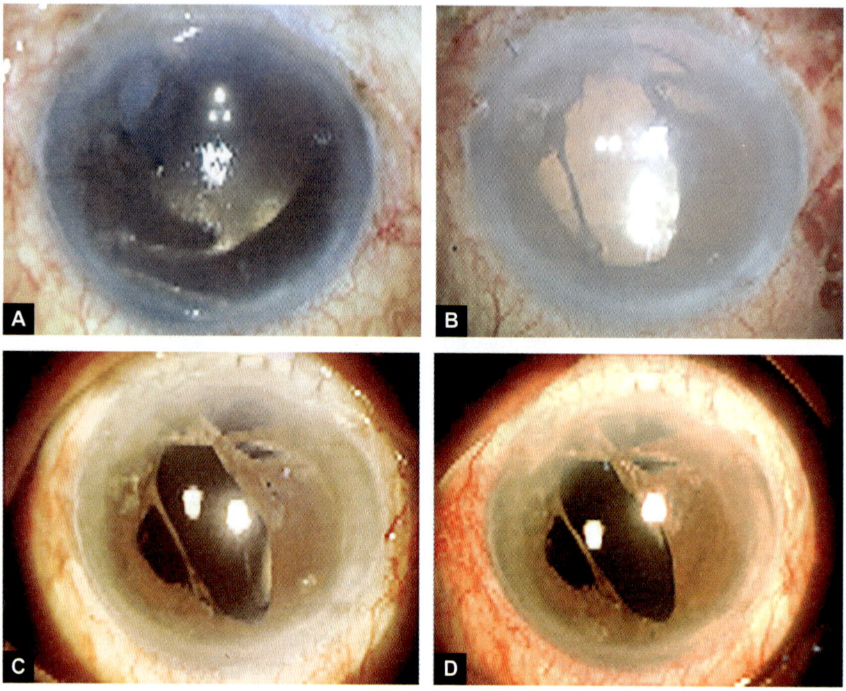

Figs. 13.3A to D: Pre-Descemet's endothelial keratoplasty (PDEK) with glued IOL (Part 3). (A) Preoperative: Pseudophakic bullous keratopathy with an AC IOL; (B) One month after glued IOL; (C) 2 months postoperative after PDEK-Vision 6/12; (D) 4 months postoperative after PDEK-Vision 6/6.
(IOL: Intraocular lens)

dislocated three piece IOL needing PDEK, a closed chamber translocation of the subluxated IOL into a glued IOL may be done using the handshake technique. This is followed by single pass 4 throw pupilloplasty if required and PDEK.

Cases with malpositioned single piece IOL requiring explantation or AC IOL need an enlargement of the wound followed by explantation of the IOL. Construction of a scleral tunnel for IOL explantation or a 3 mm L-shaped sclera tunnel incision gives very good wound closure and excellent AC stability.

A potential complication that may occur on combining glued IOL with PDEK is the risk of hypotony and subsequent graft detachment in the postoperative period. Hypotony can lead to detachment of the PDEK graft from the eyelids pushing on the cornea with normal lid movements. This risk can be decreased by making sure that the globe is adequately pressurized at the end of surgery. As noted, this is done by achieving an adequately tight air bubble in the AC. If the globe still feels hypotonic, air is injected through the pars plicata into the vitreous cavity with a 30 G needle under direct visualizing of the needle tip in the vitreous cavity. At the conclusion of surgery, it should also be made sure that the sclerotomies are well sealed by the scleral flaps using fibrin glue. All corneal incisions should be leak-proof and may also be sealed using fibrin glue to avoid any postoperative leak of aqueous or escape of air which could increase the risk of detachment. Patients undergoing the procedure therefore need to be watched more closely after surgery to look for any evidence of partial or total graft detachments and taken for rebubbling if required.

A properly positioned IOL and a good iridoplasty decrease the chances of the graft slipping into the vitreous cavity during surgery. However, this possibility should be kept in mind and care should be taken to avoid any inappropriate fluidics, which may cause a graft drop (Figs. 13.4 to 13.6).

IT TAKES TWO TO TANGO: PRE-DESCEMET'S ENDOTHELIAL KERATOPLASTY WITH GLUED IOL

In PDEK, the newly described pre-Descemet's layer, the Descemet's membrane, and the endothelium are transplanted after host Descemet's membrane stripping. The combination of PDEK with glued IOL (Figs. 13.7 and 13.8) serves the purpose of handling corneal endothelial dysfunction and secondary IOL fixation simultaneously.

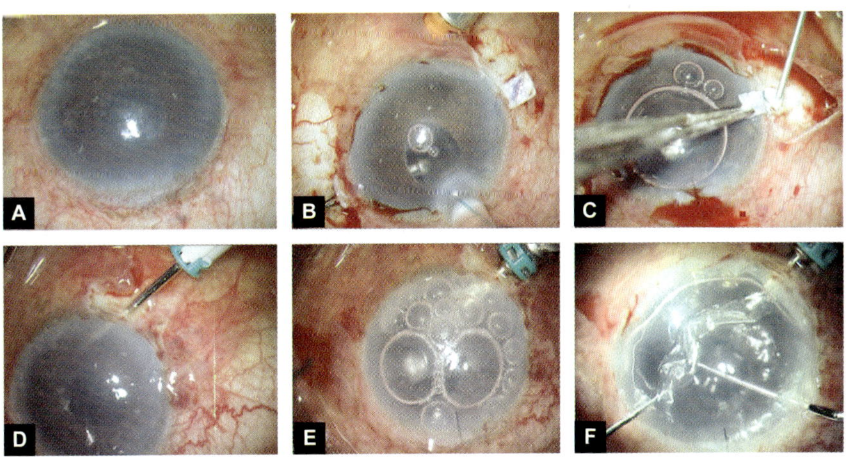

Figs. 13.4A to F: PDEK with glued IOL in a one eyed patient (Part 1). (A) Aphakic bullous keratopathy; (B) Two partial scleral thickness limbal-based scleral flaps of 2.5 mm × 2.5 mm are created 180° opposite to each other followed by placement of infusion cannula. Glued IOL is performed, (C) Fibrin glue is applied; (D) One week after glued IOL, trocar AC maintainer is fixed; (E) Air pump is connected to the trocar AC maintainer; (F) Descemetorhexis.

(PDEK: Pre-Descemet's endothelial keratoplasty; IOL: Intraocular lens; AC: Anterior chamber)

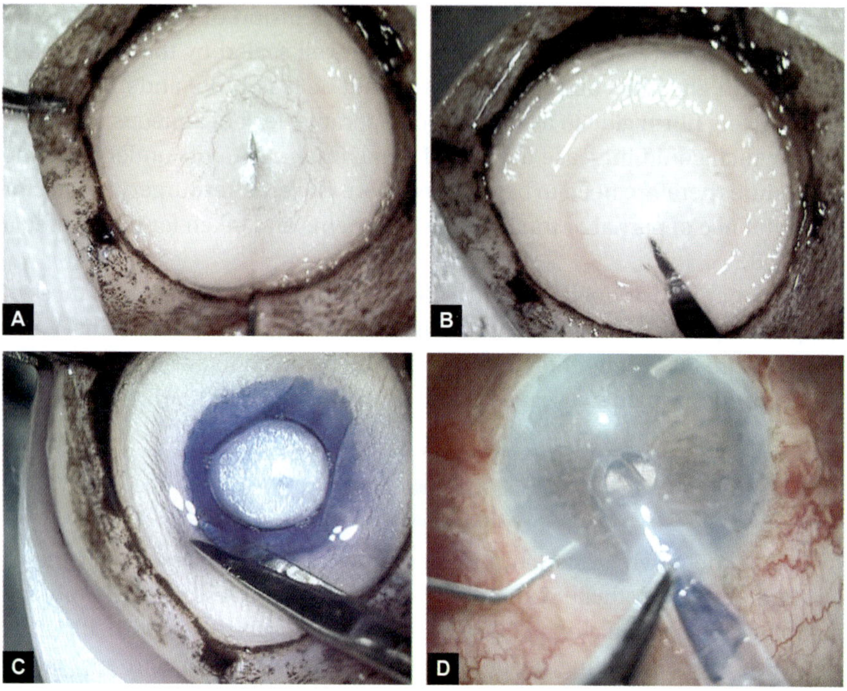

Figs. 13.5A to D: PDEK with glued IOL in a one eyed patient (Part 2). (A) 30-G needle injecting air into the stroma to create a type-1 big bubble; (B) Type-1 big bubble is created; (C) PDEK graft is stained with trypan blue and dissected; (D) PDEK graft is injected into the AC.
(PDEK: Pre-Descemet's endothelial keratoplasty; IOL: Intraocular lens; AC: Anterior chamber)

TECHNIQUE

The PDEK graft is prepared. A 30 G needle attached to an air-filled 5 mL syringe is introduced in a bevel up position into the donor corneoscleral rim placed endothelial side up. Air is then injected to form a type-1 bubble of the desired diameter. The type-1 bubble consists of the pre-Descemet's layer, the Descemet's membrane, and the endothelium and is seen as a dome-shaped elevation that is around 7–8 mm in diameter. It typically enlarges from center to periphery and has a distinct edge all around. Trypan blue is then used to stain the graft with a 26 G needle introduced into the edge of the bubble. A Vannas scissor is used to cut the graft all around the edges of the bubble and the graft is harvested. It is placed into a bowl containing the storage medium. If a type-2 bubble consisting of only Descemet's membrane and endothelium is formed, surgery may be continued as a DMEK. The type-2 bubble is larger and enlarges from periphery to center. It does not have a clearly defined edge and is more likely than a type-1 bubble to burst; therefore, care should be taken while expanding it.

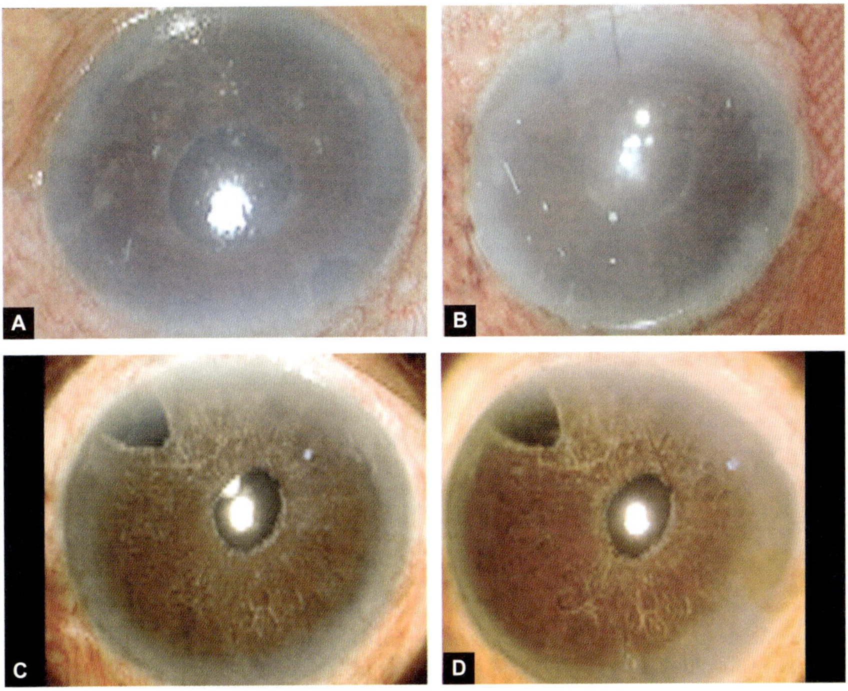

Figs. 13.6A to D: PDEK with glued IOL in a one eyed patient (Part 3). (A) Preoperative; (B) 1 week after glued IOL; (C) 2 months postoperative after PDEK-Vision 6/9; (D) 7 months postoperative after PDEK-Vision 6/6.
(PDEK: Pre-Descemet's endothelial keratoplasty; IOL: Intraocular lens; AC: Anterior chamber)

The recipient eye is prepared by stripping the Descemet's membrane. When combining with glued IOL, the IOL implantation is completed followed by single pass 4 throw pupilloplasty and PDEK graft implantation. The graft is loaded into an IOL injector as described by Francis Price and injected into the AC. Graft orientation is confirmed followed by unfolding and floating up of the graft using an air bubble.

The PDEK graft has advantages over DMEK graft in being more robust, stronger, and less likely to tear. It also allows the use of young donor grafts of any age, thereby allowing the transfer of greater quantity of endothelial cells. This allows the use of better quality of donor grafts as compared to DMEK.

If an AC IOL is there that should be explanted followed by vitrectomy, glued IOL and if necessary pupilloplasty and finally PDEK.

ADVANTAGES

The glued IOL can be done in much lesser open sky time as compared to other secondary IOL fixation techniques. Once the haptics have been exteriorized,

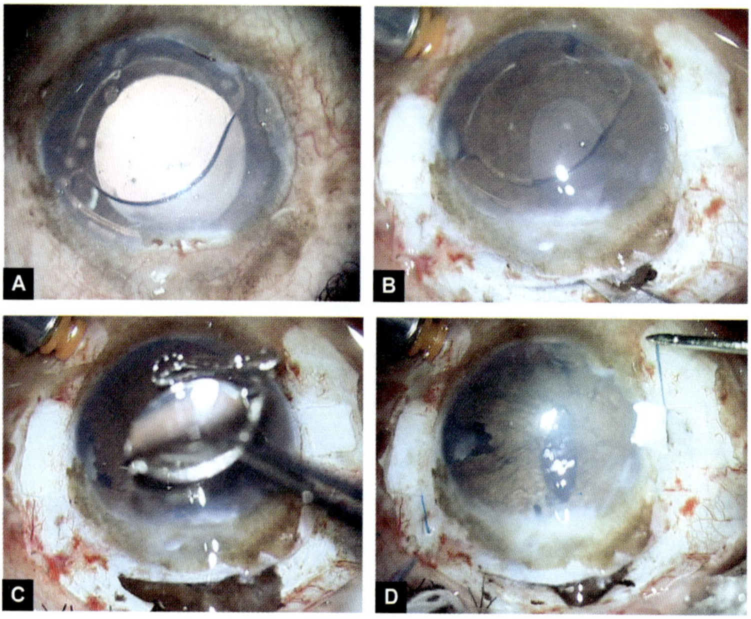

Figs. 13.7A to D: It takes two to tango—pre-Descemet's endothelial keratoplasty (PDEK) with glued IOL (Part 1). (A) Preoperative photograph of the cornea of the patient with pseudophakic bullous keratopathy. AC IOL tilted and partly protruding out of the sclera; (B) Scleral tunnel incision is done. Scleral flaps are created for glued IOL; (C) AC IOL is explanted; (D) Glued IOL is done. Note the haptics externalized.
(IOL: Intraocular lens; AC: Anterior chamber).

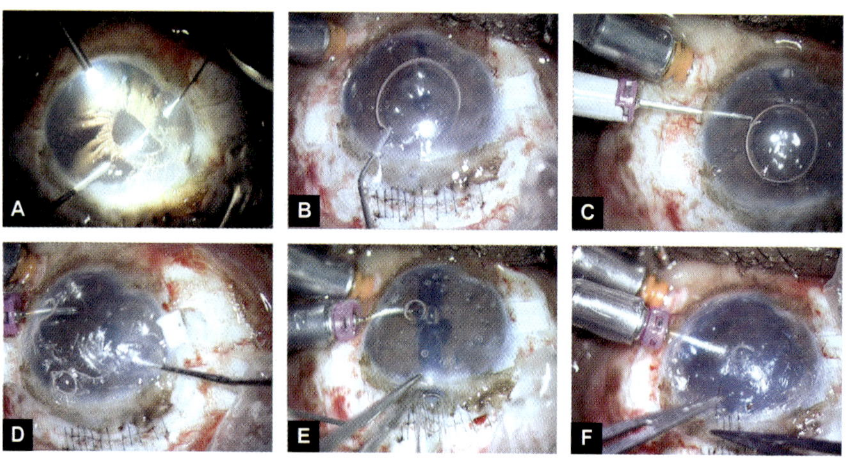

Figs. 13.8A to F: It takes two to tango—pre-Descemet's endothelial keratoplasty (PDEK) with glued IOL (Part 2). (A) Single-pass four-throw pupilloplasty (SFT) is done; (B) Air remains in the AC; (C) Trocar AC maintainer is fixed. Note the retina trocar infuses fluid into the vitreous cavity pushing iris IOL diaphragm anteriorly. Double infusion cannula technique (DICT); (D) Descemetorhexis; (E) PDEK graft is injected in the AC; (F) Graft is attached.
(IOL: Intraocular lens; AC: Anterior chamber).

the optic acts as a tamponade and is helpful in preventing expulsive hemorrhage. It can also be done with any three piece IOL available without the need for special IOL with eyelets on the haptic. The glued IOL may be done even in hypotonous eyes and centration can be adjusted once the graft is sutured and the globe is formed. Lack of pseudophacodonesis is another advantage in glued IOL as compared to other secondary IOL fixation techniques.

While doing scleral fixation with sutures, the surgeon must readjust the knots to maintain the central position of the IOL. In our procedure, simply manipulating the amount of externalization can cause proper centration of the IOL. The final tucking of the haptic provides further stabilization. A sutured scleral-fixated IOL hangs in the posterior chamber, with the sutures passing through the haptic eyes, similar to a hammock, causing dynamic torsional and anteroposterior oscillation. This pseudophacodonesis may result in progressive endothelial loss. However, in this technique, haptics are used for fixation on the scleral side and the stable optic–haptic junction prevents torsional and anteroposterior instability. Therefore, there is much less pseudophacodonesis. The haptics are covered in the scleral flap and tucked well inside the scleral pocket. There is an additional well-apposed layer of conjunctiva over the sclera. This further reduces the chances of haptic extrusion. Better dynamic stability of the glued IOL prevents pseudophacodonesis and may reduce endothelial cell loss or repositioning surgery. Combined, these two surgical modalities may improve results.

IPHONE-ASSISTED HIGH-SPEED PHOTOGRAPHY FOR GLUED IOL UNDERSTANDING

High-speed photography is a procedure of capturing images with a remarkably quick shutter speed, and it is mostly used for capturing moments that are not appreciated with naked eyes. It is the art of photographing a rapidly occurring event. Scientists have used high-speed photography to study physical movement, measuring phenomena like surface tension and gravitational effects. It is also employed for tracking the accuracy of missiles and rockets, and also to record sequence of events at the core of nuclear explosions. Sports photographers also use high-speed photography to shoot fast-moving sporting events and also to enhance the performance of the athletes by analyzing their speed and movements.

Human eyes are accustomed to viewing videos at 24–25 frames per second (fps), and it is believed that 30 fps is the final limit of a human eye to appreciate the sequence of movements. "fps" states the number of images recorded per second. High-speed cameras with much faster shutter speed are usually employed for recording videos to assess the fine details of any special event. iPhone 5S and the newer models thereafter have an inbuilt native feature of recording videos at 120 fps (iPhone 5S) and 240 fps (iPhone 6). Attaching an iPhone to the slit lamp or to a microscope with the help of an adaptor can help in recording videos at higher fps on "SLO-MO" mode of video recorder. These videos capture 120 frames in one second; in other words, 120 images are being recorded in a second of a particular event. This provides a detailed analysis of the sequence of events that a normal human eye fails to appreciate. Clinically, the surgeon switches on the "camera" and goes to "SLO-MO" mode written just adjacent to "video" recording. The video at SLO-MO mode is recorded just as a normal video recording is done by pressing the concerned button. When this video is recorded at high fps and is later played then it runs at an eye-friendly rate of 25–30 fps. Thus, it helps the surgeon to appreciate every minute detail that a normal eye fails to appreciate.

The presence of subtle movements of intraocular structures like iris, lens, and the capsular bag IOL complex has crucial clinical implications. Preoperative detection of these subtle intraocular movements often goes unnoticed and the surgeon comes across the surgical challenge intraoperatively. In our practice, we have utilized and exploited this scenario to detect subtle intraocular movements like iridodonesis, phacodonesis, and pseudophacodonesis. Presence of iridodonesis in an otherwise normal looking eye should raise the suspicion of compromised zonules or lens instability and the surgeon can get apprised of the impending complication that may be encountered in the intraoperative period. We recommend that all cases of traumatic cataract or those associated with pseudoexfoliation or connective tissue disorders should be evaluated with high fps recording to detect subtle intraocular movements as this allows the surgeon to be ready with contingency plans if required. Detection of pseudophacodonesis is another important aspect of SLO-MO recording as it goes a long way in explaining the process of vitreous disturbance in the eye following a secondary IOL implantation that can eventually lead to cystoid macular edema. Higher fps recording allows predetection and warns the surgeon of the possible challenges inherent in such cases. Apprehending and anticipating a clinical entity and its subsequent repercussions allows the case to be handled in a better way and allows a thorough preparation for and consideration of adjunctive surgical devices before surgery and simultaneously it often curbs the intraoperative surprise and makes the surgery more predictable.

Surgeons who have an older version of iPhone can use third-party applications that are available on iTunes, e.g. "SLO-PRO" is an app that can be downloaded and videos at high fps can be recorded with its help. Various apps are also available for android phone users too. The use of smartphones obviates the need to purchase a high-speed camera and is comparatively cost effective. Glued IOL fixation demonstrates iridodonesis but no pseudophacodonesis is seen due to intrascleral haptic tuck. AC IOL or a sutured IOL demonstrates pseudophacodonesis.

CONCLUSION

Thus, we see that glued IOL can be combined with PDEK in a safe and effective manner. An iridoplasty should be done when required. In complete aniridia, it may be required to be combined with an aniridia IOL or with artificial iris.

REFERENCES

1. Agarwal A, Kumar DA, Jacob S, et al. Fibrin glue-assisted sutureless posterior chamber intraocular lens implantation in eyes with deficient posterior capsules. J Cataract Refract Surg. 2008;34:1433-8.
2. Prakash G, Jacob S, Kumar DA, et al. Femtosecond-assisted keratoplasty with fibrin glue assisted sutureless posterior chamber lens implantation: new triple procedure. J Cataract Refract Surg. 2009;35:973-9.
3. Prakash G, Agarwal A, Jacob S, et al. Femtosecond-assisted Descemet stripping automated endothelial keratoplasty with fibrin glue-assisted sutureless posterior chamber lens implantation. Cornea. 2010;29:1315-9.
4. Jacob S, Agarwal A, Kumar D, et al. Modified technique for combining DMEK with glued intrascleral haptic fixation of a posterior chamber IOL as a single-stage procedure. J Refract Surg. 2014;30:492-6.
5. McKee Y, Price Jr FW, Feng MT, et al. Implementation of the posterior chamber intraocular lens intrascleral haptic fixation technique (glued intraocular lens) in a United States practice: outcomes and insights. J Cataract Refract Surg. 2014;40(12):2099-105.
6. Agarwal A, Dua HS, Narang P, et al. Pre-Descemet's endothelial keratoplasty (PDEK). Br J Ophthalmol. 2014;98(9):1181-5.
7. Osher RH, Snyder ME, Cionni RJ. Modification of the Siepser slipknot technique. J Cataract Refract Surg. 2005;31:1098-100.
8. Dua HS, Faraj LA, Said DG, et al. A novel pre-Descemet's layer (Dua's layer). Ophthalmology. 2013;120:1778-85.
9. Agarwal A, Jacob S, Kumar DA, et al. Handshake technique for glued intrascleral fixation of a posterior chamber intraocular lens. J Cataract Refract Surg. 2013;39:317-22.
10. Gabor SGB, Pavilidis MM. Sutureless intrascleral posterior chamber intraocular lens fixation. J Cataract Refract Surg. 2007;33:1851-4.
11. Price FW Jr, Price MO. Descemet's stripping with endothelial keratoplasty in 200 eyes: early challenges and technique to enhance donor adherence. J Cataract Refract Surg. 2006;32:411-18.
12. Jacob S, Agarwal A, Agarwal A, et al. Endoilluminator-assisted transcorneal illumination for Descemet's membrane endothelial keratoplasty: enhanced intraoperative visualization of the graft in corneal decompensation secondary to pseudophakic bullous keratopathy. J Cataract Refract Surg. 2014;40:1332-6.
13. Schoenberg ED, Price FW Jr. Modification of Siepser sliding suture technique for iris repair and endothelial keratoplasty. J Cataract Refract Surg. 2014;40:705-8.

CHAPTER 14

Double Infusion Cannula Technique: Pre-Descemet's Endothelial Keratoplasty in Eyes without a Capsule

Priya Narang, Amar Agarwal

INTRODUCTION

Endothelial keratoplasty (EK) helps to restore the sanctity of the corneal endothelium both from the functional and structural aspects. Graft tissue adherence to the corneal surface is a matter of concern in eyes with pseudophakic bullous keratopathy (PBK) and aphakia that need either an intraocular lens (IOL) explanation or an IOL placement respectively along with an EK procedure. Hypotony and graft adherence are the two major concerns in eyes undergoing secondary IOL placement with an EK procedure. Double infusion cannula technique (DICT) is a method where two infusion cannulas are introduced inside the eye.[1-8] The primary one is introduced for fluid infusion at pars plana level and the second one at the level of limbus as a trocar anterior chamber maintainer (T-ACM) that is employed for air infusion inside the eye. DICT (Figs. 14.1 and 14.2) is aimed at solving both the issues simultaneously thereby decreasing the chances of complications and optimizing the surgical outcomes.

DOUBLE INFUSION CANNULA TECHNIQUE (DICT)

Endothelial keratoplasty presents with the surgical challenge of increased incidence of graft dislocation, loss of air tamponade, and loss of donor tissue in the posterior cavity of aphakic eyes. Fluid infusion at pars plana serves as an effective site for performing vitrectomy along with secondary IOL fixation. Once secondary IOL is fixated and pupil shape and size is conformed to, it almost leads to isolation and compartmentalization of the anterior chamber (AC) and posterior chamber in an aphakic eye. In EK, introduction of air into the AC facilitates adhesion of the donor disk to the recipient endothelium. Maintenance of air tamponade in aphakic eyes is difficult to attain, as there is a communication between the anterior and the posterior chamber. Therefore, it is essential to perform secondary IOL fixation procedure that helps to compartmentalize the posterior chamber followed by an EK procedure. Controlled pressurized air infusion in the AC for graft adherence in EK has been described before. In the DICT wherein two infusion cannulas (Figs. 14.3 to 14.5)

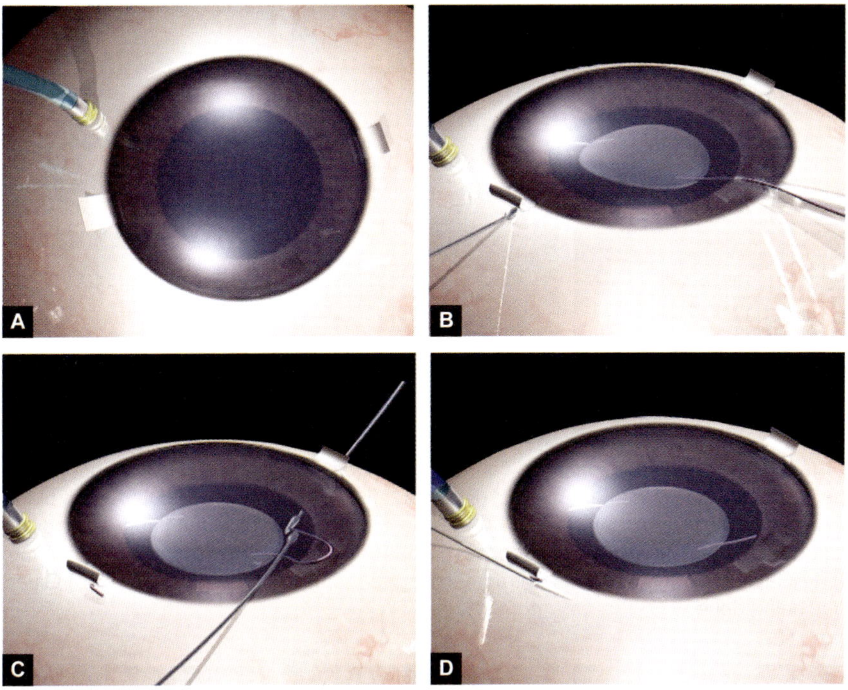

Figs. 14.1A to D: Animation of double infusion cannula technique (DICT): Glued intraocular lens (IOL) implantation. (A) Retina trocar cannula fixed. Scleral flaps for glued IOL prepared; (B) Glued IOL implantation. Leading haptic externalized; (C) Handshake technique for trailing haptic; (D) Scharioth pocket created and haptic tucked.

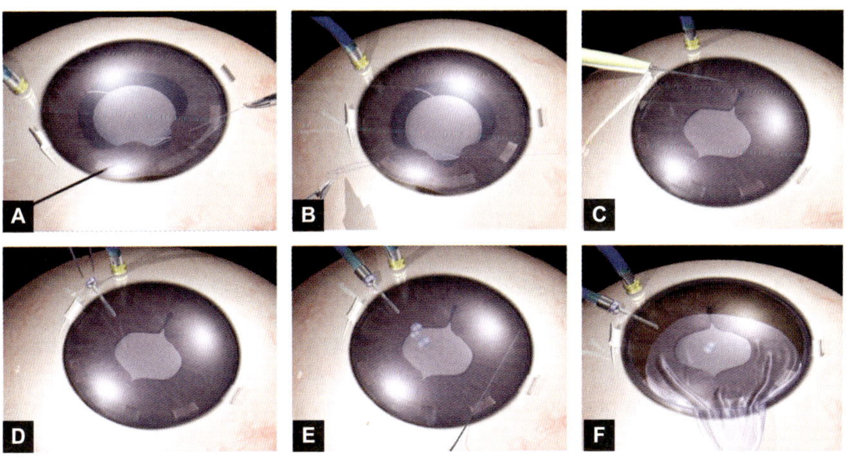

Figs. 14.2A to F: Animation of double infusion cannula technique (DICT): (A) Single-pass four-throw (SFT) pupilloplasty started; (B) SFT pupilloplasty knot tied; (C) SFT pupilloplasty completed. Trocar anterior chamber (AC) maintainer entering the AC, (D) Trocar AC maintainer getting fixed; (E) Trocar AC maintainer fixed in place. *Note*: Double infusion cannula present. Air infused through the trocar AC maintainer; (F) Descematorhexis done while continuous air is being infused in the AC. Now it is easy to inject the PDEK graft and unroll it as the fluid from the pars plana trocar pushes the iris IOL diaphragm anteriorly.

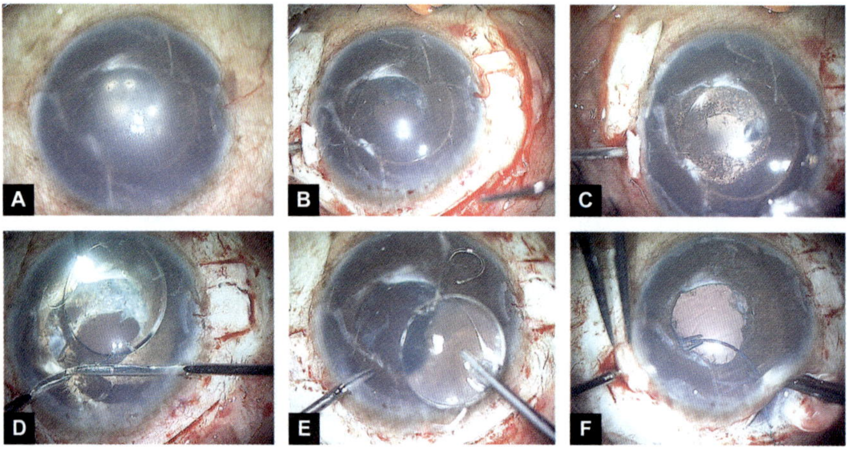

Figs. 14.3A to F: Double infusion cannula technique—DICT- Part 1. (A) Pseudophakic bullous keratopathy with an AC IOL; (B) Scleral flaps made for glued IOL. A pars plana trocar is fixed for fluid infusion. 22 G needle creates a sclerotomy 1 mm behind the limbus under the scleral flaps. The epithelium has been removed for clarity; (C) Vitrectomy; (D) AC IOL dislodged from its entrapment to the iris; (E) AC IOL explanted; (F) Glued IOL being done.

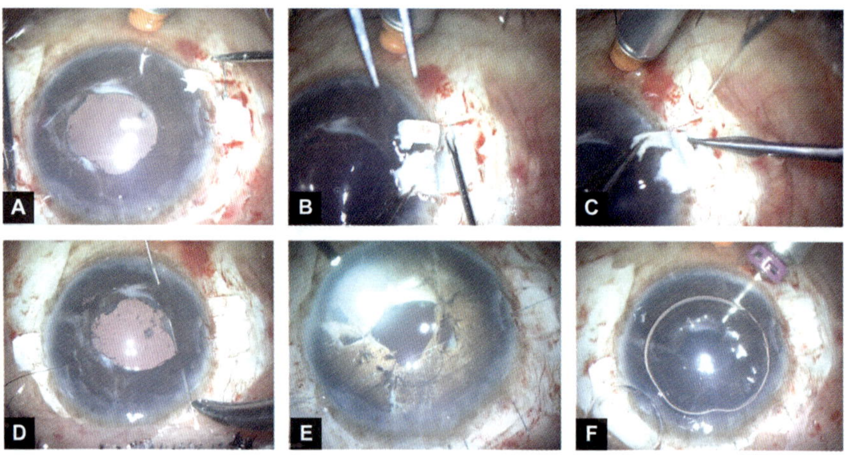

Figs. 14.4A to F: Double infusion cannula technique—DICT-Part 2. (A) Glued IOL in place, note both haptics externalized; (B) 26 G needle creates Scharioth pocket; (C) Haptic tuck; (D) Single pass 4 throw pupilloplasty started; (E) Single pass 4 throw pupilloplasty completed; (F) Trocar AC maintainer (TACM) fixed infusing air.

Note: Double cannula present. One is the pars plana trocar for fluid and the other is the TACM for air.

are placed in the eye; the initial being for fluid infusion at pars plana site for performing vitrectomy and secondary IOL placement with glued intrascleral fixation technique and the latter at the limbus level for air infusion that facilitates descemetorhexis along with the graft unrolling and its adherence to the recipient bed.

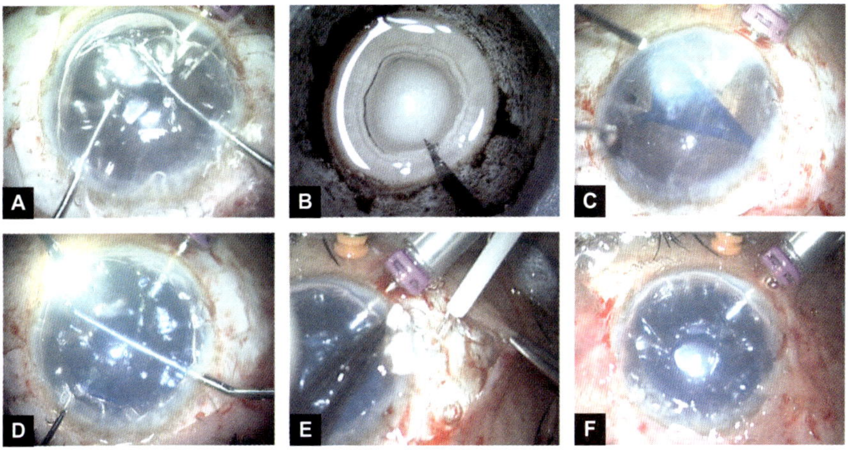

Figs. 14.5A to F: Double infusion cannula technique—DICT-Part 3. (A) Descemetorhexis. Note the continous air infusion in the AC through the TACM; (B) Type 1 big bubble created in a young donor cornea for PDEK graft preparation; (C) PDEK graft injected; (D) PDEK graft unrolled. Continuous air infusion through the TACM helps in unrolling the graft. A reverse Sinskey is used to unroll the peripheral edges of the PDEK graft; (E) Fibrin glue applied; (F) Both the trocars finally will be removed.

Note: The PDEK graft well attached.

SURGICAL TECHNIQUE

The initial procedure comprises of making two partial thickness scleral flaps 180° opposite to each other followed by introduction of fluid infusion cannula at pars plana site about 3–3.5 mm away from the limbus. Glued IOL procedure is performed and the IOL is securely tucked into the intrascleral pockets.

Once the IOL is fixed, a T-ACM is introduced inside the eye at a distance of 0.5 mm away from the limbus creating a biplanar wound. The T-ACM is introduced in a way that it enters the eye in front of the iris tissue into the AC. The T-ACM is attached to the tubing of the constellation machine and air infusion is switched on with a pressure of 30 mm Hg. Descemetorhexis is performed and the donor graft of pre-Descemet's endothelial keratoplasty (PDEK) is loaded onto the cartridge of a foldable IOL and is injected inside the AC. The graft is gently unfolded by tapping the anterior surface of cornea and once it is totally unfolded, air infusion is switched on with a pressure of 50 mm Hg for 30–45 seconds (Figs. 14.3 to 14.5). Following this, the pressurized air infusion is stopped and no specific attempt to burp the air from the AC is attempted or is needed as the posterior infusion cannula replaces some amount of air with fluid in a controlled way. The TACM is removed and the air connected to the pars plana trocar. This way both the vitreous cavity and the AC have air. Finally the pars plana trocar is also removed. Pressure is applied over the entry site with a cotton tip applicator to avoid egress of air or fluid from the eye. Fibrin glue is then applied to seal the scleral flaps and the conjunctival wounds. After the placement of first infusion cannula and performance of secondary IOL glued fixation, the eye gets effectively compartmentalized into the anterior and posterior chamber. The fluid infusion helps to maintain the tonicity of the eye and prevents the globe from collapsing. Pressurized air infusion in the eye from T-ACM helps to vault the graft and adhere it to the recipient bed.

Performing DICT has various advantages like there is no seepage of air into the vitreous cavity in both intraoperative and postoperative period as the posterior chamber is continuously maintained with fluid seeping into the eye from pars plana infusion cannula. This helps in graft adherence. Moreover, when after descemetorhexis air infusion from the T-ACM is stopped, the AC does not collapse as gentle fluid seepage occurs into the AC from the fluid infusion from the posterior vitreous cavity. This facilitates graft unfolding and maneuvering. Pressurized air infusion is switched on only when the entire graft has unfolded. DICT provides internal globe stability, prevents pressure fluctuations, and enhances the graft stability and adherence thereby making the surgery more surgeon's dependent.

DISCUSSION

Aphakic eyes are prone to globe collapse in the absence of posterior segment infusion and this directly reflects on the outcomes of the EK surgery. The infusion fluid in the vitreous cavity prevents globe collapse and helps to maintain adequate pressure in the posterior segment thereby preventing the issue of air seepage posteriorly and maintaining an adequate air tamponade anteriorly that facilitates graft adherence intraoperatively as well as in the postoperative period too.

Pressurized air infusion has been suggested as a technique to overcome the issue of graft dislocation that has been a major concern in EK with both phakic and aphakic eyes. In our technique, air was infused in a similar fashion where the T-ACM or an ACM is effectively connected to the constellation vitrectomy (Alcon) machine with flexible tubing. We used this site for only air injection and we did not feel the need for an air-fluid exchange as the fluid from the posterior segment continuously and gently seeped into the AC and prevented any gross pressure fluctuations in the eye that could be detrimental to the graft stability or would promote striae formation. At this stage, a steady pressure of 30 mm Hg was fixed so as to make the cornea adequately taut to facilitate the stripping and scoring of Descemet's membrane. In DICT, we switched off the air infusion once descemetorhexis was achieved. Gentle flow of fluid seepage was seen in AC from the posteriorly placed cannula and this prevented the collapsing of AC and also facilitated graft insertion and unfolding. Graft was then injected and unfolded by tapping/stroking the corneal surface with blunt instrument. Air was injected beneath the graft with the help of an air-filled syringe and the air infusion was switched on only when the graft had adequately unrolled and was properly centered and rightly oriented. This promoted the vaulting of the graft against the recipient bed and graft adherence.

The authors believe that the intact iris diaphragm and pupil reconstruction helped to contain air in AC and also contributed to the prevention of air loss into the vitreous cavity. The technique of DICT can also be applied for sutured posterior chamber IOL fixation and retro-iris fixation as it targets the stabilization of the posterior chamber cavity too along with the AC. This technique can also be performed in cases of PBK that need an IOL exchange along with endothelial replacement procedure.

CONCLUSION

To conclude, our technique of DICT allows performing posterior chamber intrascleral glued IOL fixation with EK [PDEK, Descemet's membrane endothelial keratoplasty (DMEK)] in a controlled way with a well-formed anterior and posterior chamber with no incidence of globe collapse.

REFERENCES

1. Prakash G, Jacob S, Ashok Kumar D, et al. Femtosecond-assisted keratoplasty with fibrin glue-assisted sutureless posterior chamber lens implantation: new triple procedure. J Cataract Refract Surg. 2009;35(6):973-9.
2. Prakash G, Agarwal A, Jacob S, et al. Femtosecond-assisted descemet stripping automated endothelial keratoplasty with fibrin glue-assisted sutureless posterior chamber lens implantation. Cornea. 2010;29(11):1315-9.
3. Jacob S, Agarwal A, Kumar DA, et al. Modified technique for combining DMEK with glued intrascleral haptic fixation of a posterior chamber IOL as a single-stage procedure. J Refract Surg. 2014;30(7):492-6.
4. McKee Y, Price FW, Feng MT, et al. Implementation of the posterior chamber intraocular lens intrascleral haptic fixation technique (glued intraocular lens) in a United States practice: outcomes and insights. J Cataract Refract Surg. 2014;40(12):2099-105.
5. Narang P, Agarwal A, Dua HS, et al. Glued intrascleral fixation of intraocular lens with pupilloplasty and pre-Descemet endothelial keratoplasty: a triple procedure. Cornea. 2015;34(12):1627-31.
6. Agarwal A, Kumar DA, Jacob S, et al. Fibrin glue-assisted sutureless posterior chamber intraocular lens implantation in eyes with deficient posterior capsules. J Cataract Refract Surg. 2008;34(9):1433-8.
7. Agarwal A, Dua HS, Narang P, et al. Pre-Descemet's endothelial keratoplasty (PDEK). Br J Ophthalmol. 2014;98(9):1181-5.
8. Agarwal A, Narang P, Kumar DA, et al. Trocar anterior chamber maintainer: Improvised infusion technique. J Cataract Refract Surg. 2016;42(2):185-9.

CHAPTER 15

Pre-Descemet's Endothelial Keratoplasty in Failed Keratoplasties

Dhivya Ashok Kumar, Amar Agarwal

INTRODUCTION

Endothelial keratoplasties have progressed widely in terms of results and technology in the recent years. Endothelial keratoplasties have nearly replaced the pennetrating keratoplasty. Corneal graft failure in any circumstances can ensue due to inherent defects in the donor graft or pre-existing pathology in the recipient.[1,2] Graft rejection is one of the key causes for secondary failure whose prevalence is high following the full thickness keratoplasty.[3,4] On the other hand, the lamellar keratoplasties, where the diseased cornea alone is transplanted, have shown fewer incidences of rejection. Endothelial grafts have the advantage of harboring less or no stromal tissue adherent to the endothelium; hence the incidence of failure due to immune rejection has been reported to be less.[3-5] With the introduction of pneumatic dissection, the donor tissue harvesting has been made simpler for the surgeons without the advanced instrumentation.[6,7] Restoring the function in a decompensated graft by means of Descemet's membrane endothelial keratoplasty (DMEK) or Descemet stripping automated endothelial keratoplasty (DSAEK) has been known.[8-15] In this chapter, we would like to share the outcomes of PDEK on preexisting failed keratoplasties.

PDEK ON FAILED KERATOPLASTY

Patients with failed keratoplasties due to endothelial decompensation who were posted for PDEK were included. Standard PDEK procedure has to be followed even in already failed graft patients. A 30 G needle attached to a 5 mL syringe was inserted from the limbus into the mid peripheral stroma. The air was slowly injected into the donor stroma until a type 1 big bubble was formed. The bubble wall was penetrated at the extreme periphery and trypan blue was injected to stain the graft, which was then cut with a pair of corneoscleral scissors and covered with the tissue culture medium. Those eyes in which type 2 bubble was obtained instead of type 1 during donor graft harvesting were proceeded as DMEK technique.

Under peribulbar anesthesia, initially a trocar anterior chamber maintainer (TACM) was placed at the limbus. The Descemet's membrane (DM) was scored all around [diameter smaller than the penetrating keratoplasty (PK) graft]. The graft host junction should not be disturbed with undue force or manipulation. The DM was then stripped off gently removed via the main port. Donor PDEK lenticule was inserted into the anterior chamber (AC) with customized injector. It was attached to the recipient bed by careful unrolling with air bubble, and attached to the overlying recipient stroma. Margins were swept in case of tight roll on the endothelial side under air with reverse Sinskey. Intrachamber positive pressure was maintained thereafter for a short time by air pump connected TACM. Main wound was closed with 10-0 monofilament nylon interrupted sutures and the previous graft host interface is rechecked for any leak.

DEMOGRAPHICS AND OBSERVATIONS

There were 23 eyes analyzed. It included 9 (34.7%) failed penetrating keratoplasty, 8 (34.7%) DMEK, 4 (17.30%) PDEK, 2 (8.7%) Descemet's stripping automated endothelial keratoplasty (DSAEK). The mean donor age was 32.4 ± 20.2 years. Out of 23, 9 (39.1%), 11 (47.8%) and 3 (13%) had donor less than 30 years, 30–50 years, and more than 50 years, respectively. The mean graft diameter in 23 eyes was 7.6 ± 1.3 mm.

Out of 23 eyes, 18 eyes (78.2%) obtained type 1 bubble intraoperatively and proceeded with PDEK and 5 eyes (21.7%) who obtained type 2 bubble intraoperatively underwent DMEK procedure. The mean donor age of those eyes with PDEK was 32.8 ± 18.3 years. Out of the 18 eyes which underwent PDEK, there were 6 (33.3%) failed PKs, 8 (44.4%) failed DMEKs, 2 (11.1%) failed PDEKs, and 2 (11.1%) failed DSAEK.

VISUAL AND CLINICAL OUTCOMES

There was significant change in visual acuity (Fig. 15.1). The mean preoperative CDVA in eyes with PDEK was 0.15 ± 0.2. At 18 months, a significant difference ($p = 0.012$) in CDVA was noted. There was no significant correlation ($p = 0.936$, $r = 0.018$) between the postoperative CDVA and donor age. Loss of CDVA was noted in 2 (8.6%) eyes and nonimprovement of CDVA was seen in 9 eyes (39.1%). The mean preoperative and 3 months postoperative central corneal thickness (CCT) was 727.8 ± 84.9 μm and 585.3 ± 72.7 μm, respectively. There was significant reduction in CCT at 3 months ($p = 0.000$) (Fig. 15.2). Superficial vascularization more than 3 clock hours were noted in 4 out of 23 eyes (17.3%) at 18 months follow-up. There was no graft infection or graft dislocation observed. Corneal clarity of grade 4, 3 and 2 was noted in 6 (26%), 4 (17.3%), and 2 (8.6%) eyes, respectively (Figs. 15.3A and B). Good graft adhesion was seen in postoperative period (Figs. 15.4A and B). The mean specular count of donor eyes was 2951.9 ± 399.8 cells/mm^2 and the postoperative specular at 6 months in the host was 1,319 ± 312.7 cells/mm^2.

COMPLICATIONS

Loss of CDVA in 2 eyes was due to graft rejection which proceeded to secondary graft failure and 9 eyes that showed no improvement in visual acuity had persistent corneal edema. Out of 9 eyes with persistent corneal edema, 4 eyes (57.1%) underwent PK and one eye (14.2%) underwent keratoprosthesis. There were 3 PDEK eyes with immediate postoperative graft detachment for which rebubbling was performed. Two (8.6%) out of 23 eyes had inverse orientation which required reorientation and one (4.3%) had large graft with folds. Postoperative glaucoma was seen in 2 (8.6%) eyes which required medical management.

PRE-DESCEMET'S ENDOTHELIAL KERATOPLASTY IN FAILED KERATOPLASTY

Compared to repeat PK, secondary endothelial keratoplasty offers lesser trauma by avoiding deep incisions and multiple sutures. During the PDEK in failed graft surgery, PDEK procedure in a failed graft, the DM stripping can slacken the adhesion of old DSAEK graft and hence care was taken not to give excess pressure. Loose adhesion of the pre-existing graft and early postoperative secondary procedure aggravate the challenges. Good intraoperative air pressure and proper postoperative positioning will aid in strong adherence in a pre-existing endothelial graft like DSAEK. Though the initial donor

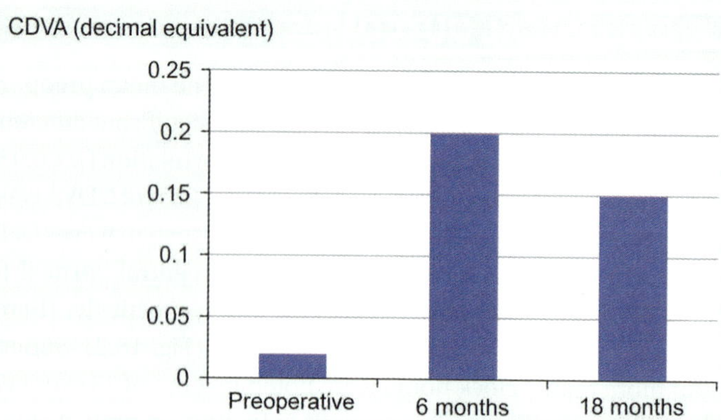

Fig. 15.1: Bar diagram showing the change in corrected distant visual acuity (CDVA) over the time period.

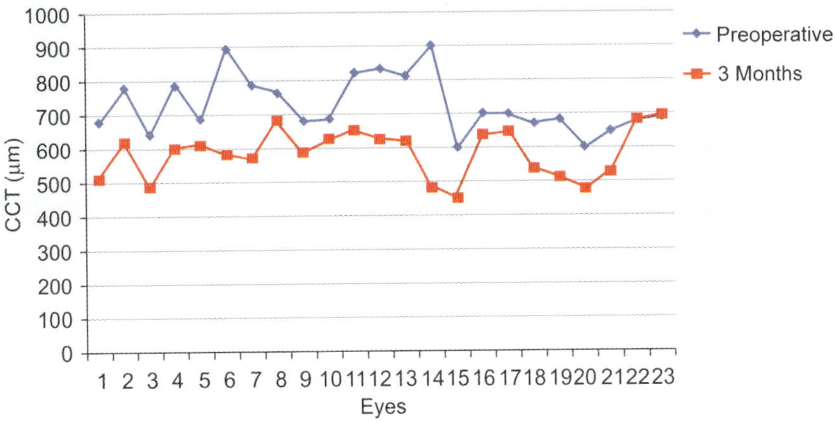

Fig. 15.2: Line diagram showing the decrease in central corneal thickness (CCT) at 3 months in operated eyes.

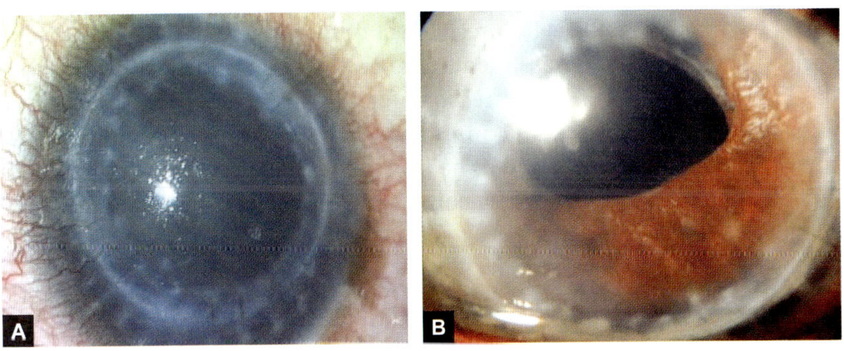

Figs. 15.3A and B: Preoperative failed penetrating keratoplasty (A) and postoperative PDEK (B) at 6 months. (*Courtesy:* Agarwal/Kim book Endothelial Keratoplasty by Thieme, USA).

endothelial cells were abundant, there was significant loss noted over the time period which was higher than the reported loss in PDEK.[14-16]

The size of the PDEK graft is preferred to be smaller than the PK graft, because there can be rolled edges or folds in large grafts which may not fit into the curvature of the original stroma. If the primary PK graft gives way intraoperatively, the wound has to be sutured to maintain wound stability. Nonvisualization during surgery has been one of the challenges faced by surgeon in operating on failed grafts; however the advantage of PDEK with endoilluminator helps in visualization of graft even in cases with corneal edema. [17] Descemet stripping automated endothelial keratoplasty has shown faster visual outcome in failed grafts, however the graft dislocations were common.[18] Pre-existing endothelial dysfunction, faster endothelial cell failure

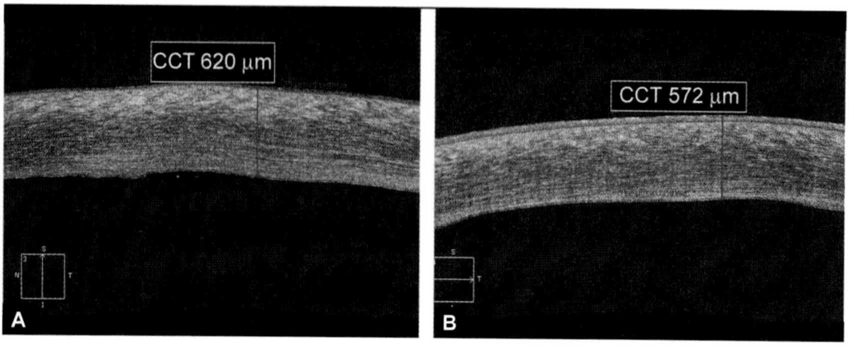

Figs. 15.4A and B: Anterior segment optical coherence tomography of PDEK in failed graft patient on day 1 (A) and day 7 (B) postoperative periods.

and corneal scattering can affect the final outcomes in secondary EK's.[19-21] Timing of the secondary surgery forever been the diagnostic dilemma in failed grafts. In long-standing corneal edema, stromal fibrosis and anterior surface irregularities might occur that limit the visual outcome of repeat surgery. Loss of endothelial cells, presence of fibrocellular tissue on the stromal surface, retained Descemet's membrane on the stromal surface and epithelial in growth are some of the reasons for primary endothelial graft failure after PDEK. Though the visual improvement was noted in all the eyes, the mean survival time was noted to be less. Our experience showed that there can be significant challenges in secondary PDEK in failed grafts similar to any other EK.

CONCLUSION

Pre-Descemet's endothelial keratoplasty can be performed as a secondary procedure in failed keratoplasties including primary penetrating keratoplasty or primary endothelial keratoplasty with favorable outcome. However, there is risk of graft failure. Nevertheless, when meticulous surgical steps, good donor selection, and intraoperative precautions are followed, good surgical outcomes can be achieved.

REFERENCES

1. Halliday BL, Ritten SA. Effect of donor parameters on primary graft failure and the recovery of acuity after keratoplasty. Br J Ophthalmol. 1990;74:7-11.
2. Williams KA, Lowe M, Bartlett C, et al. Risk factors for human corneal graft failure within the Australian corneal graft registry. Transplantation. 2008;86:1720-4.
3. Price MO, Gorovoy M, Price FW Jr, et al. Descemet's stripping automated endothelial keratoplasty: three-year graft and endothelial cell survival compared with penetrating keratoplasty. Ophthalmology. 2013;120:246-51.
4. Zhang YM, Wu SQ, Yao YF. Long-term comparison of full-bed deep anterior lamellar keratoplasty and penetrating keratoplasty in treating keratoconus. J Zhejiang Univ Sci B. 2013;14:438-50.

5. Kymionis GD, Mikropoulos DG, Portaliou DM, et al. New perspectives on lamellar keratoplasty. Adv Ther. 2014;31:494-511.
6. Anwar M, Teichmann KD. Deep lamellar keratoplasty: surgical techniques for anterior lamellar keratoplasty with and without baring of Descemet's membrane. Cornea. 2002;21:374-83
7. Yoeruek E, Bayyoud T, Hofmann J, et al. Comparison of pneumatic dissection and forceps dissection in Descemet membrane endothelial keratoplasty: histological and ultrastructural findings. Cornea. 2012;31:920-5.
8. Weller JM, Tourtas T, Kruse FE, et al. Descemet membrane endothelial keratoplasty as treatment for graft failure after descemet stripping automated endothelial keratoplasty. Am J Ophthalmol. 2015;159:1050-7.
9. Kymionis GD, Kankariya VP, Diakonis VF, et al. Descemet stripping automated endothelial keratoplasty in a child after failed penetrating keratoplasty. J AAPOS. 2012;16:95-6.
10. Yoeruek E, Bartz-Schmidt KU. Secondary descemet membrane endothelial keratoplasty after failed primary descemet membrane endothelial keratoplasty: clinical results. Cornea. 2013;32:1414-7.
11. Price MO, Feng MT, McKee Y, et al. Repeat Descemet membrane endothelial keratoplasty: secondary grafts with early intervention are comparable with fellow-eye primary grafts. Ophthalmology. 2015;122:1639-44.
12. Anshu A, Price MO, Price FW Jr. Descemet membrane endothelial keratoplasty and hybrid techniques for managing failed penetrating grafts. Cornea. 2013;32:1-4.
13. Agarwal A, Dua HS, Narang P, et al. Pre-Descemet's endothelial keratoplasty (PDEK). Br J Ophthalmol. 2014;98:1181-5.
14. Kumar DA, Dua HS, Agarwal A, et al. Postoperative spectral-domain optical coherence tomography evaluation of pre-Descemet endothelial keratoplasty grafts. J Cataract Refract Surg. 2015;41:1535-6.
15. Agarwal A, Narang P, Kumar DA, et al. Trocar anterior chamber maintainer: Improvised infusion technique. J Cataract Refract Surg. 2016;42:185-9.
16. Agarwal A, Agarwal A, Narang P, et al. Pre-Descemet endothelial keratoplasty with infant donor corneas: a prospective analysis. Cornea. 2015;34:859-65.
17. Jacob S, Agarwal A, Agarwal A, et al. Endoilluminator-assisted transcorneal illumination for Descemet membrane endothelial keratoplasty: enhanced intraoperative visualization of the graft in corneal decompensation secondary to pseudophakic bullous keratopathy. J Cataract Refract Surg. 2014;40:1332-6.
18. Covert DJ, Koenig SB. Descemet stripping and automated endothelial keratoplasty (DSAEK) in eyes with failed penetrating keratoplasty. Cornea. 2007; 26:692-6.
19. Tarantino-Scherrer JN, Kaufmann C, Bochmann F, et al. Visual recovery and endothelial cell survival after Descemet stripping automated endothelial keratoplasty for failed penetrating keratoplasty grafts—a cohort study. Cornea. 2015;34:1024-9.
20. Arnalich-Montiel F, Hernández-Verdejo JL, Oblanca N, et al. Comparison of corneal haze and visual outcome in primary DSAEK versus DSAEK following failed DMEK. Graefes Arch Clin Exp Ophthalmol. 2013;251:2575-84.
21. Ćirković A, Schlötzer-Schrehardt U, Weller JM, et al. Clinical and ultrastructural characteristics of graft failure in DMEK: 1-year results after repeat DMEK. Cornea. 2015;34(1):11-7.

SECTION 4

Complications and Results

CHAPTER 16

Intraoperative Complications of Pre-Descemet's Endothelial Keratoplasty

Dhivya Ashok Kumar, Amar Agarwal

BACKGROUND

Pre-Descemet's endothelial keratoplasty (PDEK) has many potential advantages over other endothelial keratoplasty's (EK) like Descemet's membrane endothelial keratoplasty (DMEK) or Descemet's stripping and endothelial keratoplasty (DSEK); however in the learning curve complications are inevitable.[1-3] **These complications are generally manageable, and the risk tends to decline as a surgeon gains experience in the new surgical technique.** Intraoperative complications have major impact on the final postoperative outcome. Hence, we have discussed the common intraoperative challenges, which can be faced during the learning curve of PDEK and the methods of management of the same.

COMPLICATIONS DURING PNEUMATIC DISSECTION

Difficulty in Bubble Creation

Type 1 bubble starts from the center and moves outward to the midperiphery (Fig. 16.1).[4] Type 2 bubble is thin and starts from the periphery and

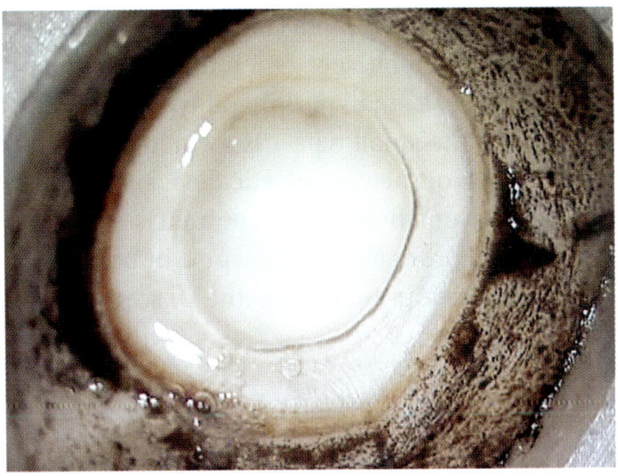

Fig. 16.1: Donor graft preparation showing a type 1 bubble formed.

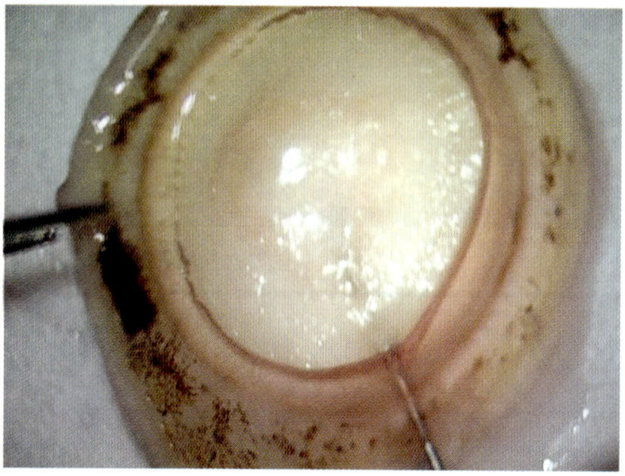

Fig. 16.2: Donor graft preparation showing a type 2 bubble formed.

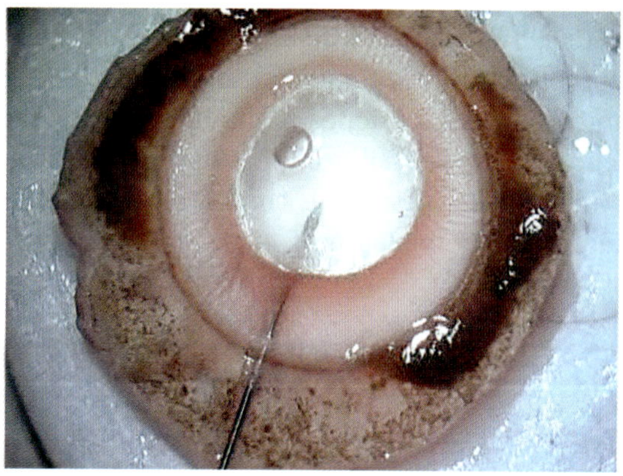

Fig. 16.3: Type 1 bubble enhanced with viscoelastic device.

is larger as compared to type 1 bubble (Fig. 16.2).[4] Failure to form the type 1 bubble can happen intraoperatively, when the correct plane of dissection is not reached. In that case, a small peripheral type 2 bubble or small type 1 bubble is formed. When the small type 1 is formed, it is enhanced by air in the same dissection plane or the viscoelastic device injection in a controlled fashion (Fig. 16.3). However when a type 2 bubble is formed, DMEK surgery can still be proceeded. In order to prevent type 2 bubble formation, one can put multiple peripheral micropunctures on the Descemet's membrane (DM) before air injection.

Double Bubble Formation

Double bubble formation or mixed bubble is also noted during donor preparation. Here there will be one central bubble and another peripheral bubble

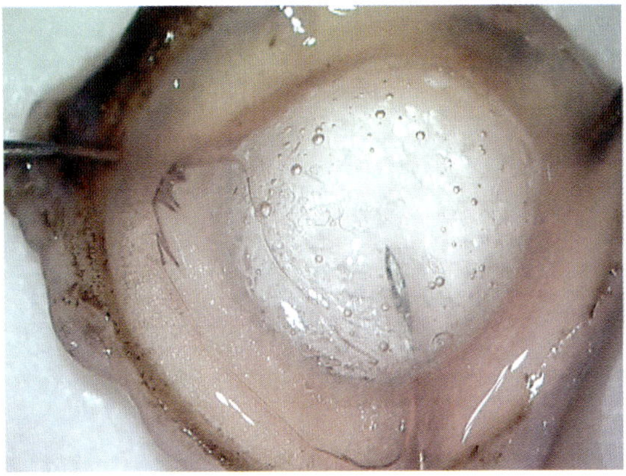

Fig. 16.4: Donor graft preparation showing double bubble where both type 1 (center) and type 2 (periphery) seen.

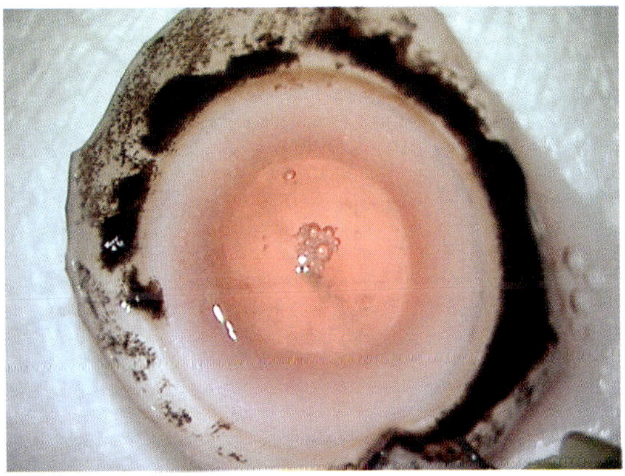

Fig. 16.5: Donor graft preparation showing the continuous injection of McCarey–Kaufman (MK) medium to enhance the type 1 bubble size.

adjacent to it in one quadrant (Fig. 16.4). Improper dissection plane during air injection is the cause for mixed bubble. Such grafts induce Descemet's detachment and hinder postoperative outcome.

No Bubble Formation with Pneumatic Dissection

Very rarely single bubble may not form on repeated attempts with air, in that case preservation medium either McCarey-Kaufman (MK) medium (Fig. 16.5) or Optisol can be used for bubble formation. If multiple attempts have ended in failure to form single bubble, it is advised to use new cornea as the stroma is pneumatically dissected at various planes and further attempts will end in failure only.

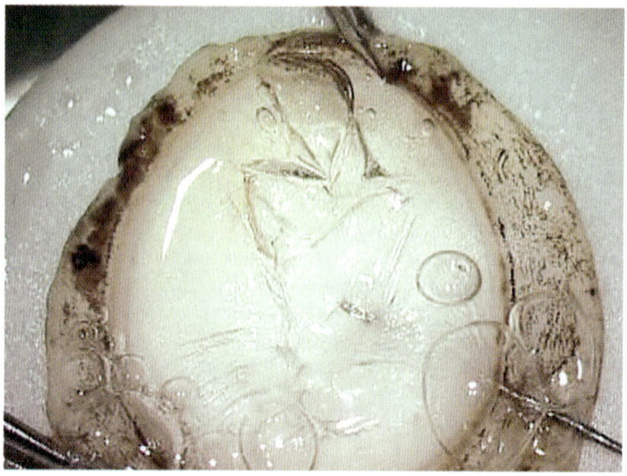

Fig. 16.6: Bubble bursts when the surgeon pushes too much air into a small space.

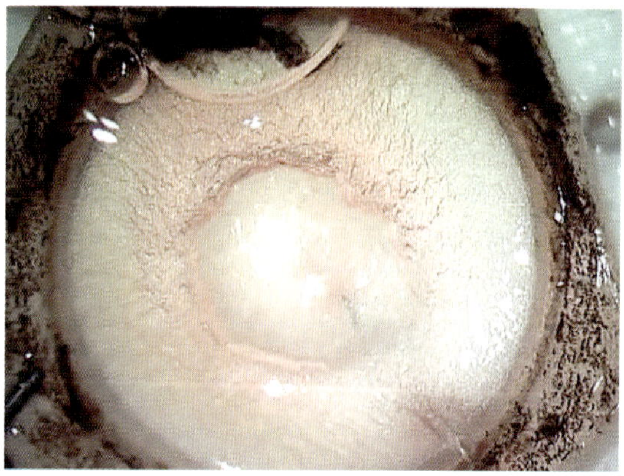

Fig. 16.7: Donor graft preparation where a small sized type 1 bubble is obtained.

Bubble Burst during Pneumatic Dissection

Bubble burst usually happen when the surgeon pushes too much air into a small space and the intrabubble pressure raises exponentially faster (Fig. 16.6). Once the bubble bursts after reaching maximum size, Vannas scissors can be used to excise the graft uniformly along its margin. If the bubble bursts in early stage (size less than 6 mm), do rebubbling in another graft as the results are not predictable in smaller grafts.

Small Graft

Similar to any endothelial keratoplasty (EK), the size of graft is vital in PDEK. Small graft is obtained due to the formation of small diameter type 1 bubble (Fig. 16.7). Whenever a bubble less than 4 mm is seen after pneumatic dissection, viscoelastic device can be injected into the bubble to enhance the size. However, too much intrabubble pressure should be avoided which again can lead to bubble burst. The preferred graft size in PDEK is 7.5–8 mm. Grafts smaller than 6.5 mm has the risk of failure later.

GRAFT-RELATED COMPLICATIONS

Graft Injection

Pre-Descemet's endothelial keratoplasty graft though very thin, can still get stuck into the injector preventing the release into the anterior chamber. Pre-loading with storage medium namely MK medium or viscoelastic device in the cartridge can reduce the incidence. If the graft was noted to be entangled in the nozzle, it is better to dislodge the graft and do reinjection rather than attempting undue maneuvers.

Inverse Curling of Graft

Similar to any endothelial grafts, the PDEK grafts have to curl with the endothelial side facing the cornea as soon as it is injected under saline. If it curls with the endothelium away from the cornea, it has to be reoriented in the anterior chamber by saline or viscoelastic device (Fig. 16.8). Gentle jets of saline through the cannula at the wound are then directed around the graft to create swirling currents that cause the scroll to roll over.

Reverse Graft Unfolding

A surgeon can notice the reverse orientation soon after injection as above or after manipulation in the later period. It is noted as nonattaching graft which scrolls with the endothelium side outward (Fig. 16.9). This is managed by

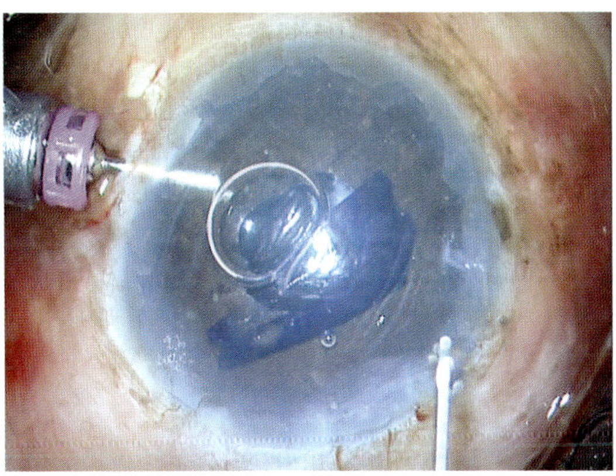

Fig. 16.8: Pre-Descemet's endothelial keratoplasty (PDEK) graft oriented reverse direction immediately after injection.

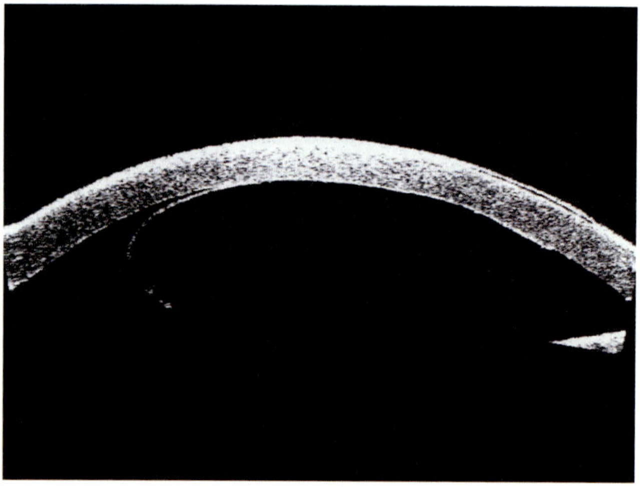

Fig. 16.9: Anterior segment optical coherence tomography showing inverted pre-Descemet's endothelial keratoplasty (PDEK) graft.

reinversion by saline in the anterior chamber or by injection of viscoelastic device. An intraoperative microscope integrated with optical coherence tomography can also guide in visualizing the real time orientation and localization of the graft.[5] Care should be taken to prevent too much manipulation on the endothelium while reinverting.

Poor Graft Visualization

Intraoperative loss of visualization can happen in eyes with chronic corneal decompensation with coexisting epithelial and anterior stromal scarring. Superficial keratectomy or epithelial debridement can be performed in many cases to improve intraoperative clarity. Another method to enhance visualization is to stain the graft with trypan blue during harvesting. If staining was not performed during donor harvesting, one can soak the graft in the diluted trypan blue for 1 minute intraoperatively before utilization. In eyes with persistent corneal edema visualization can be enhanced by external endoilluminator termed as "endoilluminator assisted" PDEK (Fig. 16.10).[6] Use of endoilluminator helps in localizing the position of graft in cases with significant edema. In addition, the intraoperative optical coherence tomography will also aid in locating grafts in eyes with significant corneal edema.

Eccentric Graft

One can also observe an eccentrically placed graft during internal air tamponade. In such situation, the surgeon can do sweeping maneuvers on the cornea to recenter the graft under air.[7]

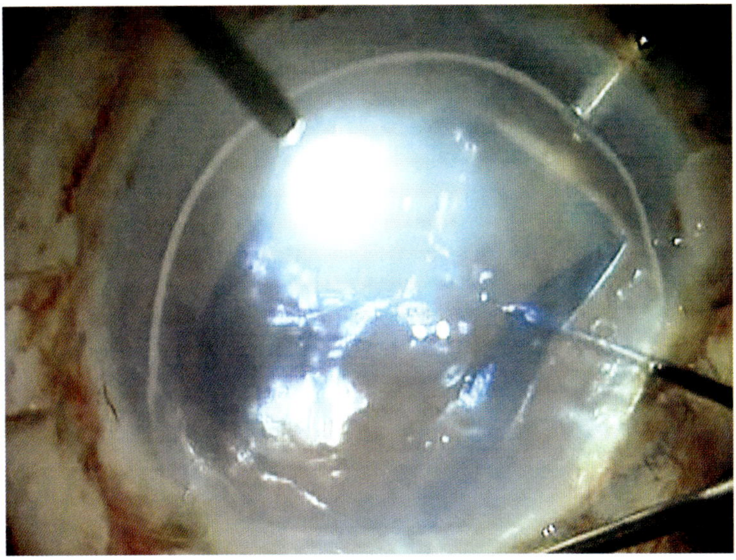

Fig. 16.10: Endoilluminator is being used to visualize the pre-Descemet's endothelial keratoplasty (PDEK) graft intraoperatively.

Folded Graft

Graft unfolding can also be challenging from time to time with persistent graft fold. A pre-existing stromal scar on the posterior cornea, the overhanging residual DM and fluctuating anterior chamber depth can create unfolding problems. Identifying the cause helps in managing the condition in early stages. Air pump-assisted PDEK can reduce chamber fluctuation and helps in unfolding of the graft edge.[7] One can also use trocar anterior chamber maintenance (Fig. 16.11) which helps in controlled infusion to maintain chamber intraoperatively.[8] It is also important to remove the unpeeled DM or DM scar overlying the unfolded graft. If there is chamber fluctuation due to the posterior capsular defect, then one has to consider stabilizing the iris-IOL (intraocular lens) diaphragm (glued IOL and pupilloplasty) before doing PDEK. Peripheral folds can happen in eyes with graft-host disproportion (large graft in small host cornea) or in eyes with previous keratoplasty due to overriding at the graft host junction.

Lenticule Loss

Intraoperative donor lenticule can get lost when it is not stained adequately as it may not be visualized due to lack of contrast. Aphakic eyes are at higher risk, where the lenticule can get dislodged into the vitreous. Hence, suitable staining of graft before injection into the eye and attaining appropriate stability of IOL-iris diaphragm is necessary to prevent lenticule drop.

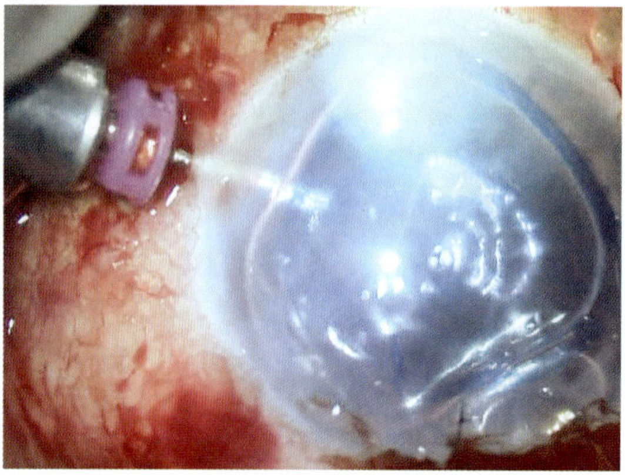

Fig. 16.11: Trocar anterior chamber maintainer cannula used intraoperatively during pre-Descemet's endothelial keratoplasty (PDEK).

OTHER INTRAOPERATIVE COMPLICATIONS

Improper Descemet's Membrane Stripping

Eye with preoperative endothelial scarring have difficult time during intra-operative peeling. Pre-existing inflammation and pigment changes also can induce challenges during DM removal. If residual DM is left, it can hinder in the adhesion of donor graft and cause graft folds. It is preferred to remove all the DM tissue before injecting the graft especially in the central cornea. Reverse Sinskey hook is used to push and pull on the fibrous tissue to release the DM.

Intraoperative Iris or Pupillary Damage

Eyes with thin atrophic iris or pre-existing pupillary abnormalities are more prone for such complication. If there is intraoperative sphincter tear or irido-dialysis, pupilloplasty has to be performed.[9] Pupilloplasty in such eyes helps in maintaining the air bubble from escaping into the posterior chamber behind the IOL, which may happen in widely dilated pupil. Large pupil due to trauma, previous complicated surgery or congenital abnormalities can prevent stable air bubble maintenance in PDEK (Fig. 16.12). Therefore, pupil abnormality should be addressed in all such cases.

Intraocular Lens Decentration

An existing IOL can get decentered due to unstable pre-existing zonules or because of previous complicated cataract surgery. In such situation when, one notices a defective zonule or defective posterior capsule intraoperatively, the IOL has to be centered by transscleral fixation (Fig. 16.13) by Glued

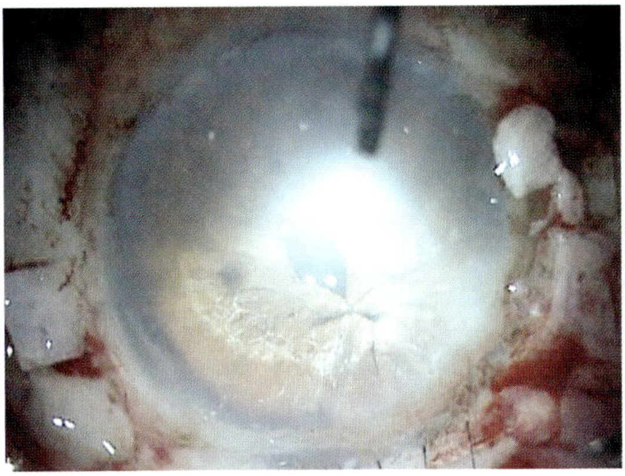

Fig. 16.12: Single-pass four-throw pupilloplasty performed before pre-Descemet's endothelial keratoplasty (PDEK) graft injection.

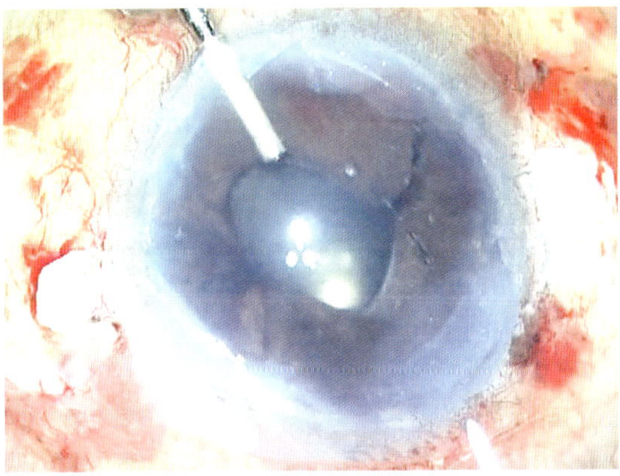

Fig. 16.13: Glued intraocular lens implantation in an eye with defective capsule performed before pre-Descemet's endothelial keratoplasty (PDEK) graft injection.

IOL method.[10] Do not use anterior chamber IOL or iris claw lenses as it might occupy the anterior chamber and further hinder the surgical field and also lead to postoperative endothelial cell loss. Any existing damaged or malpositioned IOL need to be corrected intraoperatively itself in such eyes.

Chamber Collapse

Loss of anterior chamber pressure can happen due to wide incision causing excess fluid outflow. Either use of trocar anterior chamber maintainer or air pump-assisted anterior chamber maintainer (Fig. 6.14) can help in assisting the chamber pressure control.[7,8] Avoiding too large incisions and proper closure of main wound immediately after graft injection can prevent intraoperative hypotony.

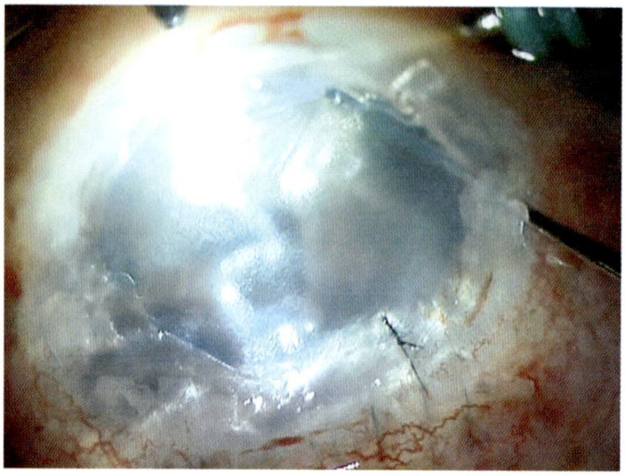

Fig. 16.14: Air pump-assisted pre-Descemet's endothelial keratoplasty (PDEK) surgery where graft is unfolded under pressurized air chamber.

Intraoperative High Intraocular Pressure

Eyes with uncontrolled preoperative intraocular pressure (IOP) are the high-risk candidates for intraoperative pressure changes. Preoperative antiglaucoma medications and intravenous osmotic agents like mannitol can reduce the IOP spike due to peribulbar block effectively. If intraoperatively, there is excess posterior pressure before making the incision, it is advisable to start intravenous mannitol and do avoid sudden decompression under high IOP to prevent suprachoroidal hemorrhage.

Intraoperative Hyphema

Eyes with pre-existing neovascularization (iris or angle) are more prone for intraoperative hyphema. Excess tissue manipulation and iris injury can also predispose to this. However, hemorrhage from the limbal wound can also enter into the anterior chamber. Hence, proper cautious cauterization of limbal wound is required. Air pump-assisted PDEK helps in preventing further internal hemorrhage by providing adequate tamponade. Use of the trocar anterior chamber maintainer will also help in continous fluid exchange and therby flushing the blood in anterior chamber.

SUMMARY

It is extremely necessary to understand the surgical steps methodically in PDEK especially in the early learning curve so as to reduce the inadvertent complications. By following proper preoperative patient selection and meticulous deployment of surgical steps one can achieve the desired results without surgical hindrances. I believe the above discussion has put some limelight on theimportant intraoperative challenges one can face during surgery and their appropriate prevention.

REFERENCES

1. Agarwal A, Dua HS, Narang P, et al. Pre-Descemet's endothelial keratoplasty (PDEK). Br J Ophthalmol. 2014;98(9):1181-5.
2. Dirisamer M, van Dijk K, Dapena I, et al. Prevention and management of graft detachment in Descemet membrane endothelial keratoplasty. Arch Ophthalmol. 2012;130(3):280-91.
3. Guerra FP, Anshu A, Price MO, et al. Descemet's membrane endothelial keratoplasty: prospective study of 1-year visual outcomes, graft survival, and endothelial cell loss. Ophthalmology. 2011;118(12):2368-73.
4. Dua HS, Faraj LA, Said DG, et al. Human corneal anatomy redefined: a novel pre-Descemet's layer (Dua's layer). Ophthalmology. 2013;120(9):1778-85.
5. Titiyal JS, Kaur M, Falera R, et al. Evaluation of time to donor lenticule apposition using intraoperative optical coherence tomography in descemet stripping automated endothelial keratoplasty. Cornea. 2016;35(4):477-81.
6. Jacob S, Agarwal A, Kumar DA. Endoilluminator-assisted Descemet membrane endothelial keratoplasty and endoilluminator-assisted pre-Descemet endothelial keratoplasty. Clin Ophthalmol. 2015;9:2123-5.
7. Jacob S, Narasimhan S, Agarwal A, et al. Air pump-assisted graft centration, graft edge unfolding, and graft uncreasing in young donor graft pre-Descemet endothelial keratoplasty. Cornea. 2017;36(8):1009-13.
8. Agarwal A, Narang P, Kumar DA, et al. Trocar anterior chamber maintainer: improvised infusion technique. J Cataract Refract Surg. 2016;42(2):185-9.
9. Narang P, Agarwal A. Single-pass four-throw technique for pupilloplasty. Eur J Ophthalmol. 2017;27(4):506-8.
10. Narang P, Agarwal A, Dua HS, et al. Glued intrascleral fixation of intraocular lens with pupilloplasty and pre-Descemet endothelial keratoplasty: A triple procedure. Cornea. 2015;34(12):1627-31.

CHAPTER 17

Postoperative Complications of Pre-Descemet's Endothelial Keratoplasty

Dhivya Ashok Kumar, Amar Agarwal

INTRODUCTION

As in our previous chapter, we have discussed on the intraoperative complications; there are few postoperative complications which the surgeons need to understand and anticipate. Unless the surgeon understands the etiopathogenesis of the complications, it is otherwise difficult to manage them. Therefore, we classify the postoperative complications as immediate (seen on day 1–30) and late postoperative (seen after 1 month) depending upon the time of onset.

IMMEDIATE POSTOPERATIVE COMPLICATIONS

Corneal Edema

Once graft in position, the endothelial pump usually starts functioning as early as possible depending upon the intraoperative loss. If there was excess intraoperative manipulation, there can be early postoperative edema due to delayed endothelial pump function (Fig. 17.1). However usually within 1 week,

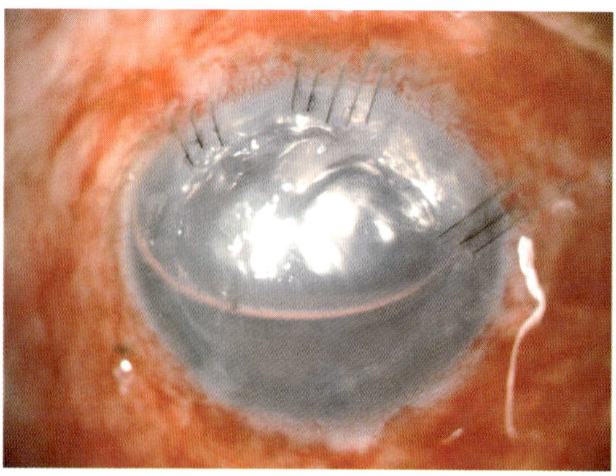

Fig. 17.1: Clinical slit lamp photograph of an eye having immediate postoperative edema after pre-Descemet's endothelial keratoplasty (PDEK).

the existing endothelial cells start functioning to recover the corneal edema. If the loss of endothelium had been significant and the donor graft already had less endothelial cell count, there can be primary graft failure which can present as persistent corneal edema. Topical hyperosmolar agent like 5% sodium chloride formulations can be added along with regular post-operative medications like steroids and antibiotics. Transient corneal edema due to manipulation usually resolves within 2 weeks. Serial anterior segment optical coherence tomography (OCT) the noncontact method to quantify pachymetry and slit lamp photography will help in assessment during the follow-up.

Descemet's Folds

Smooth concave configuration of posterior cornea should be obtained in all the eyes with good graft adherence. Descemet's fold can occur when there was excess tissue manipulation intraoperatively (Fig. 17.2). Avoiding too much endothelial handling and following the "no-touch" technique would definitely reduce this complication on the immediate postoperative period. This usually resolves with medical management and no additional treatment is required except for the maintenance of the supine position for the next 24 hours. Air pump-assisted surgery helps in maintaining intraoperative chamber pressure and aids in adhesion.[1]

Loss of Air Bubble

We expect 80% of the anterior chamber (AC) to be filled with air bubble on the immediate postoperative period. When the surgeon has put enough air at the

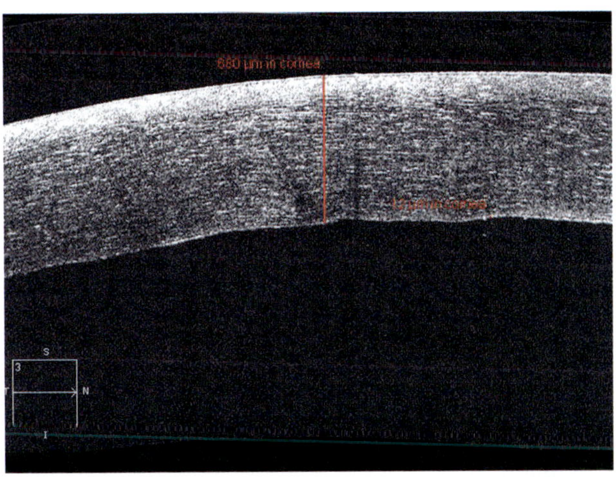

Fig. 17.2: Spectral domain OCT showing Descemet's fold after PDEK.
(OCT: Optical coherence tomography; PDEK: Pre-Descemet's endothelial keratoplasty).

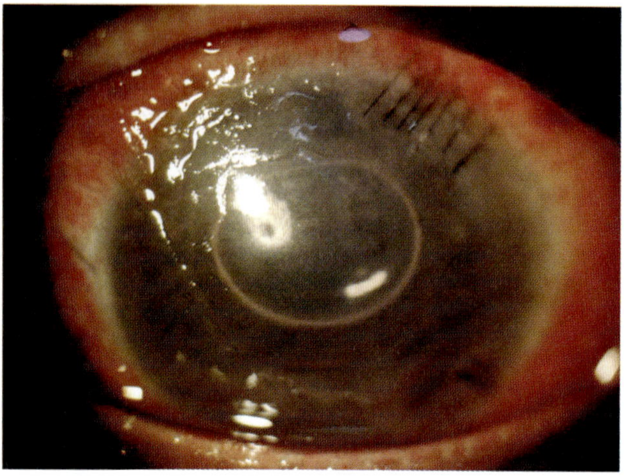

Fig. 17.3: Decreased air bubble size due to loss of air through wound and subsequent shallow anterior chamber after pre-Descemet's endothelial keratoplasty (PDEK).

end of the procedure and noticed less air on day 1, there could be two reasons why it has occured. The air has the tendency to move or shift depending on the pressure gradient (either the ocular or the atmosphere). In ocular causes, large pupil, posterior capsular rupture, scleral fixated intraocular lens (IOL), or previous iridectomy; the air enters the posterior chamber (PC) or the vitreous. In leaky wound or loose sutures, the air escapes into the atmosphere (Fig. 17.3). In both the cases, there is less air in the AC to aid graft adherence. This can lead to spontaneous graft detachment and hence it is recommended to reinject air in cases when there is no air on the immediate postoperative day 1 and there is associated detachment.

Folded Graft

Improper intraoperative sweeping of the graft can present as postoperative graft fold. Clinically it is seen as marks or striated endothelial lines and on OCT it can be clearly delineated as folded layers (Fig. 17.4). If it is in periphery and there is air filling 80% of the chamber, there is no intervention required. Only supine position maintenance and withholding any hypotensive medications can help. When the folded region is more and there is minimal air fill, it is recommended to reposition it surgically.

Inverted Graft

Immediate postoperative period, one can notice persistent edema with partial graft detachment. There can be an entity called "inverted flap", where the endothelial side is towards the stroma in reverse fashion. We have noticed

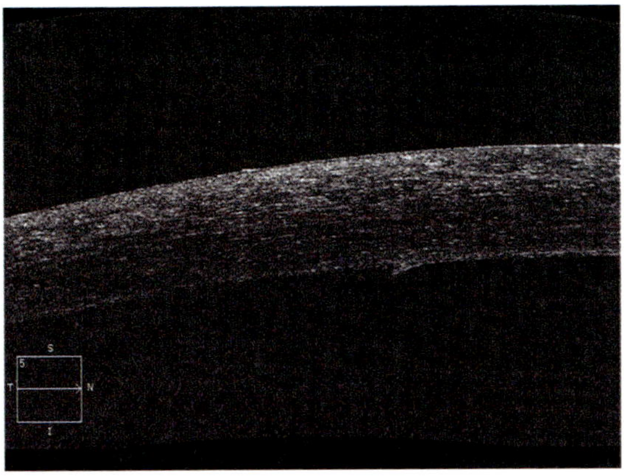

Fig. 17.4: Graft fold seen in the immediate postoperative period after pre-Descemet's endothelial keratoplasty (PDEK).

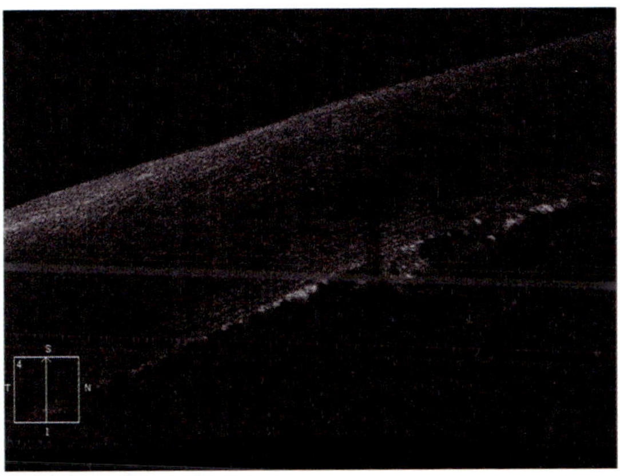

Fig. 17.5: An inverted PDEK graft in OCT. *Note*: The graft curling away from the host cornea in computer mouse fashion.
(OCT: Optical coherence tomography; PDEK: Pre-Descemet's endothelial keratoplasty).

"computer mouse sign" in eyes with inverted graft seen as convex graft configuration on OCT (Fig. 17.5). Such inverted flaps need to be replaced.[2]

Graft Detachment

Due to improper air injection or leaking wound, the pressure inside the chamber may not be sufficient for graft adhesion. Prolonged graft hydration which induces change in intracorneal pressure, is known to affect the immediate graft attachment. The initial 30 minutes after air injection is crucial in maintaining the graft attached. In a short series of pre-Descemet's endothelial keratoplasty (PDEK) (n = 12), we noted graft detachment in four eyes.[3]

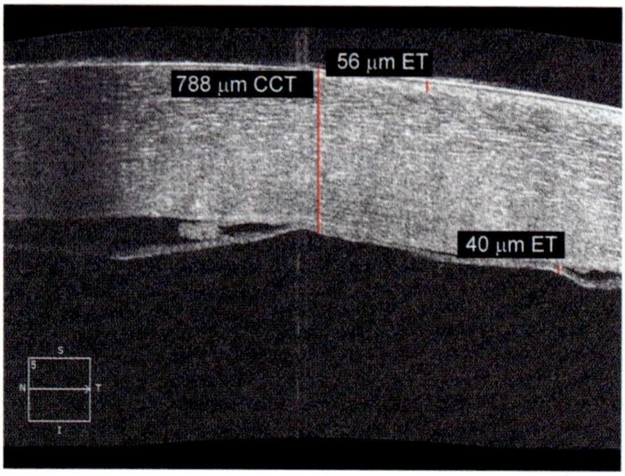

Fig. 17.6: Grade III graft detachment after pre-Descemet's endothelial keratoplasty as seen in optical coherence tomography (OCT). (CCT: Central corneal thickness; ET: Epithelial thickness; GT: Graft thickness).

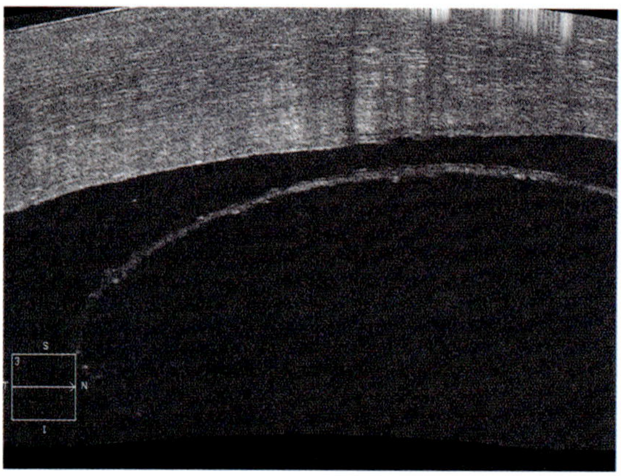

Fig. 17.7: Total detachment of PDEK graft in the early postoperative period as seen in spectral domain OCT. (OCT: Optical coherence tomography; PDEK: Pre-Descemet's endothelial keratoplasty)

Graft detachment was classified similar to Descemet's membrane endothelial keratoplasty (DMEK) grafts[4] as: grade I—when there was a minimal peripheral edge detachment with the remainder of the graft being well attached; grade II—graft detachments less than one-thirds of the graft surface area, not affecting the visual axis; grade III—graft detachment affecting more than one-thirds of the graft surface area (Fig. 17.6); and grade IV—completely detached grafts (Fig. 17.7). Out of four eyes with graft detachment, there were group I (n = 2), group II (n = 1), and group III (n = 1). In group I detached grafts, shallow peripheral detachment inferiorly (n = 1) and nasally (n = 1) was observed. Both the group I and II detachments did not require any further intervention. One eye with group III detachment underwent air injection on day 1 postoperative period. Graft was noted to be apposed after air injection in that one eye with group III detachment. However, there was redetachment on day 12 in the same eye and rebubbling was done subsequently with success on day 12.

Lenticule Drop

When there is hindrance for graft attachment or when the chamber pressure is not sufficient to maintain graft apposed, lenticule drop can happen. Especially in eyes with complicated surgery, which had posterior capsular rupture or deficient capsule, there is always difficulty in maintaining the air in the AC. In such eyes, one can implant a transscleral fixated IOL and do a pupilloplasty if the pupil was large. Giving strict supine position and following the earlier surgical steps can prevent lenticule drop. By combining glued IOL procedure with PDEK in eyes with deficient capsules, the PCIOL aids in maintaining the air in place as compared to an aphakic eye.

Ocular Hypertension

Raised intraocular pressure (IOP) recorded for the first time after PDEK on day 1 postoperative period in an eye without any clinical signs of glaucoma is termed as ocular hypertension due to surgery. The common cause is the high bubble pressure due to 100% air bubble filling the AC. In that case, anti-osmotic medications (both topical and systemic) should be given. If the IOP is not controlled by that, the AC can be decompressed surgically by reducing the air bubble size.

Hyphema

Postoperative hyphema is seen in eyes with intraoperative iris tissue manipulation and combined surgeries. Usually it is mild and resolves spontaneously. Very rarely, it can affect graft attachment.

Sterile Hypopyon or Fibrin

This is seen in eyes with prolonged surgeries especially, in eyes with combined procedures like pupilloplasty or in eyes with predisposition to uveitis. It is always sterile and resolves with intense topical steroids and rarely oral steroids. Nonresolving fibrin in the AC can induce traction and can affect graft adherence. Hence, it is very essential to treat these eyes in priority. Subconjunctival steroids along with hyalase can help in some cases; topical cycloplegic is required in all the eyes (Figs. 17.8A and B).

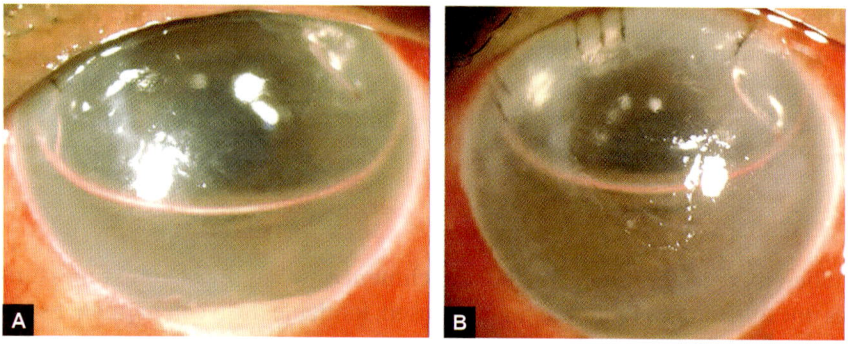

Figs. 17.8A and B: (A) Immediate postoperative inflammatory reaction; and (B) Subsequent resolution after medical management.

LATE POSTOPERATIVE COMPLICATIONS

Graft Rejection

Graft rejection is identified by the formation of acute onset endothelial keratic precipitates "Khodadoust line" and sudden AC reaction with corneal edema. The incidence of rejection in PDEK is expected to be similar to DMEK as there is no stroma seen in both the grafts.[5] However, this needs to be compared by further study in the future. When the endothelial rejection is diagnosed, immediate intense topical (1% prednisolone acetate hourly) and systemic steroids (oral prednisolone 1 mg/kg for 1st week and followed by tapering dose) are recommended. Regular follow-up with good compliance of medication is required to prevent rejection in some cases. Early cessation of steroids can be a risk factor in few cases to trigger graft rejection.

Graft Failure

This is a rare complication after endothelial keratoplasty and seen in eyes in which donor endothelium was less than 2,500 cells/sq. mm^2 or elderly more than 60 years. Since PDEK is done in both young and adult donor corneas, the risk of primary graft failure due to donor age will be less. Nonresolving corneal edema after endothelial keratoplasty with recurrence of bullous keratopathy is a sign of graft failure (Fig. 17.9). Profound deep and superficial vascularization in an opacified graft also indicates graft failure. Incidence of graft failure and the factors determining it will be similar to other endothelial keratoplasty. If there are failure and recurrent corneal decompensation noted, repeat PDEK (Figs. 17.10A and B) or penetrating keratoplasty can be planned accordingly. Our early results of repeat PDEK on failed endothelial keratoplasty has been satisfactory.

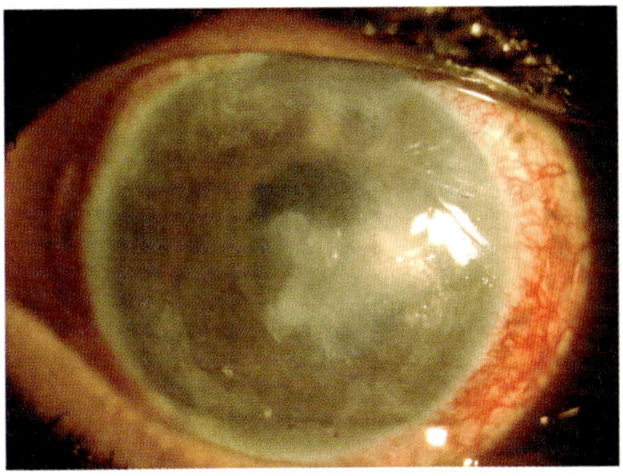

Fig. 17.9: Persistent corneal edema in an eye after pre-Descemet's endothelial keratoplasty (PDEK) indicating graft failure.

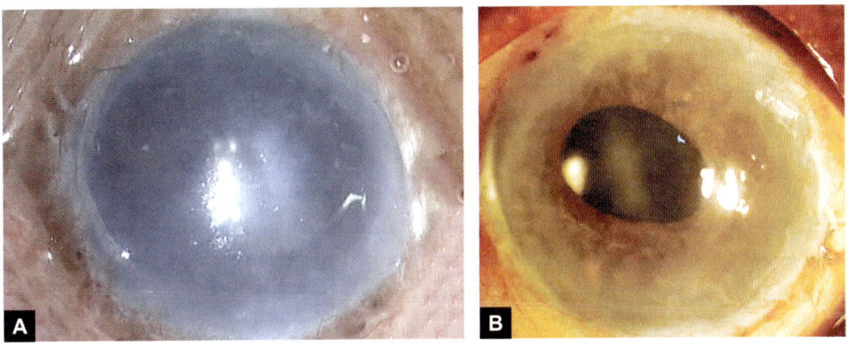

Figs. 17.10A and B: Preoperative previous failed pre-Descemet's endothelial keratoplasty (PDEK) graft which has undergone repeat PDEK.

Graft Host Interface

Graft host interface is examined for the presence of haze or opacification. It can be seen clinically in slit lamp as thin haze in between the host stroma and the donor Descemet's membrane (DM)-endothelium complex and confirmed by anterior segment OCT. 11 out of 12 eyes had smooth graft host interface in our series.[3] One eye had minimal interface haze by postoperative 1 month. After a course of intense steroid treatment, the graft host interface haze decreased in the final follow-up.

Epithelial Change

Central corneal epithelial defect on postoperative day 1 is often seen due to the intraoperative removal of epithelium. Epithelial healing completes in all eyes by 48 hours. In our short series, the mean epithelial thickness of 44.4 ± 9.8 μ on day 7, reduced to 37.5 ± 6.2 μ by day 90. There was no significant

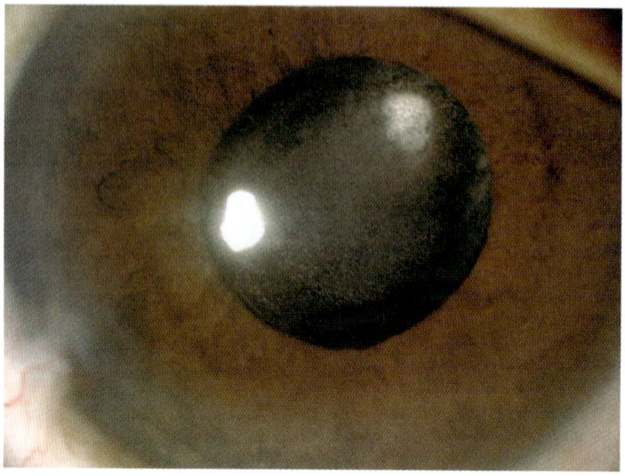

Fig. 17.11: Intraocular lens opacification after pre-Descemet's endothelial keratoplasty (PDEK) procedure.

change in the thickness ($p = 0.060$) over the time period.[6] There was no difference in the central and peripheral epithelium. Chronic epithelial haze can happen in eyes with too many topical medications with preservatives. In such situation reduce the frequency of medications or change to alternative medication without preservative. Copious ocular lubricants in the form of drops and gel are recommended for further prevention of symptoms. In some cases autologous serum may be required for a short period.

Intraocular Lens Opacification

Intraocular lens opacification after endothelial keratoplasty has been reported.[7] It usually occurs after 4–24 months after the initial surgery. Intracameral iso-expansible gases like C_3F_8 or SF_6 have been noted to be the etiology in some cases.[8] Though this is a very rare complication, it can happen even after PDEK in those eyes which required repeat gas injection. Repeated surgeries and chronic inflammation can be another risk factor in initiating opacification. Significant loss of visual acuity due to IOL opacification (Fig. 17.11) will require IOL explantation and reimplantation. Care should be taken in such cases, as many times such IOL explantation will land in explantation of the whole capsular bag. Then in that case, one has to do glued transscleral fixation of IOL. Hence, it is preferred to use, hydrophobic acrylic IOLs in such eyes to prevent recurrence of opacification to certain extent. It is better to avoid AC IOLs or iris claw lenses in eyes with PDEK surgery as there can be further damage induced by these type of IOLs. The reason being that the AC depth is reduced and there can be pseudophakodonesis in the eyes with AC or iris claw IOL, which in turn can cause endothelial injury.[9]

Infection

Infections are very rare after endothelial keratoplasty as there are no sutures or open sky manipulation as in conventional keratoplasty. However, these patients are on prolonged steroids therapy and the risk of keratitis cannot be excluded. Steroid topical drops are required in PDEK patients for minimum of 6 months and tapered subsequently. While the patients on topical steroids, it is advised to have one antibiotic cover in single dose frequency along with lubrications. Hence, regular follow-up and monitoring of symptoms in patients on steroids with or without antibiotics are necessary. Patients should be educated to report to the surgeon, if any of the symptoms like acute pain, redness, or photophobia is noted.

Postoperative Glaucoma

Persistent raised IOP and subsequent optic nerve head cupping can occur due to steroid response or in eyes with coexisting risk for glaucoma. Hence, the regular IOP screening by the noncontact method can be done in the early postoperative period. Late postoperative patients can undergo a standard applanation tonometry and optic disc examination in their follow-ups. Steroid responders should undergo cessation of steroids as soon as it is diagnosed and they have to be shifted to a nonsteroidal anti-inflammatory topical medication toreduce inflammation instead of high potent topical steroids. The initial treatment of glaucoma includes the topical antiglaucoma medications; however when the IOP is uncontrolled with maximum medications trabeculectomy or valve procedure is preferred. Secondary inflammation in eyes with multiple surgeries or pre-existing uveitis can induce secondary angle closure, and such cases will require pupilloplasty to mechanically pull the iris away from the angles can help.

SUMMARY

Detachment of grafts in the postoperative period is a known complication after endothelial keratoplasty. Though thinner grafts are more susceptible to incomplete graft adhesion after primary positioning, early and possibly better visual recovery may be possible only with thin graft. Timely identification of complications and in-depth knowledge of the cause can help in management of such complications in the postoperative period.

REFERENCES

1. Jacob S, Narasimhan S, Agarwal A, et al. Air pump-assisted graft centration, graft edge unfolding, and graft uncreasing in young donor graft pre-Descemet endothelial keratoplasty. Cornea. 2017;36(8):1009-13.
2. Kumar DA, Sood SS, Agarwal A. 'Mouse sign' in optical coherence tomography of detached endothelial graft indicate graft inversion. J Ophthalmic Vis Res. 2017. [Epub ahead of print]

3. Kumar DA, Dua HS, Agarwal A, et al. Postoperative spectral-domain optical coherence tomography evaluation of pre-Descemet endothelial keratoplasty grafts. J Cataract Refract Surg. 2015;41(7):1535-6.
4. Yeh RY, Quilendrino R, Musa FU, et al. Predictive value of optical coherence tomography in graft attachment after Descemet's membrane endothelial keratoplasty. Ophthalmology. 2013;120(2):240-5.
5. Anshu A, Price MO, Price FW. Risk of corneal transplant rejection significantly reduced with Descemet's membrane endothelial keratoplasty. Ophthalmology. 2012;119(3):536-40.
6. Jacob S, Agarwal A, Kumar DA. Endoilluminator-assisted Descemet membrane endothelial keratoplasty and endoilluminator-assisted pre-Descemet endothelial keratoplasty. Clin Ophthalmol. 2015;9:2123-5.
7. Nieuwendaal CP, van der Meulen IJ, Patryn EK, et al. Opacification of the intraocular lens after descemet stripping endothelial keratoplasty. Cornea. 2015;34(11):1375-7.
8. Werner L, Wilbanks G, Nieuwendaal CP, et al. Localized opacification of hydrophilic acrylic intraocular lenses after procedures using intracameral injection of air or gas. J Cataract Refract Surg. 2015;41(1):199-207.
9. Kumar DA, Agarwal A, Jacob S, et al. Glued trans-scleral intraocular lens exchange for anterior chamber lenses in complicated eyes: analysis of indications and results. Am J Ophthalmol. 2013;156(6):1125-33.e2.

CHAPTER 18

Mouse Sign for Inverted Pre-Descemet's Endothelial Keratoplasty Grafts

Dhivya Ashok Kumar, Amar Agarwal

BACKGROUND

Corneal endothelial decompensation has been recently treated successfully by endothelial keratoplasty techniques.[1-4] Endothelial migration and cell signaling are required for re-endothelization to draw donor endothelial cells toward the recipient posterior stroma. Intrinsic properties of the host and multiple factors in the graft play role in graft adherence.[4-7] Graft detachments and positional problems are often detected clinically or by anterior segment optical coherence tomography (OCT). Though OCT has been used for analysis of graft, there have been no clear patterns described for detachments or inverted graft. In this chapter, we have described a unique configuration in the form of a computer mouse which is seen in patients with tight scroll which often is difficult to unroll and require graft removal.

MOUSE SIGN IN OPTICAL COHERENCE TOMOGRAPHY

Mouse sign is described in relation to the configuration of a computer mouse. This sign is seen only by OCT, preferably by spectral or Fourier domain OCT. The spectral domain OCT has resolution of 5 μm and shows clear pattern with endothelial graft. We used cirrus 5000, Carl Zeiss spectral domain OCT for examining the postoperative patients after pre-Descemet's endothelial keratoplasty (PDEK). Fourier domain OCT showed detached graft involving the partial central and inferior cornea with the convex configuration (Figs. 18.1A and B) and one end attached still to cornea like a "computer mouse". The partial attachment of the graft and the end scroll together gives the mouse configuration. We noticed such pattern in 5 eyes of patients who underwent PDEK and seemed to have inverted graft. All the five patients had unsuccessful rebubbling and they all ended in graft exchange.

CASE SCENARIOS

A 60-year-old female underwent PDEK and the immediate postoperative graft period showed good graft adherence. Slit lamp examination on 10th POD revealed diffuse stromal edema, Descemet's folds and rolled graft

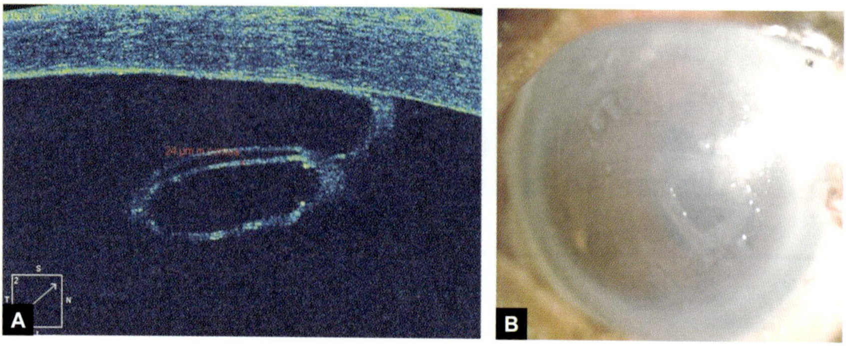

Figs. 18.1A and B: (A) Fourier domain optical coherence tomography (FDOCT) showing convex graft rolled in one end and inverted and one end attached to cornea showing the "mouse configuration"; (B) Postoperative clinical photograph after initial pre-Descemet's endothelial keratoplasty (PDEK) showing detached graft in case 1.

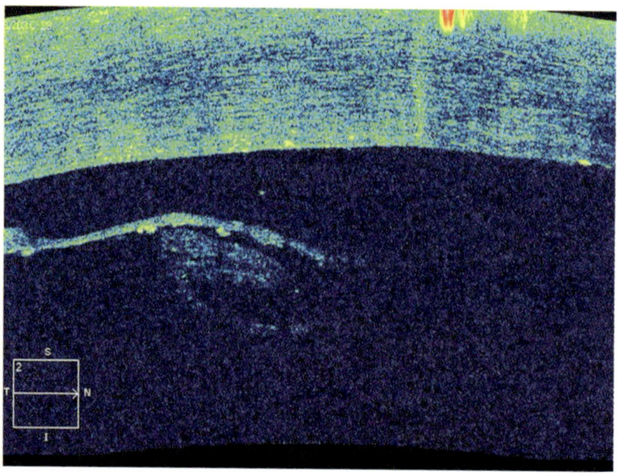

Fig. 18.2: Fourier domain optical coherence tomography (FDOCT) showing convex graft rolled in one end in "mouse configuration" in case 2.

detachment centrally. Fourier domain OCT showed detached graft involving the partial central and inferior cornea with the convex configuration (Figs. 18.1A and B) and one end attached still to cornea like a "computer mouse". Patient underwent rebubbling; however redetachment occurred which finally required graft exchange.

A 59-year-old male who underwent PDEK surgery for pseudophakic bullous keratopathy attended our outpatient follow-up. Slit lamp examination revealed diffuse stromal edema and graft detachment central and inferiorly on day 2 postoperative period. Fourier domain optical coherence tomography (FDOCT) showed detached, inverted, convex graft in the anterior chamber (mouse sign) (Fig. 18. 2). The patient underwent rebubbling with air as

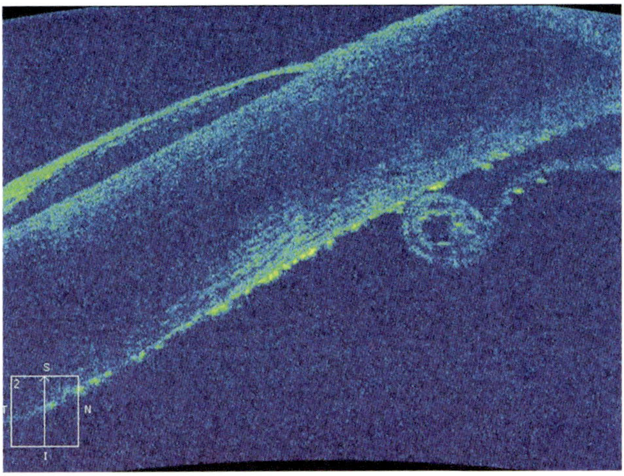

Fig. 18.3: Fourier domain optical coherence tomography (FDOCT) showing convex graft rolled central and inferior and inverted in "mouse configuration" in case 3.

an attempt to reattach the graft. Follow-up on day 8 showed epithelial defect, diffuse corneal edema, and detached graft. Patient underwent graft exchange in the same eye on follow-up.

A 67-year-old female who underwent PDEK for pseudophakic bullous keratopathy showed non-improvement of visual acuity for 1 week postoperatively. Clinical examination showed dense corneal edema and further anterior chamber details were not visible. Her OCT evaluation of the operated eye showed, detached graft with mouse sign (Fig. 18.3). The patient underwent graft exchange.

ETIOLOGY FOR MOUSE CONFIGURATION

The configuration of "mouse" was seen in all the patients with thick scroll that showed difficulty in unrolling and recurrent detachment in the same configuration after repeat air injection. The probable reasons for rolling of the grafts reported are: (1) the uncorrected rolled or curled edges in the end of surgery, (2) insufficient air support inside the chamber, (3) inverse graft positioning, and (4) stromal irregularities or incomplete recipient DM removal. Graft edema, tight scroll, and premature loss of air support may also be the probable reasons for this configuration. Early stage of mouse sign will show the convex configuration (Figs. 18.4A and B) which subsequently detaches and forms the full-fledged mouse sign. Though the influence of donor age on the graft configuration cannot be ruled out, the age in the PDEK group varied from young to adult donors. The attempts for rebubbling failed in all the cases and the graft regained the same configuration each time after manipulation.

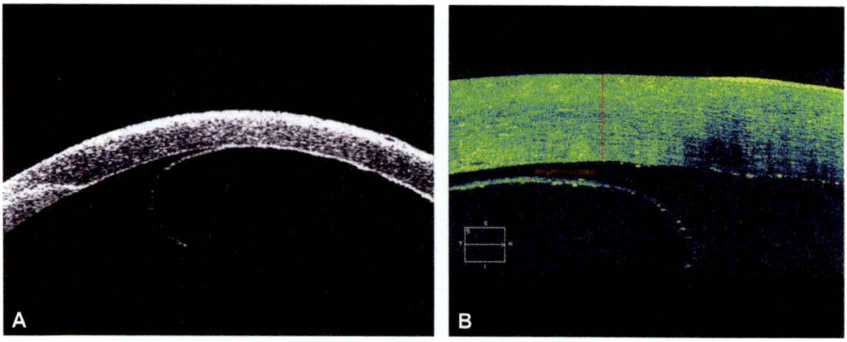

Figs. 18.4A and B: (A) Early stage of mouse sign in time domain; and (B) Spectral domain anterior segment optical coherence tomography (OCT).

GRAFT ADHESION

There are various factors which can influence graft adhesion; that can be both intraoperative and postoperative factors. Similarly, both the donor and the host conditions also contribute equally in stability of the graft. A stable well-formed anterior chamber morphology and adequate pressure in the chamber is achieved by 80% air fill. Higher donor age due to easy unrolling of graft and postoperative supine position has also been known as a factor for adherence.[6,7] Factors favoring graft displacement are incomplete host epithelial Descemet's membrane removal and residual anterior band layer fragments.[7] In situ glaucoma drainage devices, post-trabeculectomy blebs and post-vitrectomy are the additional causes for graft detachments.[8,9] Graft reversal is labeled when the endothelium side of the donor graft faces the host cornea while the Descemet's membrane faces the iris lens diaphragm. There are many techniques suggested to identify and avoid graft reversal intraoperatively. Bimanual infusion technique, endoilluminator-assisted endothelial keratoplasty, F mark, intraoperative OCT, S mark, triangular mark, taco configuration, Venn diagram, and Mourtiser's sign are the clinical methods followed.[10-16] Dirisamer et al. studied a series of graft displacements and grouped them in the following categories.[17] Even though that elderly donor had shown easy intraoperative unrolling in Descemet's membrane endothelial keratoplasty (DMEK), young age group has also favored well in graft adherence after PDEK.[3,18]

CONCLUSION

Graft detachment in the early postoperative period can happen after endothelial keratoplasty. Routine anterior segment Fourier domain OCT can be used for evaluation of these patients. "Mouse sign" can be a predictor of inverted graft and indicate that rebubbling may not be successful in such eyes. Graft exchange will be required subsequently for rapid visual rehabilitation.

REFERENCES

1. Price MO, Price FW. Descemet's stripping endothelial keratoplasty. Curr Opin Ophthalmol. 2007;18(4):290-4.
2. Busin M, Madi S, Santorum P, et al. Ultrathin descemet's stripping automated endothelial keratoplasty with the microkeratome double-pass technique: two-year outcomes. Ophthalmology. 2013;120(6):1186-94.
3. Agarwal A, Dua HS, Narang P, et al. Pre-Descemet's endothelial keratoplasty (PDEK). Br J Ophthalmol. 2014;98(9):1181-5.
4. Brockmann T, Brockmann C, Maier AK, et al. Clinicopathology of graft detachment after Descemet's membrane endothelial keratoplasty. Acta Ophthalmol. 2014;92(7):e556-61.
5. Dapena I, Moutsouris K, Ham L, et al. Graft detachment rate. Ophthalmology. 2010;117:847-847e1.
6. Brockmann T, Brockmann C, Maier AK, et al. Clinicopathology of graft detachment after descemet membrane endothelial keratoplasty. Acta Ophthalmol. 2014;92(7):e556-61.
7. Nahum Y, Mimouni M, Busin M. Risk factors predicting the need for graft exchange after descemet stripping automated endothelial keratoplasty. Cornea. 2015;34(8):876-9.
8. Ni N, Sperling BJ, Dai Y, et al. Outcomes after descemet stripping automated endothelial keratoplasty in patients with glaucoma drainage devices. Cornea. 2015;34(8):870-5.
9. Yoeruek E, Rubino G, Bayyoud T, et al. Descemet membrane endothelial keratoplasty in vitrectomized eyes:clinical results. Cornea. 2015;34(1):1-5.
10. Titiyal JS, Kaur M, Falera R, et al. Evaluation of time to donor lenticule apposition using intraoperative optical coherence tomography in descemet stripping automated endothelial keratoplasty. Cornea. 2016;35(4):477-81.
11. Güell JL, Morral M, Gris O, et al. Bimanual technique for insertion and positioning of endothelium-Descemet membrane graft in Descemet membrane endothelium keratoplasty. Cornea. 2013;32(12):1521-6.
12. Jacob S, Agarwal A, Kumar DA. Endoilluminator-assisted Descemet membrane endothelial keratoplasty and endoilluminator-assisted pre Descemet membrane endothelial keratoplasty. Clin Ophthalmol. 2015;9:2123-5.
13. Veldman PB, Dye PK, Holiman JD, et al. The S-stamp in Descemet membrane endothelial keratoplasty safely eliminates upside-down graft implantation. Ophthalmology. 2016;123(1):161-4.
14. Bhogal M, Maurino V, Allan BD. Use of a single peripheral triangular mark to ensure correct graft orientation in Descemet membrane endothelial keratoplasty. J Cataract Refract Surg. 2015;41(9):2022-4.
15. Droutsas K, Bertelmann T, Schroeder FM, et al. A simple rescue maneuver for unfolding and centering a tightly rolled graft in descemet membrane endothelial keratoplasty. Clin Ophthalmol. 2014;8:2161-3.
16. Liarakos VS, Dapena I, Ham L, et al. Intraocular graft unfolding techniques in descemet membrane endothelial keratoplasty. JAMA Ophthalmol. 2013;131(1):29-35.
17. Dirisamer M, van Dijk K, Dapena I, et al. Prevention and management of graft detachment in descemet membrane endothelial keratoplasty. Arch Ophthalmol. 2012;130(3):280-91.
18. Maier AK, Gundlach E, Pilger D, et al. Rate and localization of graft detachment in descemet membrane endothelial keratoplasty. Cornea. 2016;35(3):308-12.

CHAPTER 19

Optical Coherence Tomography Analysis and Results in Pre-Descemet's Endothelial Keratoplasty

Dhivya Ashok Kumar, Amar Agarwal

INTRODUCTION

Pre-Descemet's endothelial keratoplasty (PDEK) is a selective transplantation of the pre-Descemet's layer (PDL) along with the Descemet's membrane (DM) with endothelium. Here, the PDL provides additional thickness and support to the thin DM.[1-3] The initial results, highlighting the technique, showed good postoperative outcomes and less surgical complications.[3] The technique encompasses the basic advantages of early visual rehabilitation and lowered graft failure similar to Descemet's membrane endothelial keratoplasty (DMEK)[4,5] with the added advantage of the ability to use donor of any age and potential of less damage to endothelial cells.[3] Postoperative slit lamp examination allows a reasonable examination of the graft position but high-resolution spectral domain optical coherence tomography (SD-OCT) provides additional information on the configuration, apposition, and thickness of the graft. Anterior segment OCT has been used in DMEK for predicting postoperative graft adherence.[6,7] In this chapter, we will be discussing the SD-OCT evaluation of PDEK and results of the studies on PDEK.

ANTERIOR SEGMENT SPECTRAL DOMAIN OCT EVALUATION

Spectral domain optical coherence tomography (SD-OCT)[8] (Cirrus HD OCT, model 5000, Carl Zeiss Meditec Inc., Dublin, CA, USA) was performed on day 1, day 7, day 30, and day 90. Graft thickness (GT), graft adherence, and epithelial thickness was measured on follow-up visits. Graft host apposition, graft-host interface changes, presence or absence of graft split, and nature of detachment were assessed.

Anterior segment five line raster pattern in axis of 0–180° and 90–270° was used. The raster scan had five lines (length 3 mm) and 250 μm distance in between the lines (Fig. 19.1). The scan was centered at the corneal vertex for central 3 mm scan. Additional inferior, temporal, nasal, and superior positional scans were also taken. GT was measured in microns with the tool caliper provided with the SD-OCT software. Graft detachment was classified[6] as

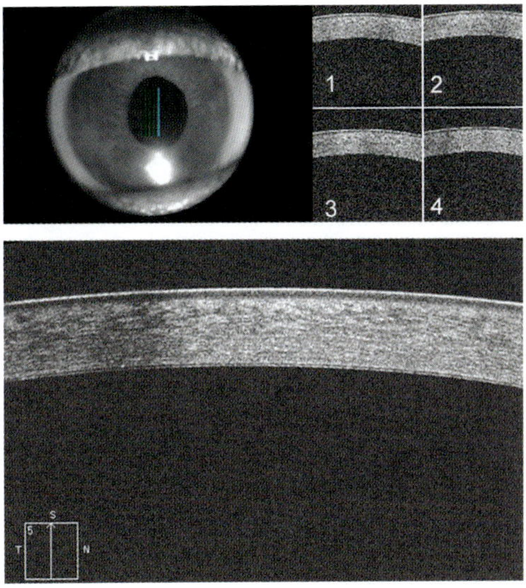

Fig. 19.1: Spectral domain OCT five line raster scan mode taken on operated PDEK patient.
(OCT: Optical coherence tomography; PDEK: Pre-Descemet's endothelial keratoplasty)

grade I when there was a minimal edge detachment with the remainder of the graft being well attached; grade II: graft detachments less than one-third of the graft surface area, not affecting the visual axis; grade III: graft detachment affecting more than one-third of the graft surface area, and grade IV: completely detached grafts. Epithelial thickness and recurrence of bulla were noted. Graft host interface was examined for presence of haze or opacification. Postoperative central corneal thickness (CCT) was also measured at all follow-up time points.

Graft Thickness

Twelve eyes of 12 patients were evaluated in the study. The mean GT of PDEK tissue on day 1 was 37.3 ± 3.5 μ (range 32–44 μ) (Fig. 19.2). The mean GT on day 7, day 30, and day 90 was 35.5 ± 3.4 μ (32–40 μ), 33 ± 1.8 μ (32–36 μ), and 30.3 ± 2.6 μ (28–36 μ), respectively. There was significant difference in the GT over the time period (Friedman test, p = 0.000). There was no significant difference (p = 1.000) between the central (3 mm) and peripheral (4–6 mm) GT.

Graft Attachment

The graft was well attached (Fig. 19.3) in 8 out of 12 eyes on day 1. Out of four eyes with graft detachment, there were grade 1 (n = 2), grade II (n = 1), and grade III (n = 1). In grade I detached grafts, shallow peripheral detachment inferiorly (n = 1) and nasally (n = 1) was observed. Both the grade I and II

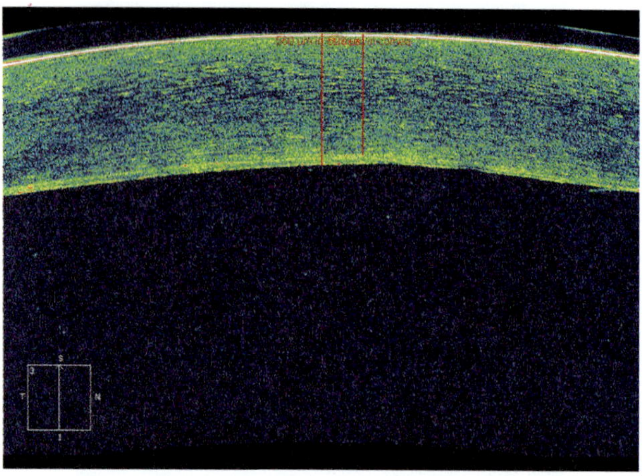

Fig. 19.2: Day 1 postoperative image showing cornea with well-attached PDEK graft in spectral domain optical coherence tomography.
(PDEK: Pre-Descemet's endothelial keratoplasty)

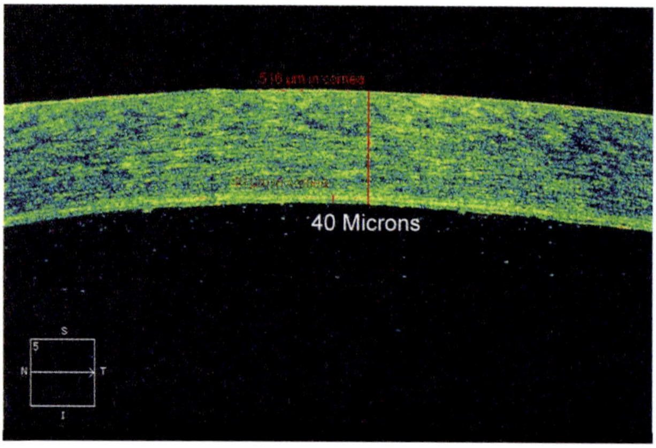

Fig. 19.3: Day one postoperative image showing 40 microns graft thickness in a patient with PDEK.
(PDEK: Pre-Descemet's endothelial keratoplasty).

detachments (Fig. 19.4) did not require any further intervention. One eye with grade III detachment underwent air injection. Graft was well apposed on the post air injection day 1; however, there was redetachment on day 12 (Figs. 19.5A and B) and re-bubbling was done subsequently with success. The mean detachment depth was 26 ± 10.3 μ. Descemet's folds were noted in two eyes on day 1 (Fig. 19.6) which resolved on day 7. Smooth concave configuration of posterior cornea was obtained in all the eyes by 1 month. Graft folds were noted in two eyes in the mid-periphery with good adherence. None of the eyes had complete graft detachment or lenticule drop.

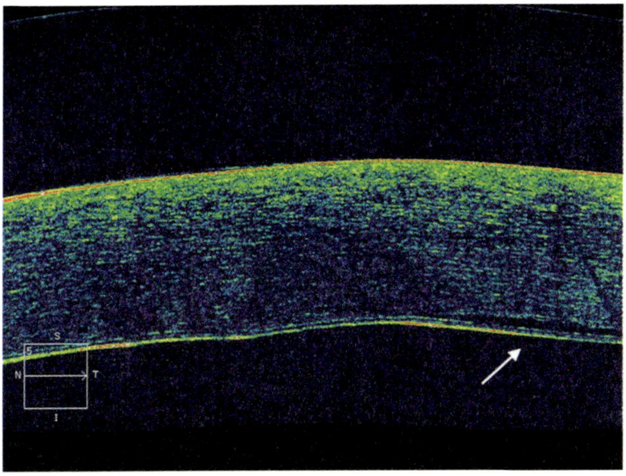

Fig. 19.4: Day 1 postoperative image showing some corneal edema shallow graft detachment (arrow) in spectral domain optical coherence tomography.

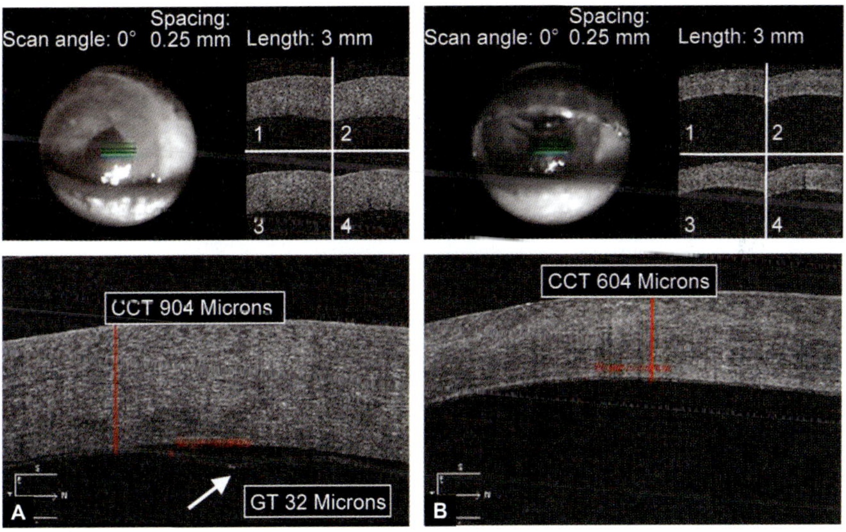

Figs. 19.5A and B: Grade III graft detachment after pre-Descemet's endothelial keratoplasty. Before (A) and after (B) air injection.

Graft Host Interface

Eleven out of 12 eyes had smooth graft host interface. One eye had minimal interface haze by postoperative 1 month. After a course of intense steroid treatment, the graft host interface haze decreased in the follow-up period.

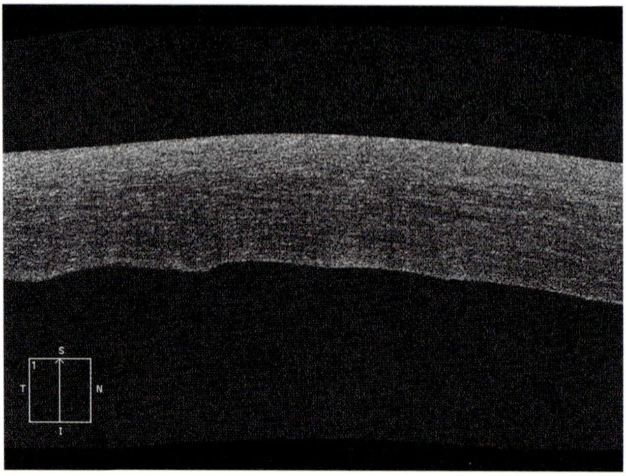

Fig. 19.6: Day 1 postoperative image as seen in spectral domain optical coherence tomography showing Descemet's membrane folds.

Graft Split

Separation of graft into two linear hyperreflective lines was seen in OCT in two eyes. The posterior layer was 16 μ and the anterior one was 12 μ. Both the eyes had mild corneal edema on day 1, which resolved with strict supine position allowing residual air in the anterior chamber to tamponade the graft against the recipient bed.

Epithelial Change

All eyes had central epithelial defect on postoperative day 1. Epithelial healing was complete in all eyes by 48 hours. The mean epithelial thickness was 44.4 ± 9.8 μ on day 7 and reduced to 37.5 ± 6.2 μ by day 90. There was no significant change in the thickness ($p = 0.060$) over the time period. There was no difference in the central and peripheral epithelium in 11 eyes. One eye had persistent peripheral epithelial edema.

Central Corneal Thickness

The mean day 1 postoperative CCT was 621 ± 46.4 μ. There was significant resolution of corneal edema by day 7 ($p = 0.000$) (Figs. 19.7A and B).

Anterior Chamber

A deep anterior chamber was noted in all the eyes. Grade 3 cellular reaction was seen in one eye and one eye had grade 4 fibrinous reaction. Shallow detachment was seen in the eye with fibrin. Intense steroid treatment (hourly

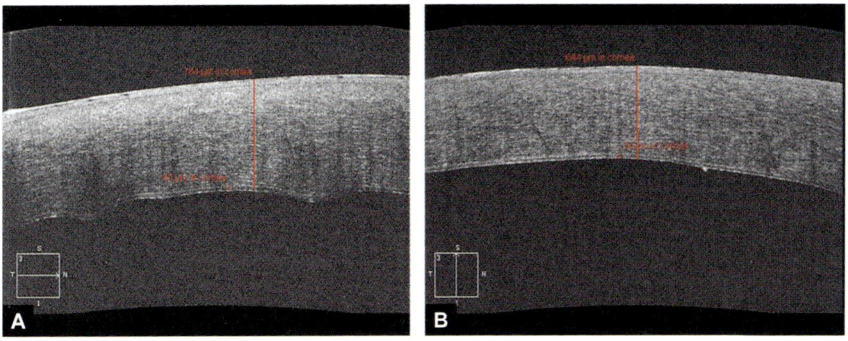

Figs. 19.7A and B: Spectral domain optical coherence tomography showing reduction in corneal edema as seen in decrease in central corneal thickness (CCT) from day 1 (A) to day 7 (B).

topical steroid and oral prednisolone in tapering doses for 1 week) with air injection attained good graft adherence by 2 weeks.

Graft Thickness and Visual Acuity

There was no significant correlation between the GT at day 1 ($p = 0.402$) and day 90 ($p = 0.649$) with the best corrected vision at the final follow-up.

Graft Thickness and Corneal Thickness

There was no correlation between the mean CCT reduction and the GT reduction from day 1 to day 90 ($p = 0.645$, $r = 0.149$). There was no correlation between the corneal edema and GT on day 1 ($p = 0.374$, $r = 0.282$).

Graft Detachment and Corneal Thickness

There was no association between the corneal thickness on day 1 and the graft detachment (Chi square test, $p = 0.285$).

Graft Thickness and Graft Detachment

There was no association between the GT on day 1 and the graft detachment (Chi square test, $p = 0.428$).

Visual Acuity and Graft Adherence

The mean best corrected visual acuity (BCVA) at the last follow-up was 0.61 ± 0.2. There was significant improvement in the visual acuity from preoperative to postoperative period ($p = 0.002$). There was association of early graft adherence (on day 1) and the BCVA (Chi square, $p = 0.017$) at the last follow-up. Sixty-six (66.6%) eyes obtained BCVA ≥ 20/20. Four eyes with detachment showed clinical improvement in vision after successful attachment. None of the eyes lost vision due to graft-related complication. The nonimprovement of BCVA to 20/20 was due to pre-existing age-related macular degeneration, epiretinal membrane, myopic degeneration, old healed macular edema, and retinal pigment epithelial changes. Visual acuity stabilization was seen by 3 months postoperatively. There was no loss of BCVA in any of the eyes.

COMPARISON OF PDEK WITH THE OTHER ENDOTHELIAL KERATOPLASTIES

The single important factor for better functional outcome after successful endothelial keratoplasty has been the graft stability and adherence.[9,10] Graft detachment has been described as a common complication after endothelial keratoplasty techniques like DMEK and DSAEK (Descemet's stripping automated endothelial keratoplasty).[9-12] Though thinner grafts are more susceptible to incomplete graft adhesion after primary positioning; early and possibly better visual recovery may be possible only with thin grafts.[13] PDEK has the advantage of thinner grafts similar to DMEK, which can aid in easy intraoperative manipulation and at the same time postoperative adherence. The mean central GT in ultrathin grafts described by Busin was 78.28 ± 28.89 μ at 3 months postoperative.[14] Shousha et al. reported the thickness of normal Descemet membrane in elderly to be about 16 ± 2 μ (range 13–20 μ) in ultrahigh-resolution OCT.[15] The mean GT in our study was 37.3 ± 3.5 μ and was stabilized by 3 months. From our study, we noticed that the PDEK grafts are thicker than DMEK grafts and thinner than ultrathin DSAEK grafts. The PDEK grafts were uniform with no difference in the thickness from center to periphery as seen in OCT.

The two main factors, which interfere with graft attachments, are the intracorneal pressure and the interposition[13] and these factors would apply to the PDEK grafts as well. Precut donor tissue over hydration, stromal edema (both donor and recipient), and irregular interface prevents graft adherence. Because of graft edema and stromal edema in the immediate postoperative period, it might be difficult to localize detachments clinically at the slit lamp. Therefore, anterior segment OCT has been utilized to better visualize endothelial grafts (DSAEK or DMEK) under such situations.[6,16,17] The absence of interface reaction is one major advantage in DMEK grafts as compared to DSAEK grafts. Similarly in our OCT analysis of PDEK grafts, there was minimal reversible or no interface opacification in the postoperative period (Figs. 19.8A and B).

RESULTS IN PDEK

In the initial reports on PDEK analysis, we reported in five eyes of five patients, with successful attachment of the graft and good postoperative visual

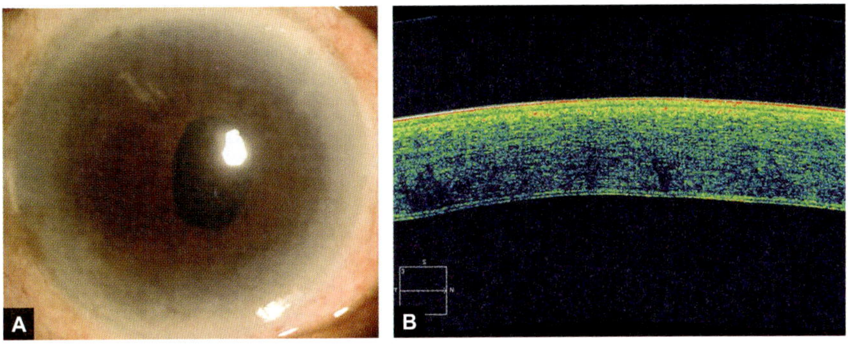

Figs. 19.8A and B: Clinical photograph (A) and spectral domain optical coherence tomography (B) 3 months postoperative eye after PDEK.
(PDEK: Pre-Descemet's endothelial keratoplasty)

recovery in all cases.[3] Postoperative optical coherence tomography showed good graft attachment without interface abnormalities and a mean GT was 28 ± 5.6 μm. There was a significant decrease in the CCT postoperatively (Friedman test, $p = 0.025$). The mean postoperative corrected distant visual acuity (CDVA) was 0.62 ± 0.07 in Snellen's decimal equivalent and there was a significant improvement in CDVA ($p = 0.025$). The mean graft size obtained was 7.6 ± 0.22 mm diameter. The mean postoperative intraocular pressure (IOP) was 12 ± 1.2 mm Hg and there was no significant change in the IOP ($p = 0.317$). The mean postoperative endothelial density was 1551.2 ± 65.2 cells/mm^2.

In a study of outcome of PDEK in infant donor, three eyes of three patients with pseudophakic bullous keratopathy who underwent the procedure were analyzed.[18] The donor age used was 12 months for case 1 and 2 whereas 9 months old for case 3. The mean BCVA preoperatively and postoperatively were 0.1 ± 0.1 and 0.5 ± 0.4 Snellen decimal equivalent, respectively. The spherical equivalent measured at the last follow-up was +0.5 D, +0.8 D, and +0.6 D for case 1, 2, and 3 respectively. The mean percentage loss of endothelial cell density (ECD) up to 6-month follow-up was 27 ± 2%. We noticed that the infant cornea can be a reliable source of donor tissue for the PDEK procedure, and no difficulties were noted in the donor lenticule preparation, insertion of the donor graft, or air bubble management.[18]

In a report ex vivo by Altaan et al., tissue for PDEK and DMEK were obtained from 10 eye bank sclerocorneal disks by trephination after air injection into corneal stroma and big bubble (BB) formation. PDEK tissue was prepared in five corneas after achieving a type-1 BB and DMEK after a type-2 BB in five corneas.[19] Five sclerocorneal disks for each group were used as controls. Endothelial cell counts were obtained from all samples before and after injection using phase-contrast microscopy with an eyepiece reticle. The average change of ECD before and after injection in the PDEK sample group was

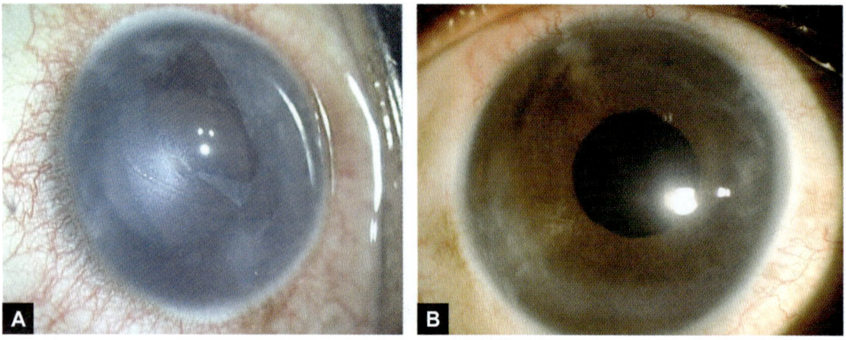

Figs. 19.9A and B: Clinical photograph showing the change in corneal clarity from preoperative (A) to the postoperative 6 months (B).

- 5.36% ± 3.8% as against −12.44% ± 8.11% of DMEK. The young donor used in PDEK has additional advantage good recovery of endothelium after surgical injury (Figs. 19.9A and B).

Pre-Descemet's endothelial keratoplasty has been combined with glued IOL implantation and pupilloplasty in eyes with defective lens capsule for IOL fixation.[20] The procedure was performed in five eyes of five patients, and the donor age ranged from 9 months to 65 years. There was a significant change in the uncorrected ($p = 0.034$) and corrected ($p = 0.043$) distance visual acuities in the postoperative period. The mean graft size was 7.6 ± 0.4 mm (range 7–8 mm). The mean preoperative and postoperative specular endothelial counts were 2,788 ± 204 cells/mm^2 and 1,898 ± 90 cells/mm^2, respectively.

SUMMARY

Our results and evaluations on PDEK demonstrate it as a viable alternative to DMEK especially as it appears to be technically less challenging. One major advantage is that it has demonstrated that tissue from donors as young as 1 year of age can be harvested successfully for PDEK, something that has not been done for DMEK. Traditionally it has been recommended that young eyes should be avoided for DMEK as risk of DM tear and loss is high, though this may be changing now with PDEK.

REFERENCES

1. Dua HS, Faraj LA, Said DG, et al. Human corneal anatomy redefined: a novel pre-Descemet's layer (Dua's layer). Ophthalmology. 2013;120(9):1778-85.
2. Dua HS, Faraj LA, Branch MJ, et al. The collagen matrix of the human trabecular meshwork is an extension of the novel pre-Descemet's layer (Dua's layer). Br J Ophthalmol. 2014;98(5):691-7.
3. Agarwal A, Dua HS, Narang P, et al. Pre-Descemet's endothelial keratoplasty (PDEK). Br J Ophthalmol. 2014;98(9):1181-5.

4. Melles GR, Ong TS, Ververs B, et al. Descemet membrane endothelial keratoplasty (DMEK). Cornea. 2006;25(8):987-90.
5. Tourtas T, Laaser K, Bachmann BO, et al. Descemet membrane endothelial keratoplasty versus Descemet stripping automated endothelial keratoplasty. Am J Ophthalmol. 2012;153(6):1082-90.
6. Yeh RY, Quilendrino R, Musa FU, et al. Predictive value of optical coherence tomography in graft attachment after Descemet's membrane endothelial keratoplasty. Ophthalmology. 2013;120(2):240-5.
7. Steven P, Le Blanc C, Velten K, et al. Optimizing Descemet membrane endothelial keratoplasty using intraoperative optical coherence tomography. JAMA Ophthalmol. 2013;131(9):1135-42.
8. Carl Zeiss Meditec. Cirrus TM HD-OCT. Details define your decisions. CIR. 1595 DS-Nr. 0-1487-872. Carl Zeiss Meditec, Dublin, CA, USA, 2012..
9. Dirisamer M, van Dijk K, Dapena I, et al. Prevention and management of graft detachment in Descemet membrane endothelial keratoplasty. Arch Ophthalmol. 2012;130(3):280-91.
10. Guerra FP, Anshu A, Price MO, et al. Descemet's membrane endothelial keratoplasty: prospective study of 1-year visual outcomes, graft survival, and endothelial cell loss. Ophthalmology. 2011;118(12):2368-73.
11. Shih CY, Ritterband DC, Rubino S, et al. Visually significant and nonsignificant complications arising from Descemet stripping automated endothelial keratoplasty. Am J Ophthalmol. 2009;148(6):837-43.
12. Suh LH, Yoo SH, Deobhakta A, et al. Complications of Descemet's stripping with automated endothelial keratoplasty: survey of 118 eyes at One Institute. Ophthalmology. 2008;115(9):1517-24.
13. Dapena I, Ham L, Melles GR. Endothelial keratoplasty: DSEK/DSAEK or DMEK--the thinner the better? Curr Opin Ophthalmol. 2009;20(4):299-307.
14. Busin M, Madi S, Santorum P, et al. Ultrathin Descemet's stripping automated endothelial keratoplasty with the microkeratome double-pass technique: two-year outcomes. Ophthalmology. 2013;120(6):1186-94.
15. Shousha MA, Perez VL, Wang J, et al. Use of ultra-high resolution optical coherence tomography to detect in vivo characteristics of Descemet's membrane in Fuchs' dystrophy. Ophthalmology. 2010;117(6):1220-7.
16. Tan GS, He M, Tan DT, et al. Correlation of anterior segment optical coherence tomography measurements with graft trephine diameterfollowing descemet stripping automated endothelial keratoplasty. BMC Med Imaging. 2012;12:19.
17. Moutsouris K, Dapena I, Ham L, et al. Optical coherence tomography, Scheimpflug imaging and slit-lamp biomicroscopy in the early detection of graft detachment after Descemet membrane endothelial keratoplasty. Cornea. 2011;30(12):1369-75.
18. Agarwal A, Agarwal A, Narang P, et al. Pre-Descemet endothelial keratoplasty with infant donor corneas:a prospective analysis. Cornea. 2015;34(8):859-65.
19. Altaan SL, Gupta A, Sidney LE, et al. Endothelial cell loss following tissue harvesting by pneumodissection for endothelial keratoplasty: an ex vivo study. Br J Ophthalmol. 2015;99(5):710-3.
20. Narang P, Agarwal A, Dua HS, et al. Glued intrascleral fixation of intraocular lens with pupilloplasty and pre-Descemet endothelial keratoplasty: a triple procedure. Cornea. 2015;34(12):1627-31.

Chapter 20

Conversion from Pre-Descemet's Endothelial Keratoplasty to Descemet's Membrane Endothelial Keratoplasty

Dhivya Ashok Kumar, Amar Agarwal

INTRODUCTION

Pre-Descemet's endothelial keratoplasty (PDEK) is a variant of endothelial keratoplasty procedure that involves the transplantation of the pre-Descemet's layer (PDL), the Descemet's membrane (DM) and the endothelium.[1,2] However, in Descemet's membrane endothelial keratoplasty (DMEK) procedure, it is the DM and the endothelial complex which is transplanted.[3,4] PDEK involves the creation of type-1 bubble that is created with a 30 G needle attached to an air-filled 5 mL syringe. This procedure has a theoretical advantage of safer manipulation of tissue and greater ease of deployment that has been encountered during traditional DMEK procedure.

BIG BUBBLE

Type-1 bubble is characterized by a central, dome-shaped bubble with distinct edges and a diameter of around 7.5–8 mm that characteristically spreads from center to periphery.[5] Its extension is limited in the extreme periphery due to the adhesions between the collagenous layers. Type-2 bubble starts from the periphery and it is thinner and larger than type-1 bubble.

INDICATIONS

- Donor eyes in which the type-2 bubble is formed where the cleavage plane is between the pre-Descemet's layer (PDL) and Descemet's membrane (DM), it has to be converted to DMEK surgery.
- Condition where there is mixed bubble formation and the DM is partially separated; it can be converted to DMEK procedure.
- During manipulation of the elderly donor graft, if there is loss of PDL or if the DM gets peeled spontaneously, it can be converted to DMEK.

ETIOLOGY

When inserted superficially the needle happens to be in between the PDL and the DM. Often the plane at which the surgeon enters is correct but due to nonmaintenance of the same plane during the procedure, it often leads to misdirection of the needle toward the endothelium. Depending upon the extent of change of plane, it may lead to accidental creation of type-2 bubble and in extreme cases it may even lead to perforation of the endothelium. When the air enters the plane between the PDL and DM, a type-2 bubble is created that spreads from periphery to center and is of larger diameter as compared to its type-1 counterpart. Elderly patients, pre-existing Descemet's membrane changes, and donor endothelial dystrophy can predispose to abnormal cleavage plane during donor graft harvesting. It then becomes essential to convert the originally planned PDEK procedure into a DMEK procedure.

CONVERSION OF PDEK TO DMEK

Conversion of PDEK to DMEK helps to avoid discarding the donor tissue. When attempts have failed to form the type-1 bubble after staining the endothelium, the surgeon can convert PDEK to a DMEK. In this, a corneal trephine is taken of about 8–8.5 mm and a mark put in the endothelium (Figs. 20.1A to D). A stripper is used to strip the endothelium from the PDL.

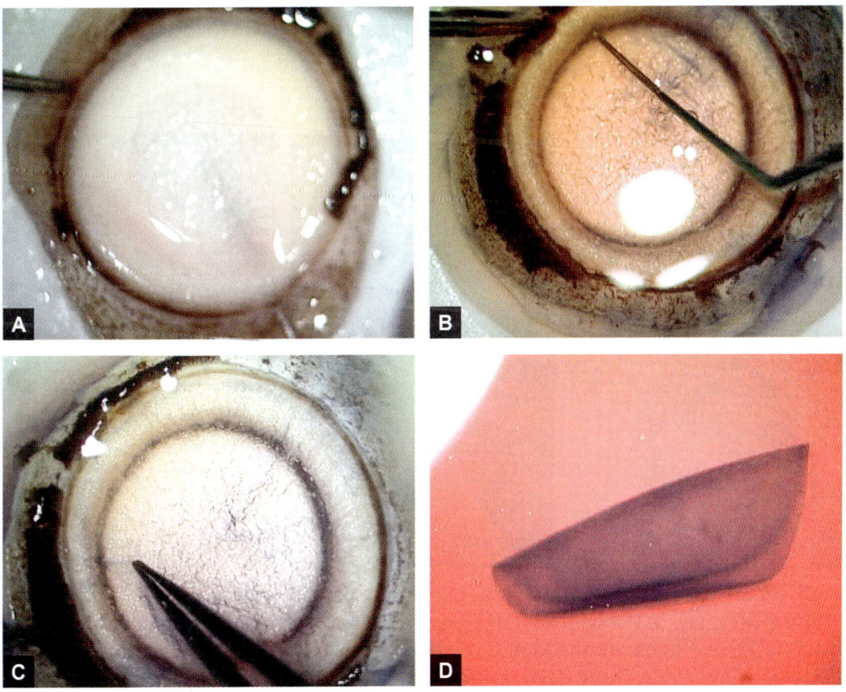

Figs. 20.1A to D. PDEK converted into a DMEK procedure. (A) A 30G needle with air-filled syringe is introduced. Type-1 bubble is not created; (B) A trephine marks the area of the endothelium to make the DMEK graft; (C) Donor DM is scored; (D) Curled DMEK graft is kept in storage media. (PDEK: Pre-Descemet's endothelial keratoplasty; DMEK: Descemet's membrane endothelial keratoplasty; DM: Descemet's membrane)

Finally, one gets a DMEK graft with DM and endothelial complex ready. The graft is loaded in the injector and injected into the anterior chamber. Similar to a PDEK surgery, the graft is unrolled inside the chamber by saline and apposed with air in anterior chamber. Excess tissue manipulation is avoided to prevent endothelial loss or tissue damage. Corneal endothelial loss was noted to be lesser with PDEK graft preparation than DMEK in pneumatic dissection.[6] DMEK can be combined with intraocular lens (IOL) explantation where the triggering anterior chamber IOL can be removed and the glued IOL procedure can be performed in the same sitting (Figs. 20.2A to F). Endoilluminator-assisted DMEK can be performed similar to PDEK where an external illumination helps in graft visualization[7] (Figs. 20.3A to F). In our short series, we have noted a good clinical and functional result in eyes where the PDEK surgery has been converted to DMEK intraoperatively. Irrespective of the type of procedure either PDEK or DMEK, maintaining the stable iris–IOL diaphragm is required before the endothelial keratoplasty. Hence, proper pupilloplasty by single-pass four-throw technique is highly essential in maintaining the pupil integrity.[8,9] Moreover, use of trocar anterior chamber maintainer (TACM) can help in maintaining the anterior chamber thereby aiding in graft manipulation and unrolling.[10] Optical coherence tomography[11] can be used for further follow analysis (Figs. 20.4A to C) for such cases.

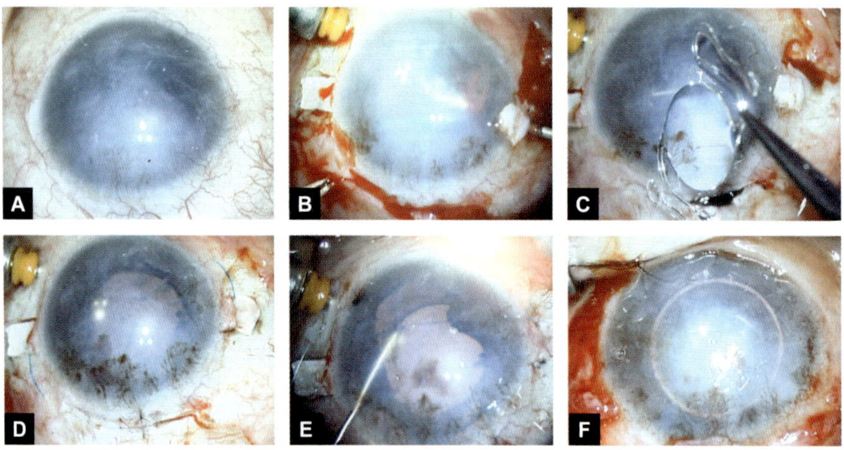

Figs. 20.2A to F: Staged procedure in decompensated cornea. Stage 1: Glued IOL with pupilloplasty. (A) Decompensated cornea with anterior chamber (AC) IOL; (B) Two diagonal scleral flaps are made and sclerostomy with port vitrectomy is done; (C) AC IOL explantation; (D) Glued IOL is performed; (E and F) Pupilloplasty is performed and air bubble is placed in the chamber to test the integrity of the pupil IOL diaphragm. (IOL: Intraocular lens)

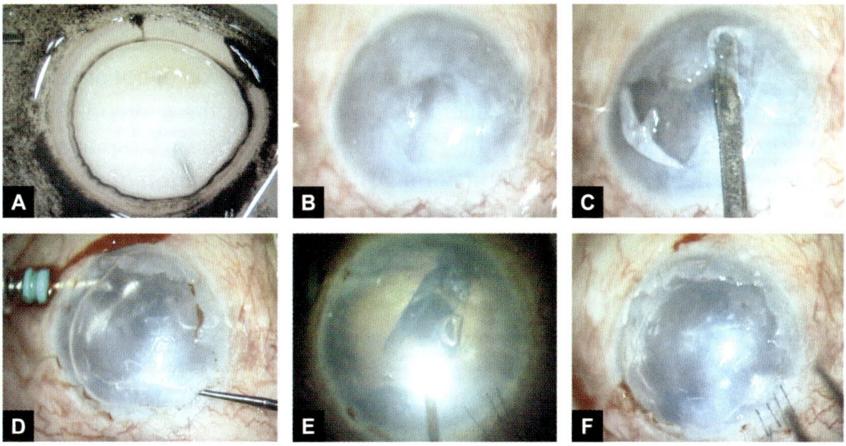

Figs. 20.3A to F: Stage 2: Descemet's membrane endothelial keratoplasty (DMEK). (A) Type-2 big bubble is obtained in donor graft; (B) Decompensated cornea with glued IOL in situ; (C) Epithelial removal; (D) Trocar anterior chamber maintainer is placed and DM is scored; (E) DMEK graft is injected in AC and visualized with endoilluminator; (F) Pneumatic adhesion of DMEK graft is done by the end of procedure.
(IOL: Intraocular lens; AC: Anterior chamber)

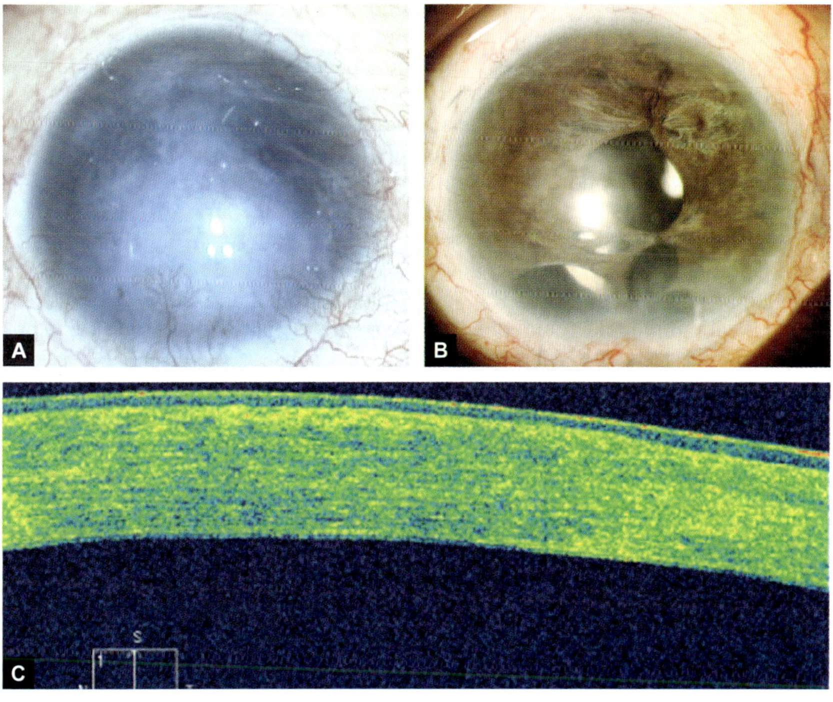

Figs. 20.4A to C: Preoperative decompensated cornea (A), postoperative image after DMEK with glued IOL and pupilloplasty (B) and the postoperative optical coherence tomography in the follow-up showing good graft adhesion (C). (IOL: Intraocular lens)

CONCLUSION

Despite good surgical practice, one may have a complication of not obtaining PDEK graft intraoperatively. Hence, it is important that the surgeon should know how to proceed further without wasting the donor graft. Despite all the surgical challenges that a surgeon comes across in the creation of a bubble, the surgical competence and the correct art of handling the corneal tissue effectively saves the loss of corneal tissue, renders economic practicality, and enhances the functional outcomes.

REFERENCES

1. Agarwal A, Dua HS, Narang P, et al. Pre-Descemet's endothelial keratoplasty (PDEK). Br J Ophthalmol. 2014;98(9):1181-5.
2. Agarwal A, Agarwal A, Narang P, et al. Pre-Descemet endothelial keratoplasty with infant donor corneas: a prospective analysis. Cornea. 2015;34(8):859-65.
3. Melles GR, Ong TS, Ververs B, et al. Descemet membrane endothelial keratoplasty (DMEK). Cornea. 2006;25(8):987-90.
4. Schlötzer-Schrehardt U, Bachmann BO, Laaser K, et al. Characterization of the cleavage plane in Descemet's membrane endothelial keratoplasty. Ophthalmology. 2011;118(10):1950-7.
5. Dua HS, Faraj LA, Said DG, et al. Human corneal anatomy redefined: a novel pre-Descemet's layer (Dua's layer). Ophthalmology. 2013;120(9):1778-85.
6. Altaan SL, Gupta A, Sidney LE, et al. Endothelial cell loss following tissue harvesting by pneumodissection for endothelial keratoplasty: an ex vivo study. Br J Ophthalmol. 2015;99(5):710-3.
7. Jacob S, Agarwal A, Agarwal A, et al. Endoilluminator-assisted transcorneal illumination for Descemet membrane endothelial keratoplasty: enhanced intraoperative visualization of the graft in corneal decompensation secondary to pseudophakic bullous keratopathy. J Cataract Refract Surg. 2014;40(8):1332-6.
8. Narang P, Agarwal A. Single-pass four-throw technique for pupilloplasty. Eur J Ophthalmol. 2017;27(4):506-8.
9. Narang P, Agarwal A, Dua HS, et al. Glued intrascleral fixation of intraocular lens with pupilloplasty and pre-Descemet endothelial keratoplasty: a triple procedure. Cornea. 2015;34(12):1627-31.
10. Agarwal A, Narang P, Kumar DA, et al. Trocar anterior chamber maintainer:-improvised infusion technique. J Cataract Refract Surg. 2016;42(2):185-9.
11. Yeh RY, Quilendrino R, Musa FU, et al. Predictive value of optical coherence tomography in graft attachment after Descemet's membrane endothelial keratoplasty. Ophthalmology. 2013;120(2):240-5.

Section 5

Miscellaneous

Chapter 21

Scarred Cornea to Clear Cornea: Avoiding Penetrating Keratoplasty and Boston Keratoprosthesis

Priya Narang, Amar Agarwal

INTRODUCTION

Cornea is a transparent structure that allows passage of light into the eye and forms the first refractive media that the ray of light embarks upon before hitting the lens and retina. Any disruption in the normal architecture of the corneal lamellae leads to scarring of the corneal stroma (Figs. 21.1A and B) that can result as a response to surgery, trauma, or by viral or bacterial keratitis. Trauma to the clear cornea often leads to opacity and scarring that varies in intensity depending on the type and duration of the episode of injury. The cells responsible for scar deposition are fibroblastic cells derived from stromal keratocytes.[1] Following trauma the proximal keratocytes undergo apoptosis and keratocytes that are distal to the wound become active fibroblasts.[1,2] Healed corneal scars are often long lasting and disrupt vision for millions of patients worldwide.

Currently, surgical replacement of the stroma is the only successful approach for restoration of vision in scarred corneas. The treatment of corneal scars depends upon the depth of the scar and fibrosis. Superficial keratectomy is performed for scar tissue that lies close to the epithelium and is quite superficial. The corneal epithelial surface cells are first removed, and then scar tissue is peeled off the front of the cornea. The epithelial cells then heal over the wound, usually in about a weeks duration. **Phototherapeutic**

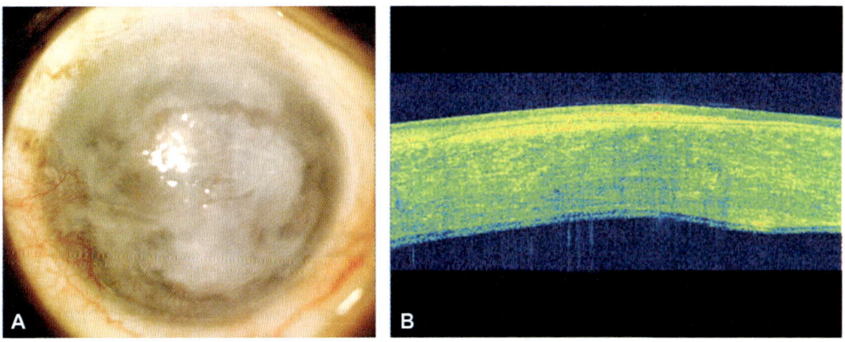

Figs. 21.1A and B: Preoperative pseudophakic bullous keratopathy with corneal scarring.

keratectomy is often employed when the corneal scar tissue extends into the upper parts of the corneal stroma, or is very irregular in nature. Anterior lamellar keratoplasty is performed for corneal scars that involve the stroma and have a healthy endothelium. Involvement of the endothelium with the stromal scar necessitates an endothelial keratoplasty (EK) procedure along with the removal of scarred corneal tissue. The surgical procedure to be performed in such a scenario depends upon the extent of corneal involvement and it may range from penetrating keratoplasty (PK) to Descemet's stripping endothelial keratoplasty (DSEK), Descemet's membrane endothelial keratoplasty (DMEK), Descemet's stripping automated endothelial keratoplasty (DSAEK), or Descemet's membrane automated endothelial keratoplasty (DMAEK). Pre-Descemet's endothelial keratoplasty (PDEK)[3,4] is a new lexicon among the variants of EK procedures that unlike other procedures of EK, facilitates the usage of infant, young, and adult donor tissue.

Penetrating keratoplasty as a procedure is faced with several difficulties, including the shortage of donor tissue, postsurgical complications associated with the use of drugs to prevent immune rejection, and a significant increase in the occurrence of glaucoma. On the other hand, EK procedures focus on the transplant of corneal endothelium, yielding better visual results but still facing the need for donor tissue. As PDEK allows the usage of infant and young donor,[4] it is believed to lead to an increase of donor tissue pool that seems to be advantageous in the current scenario (Figs. 21.2A and B).

OUR SURGICAL EXPERIENCE

The use of infant donor tissue for scarred cornea cases has helped a great deal in the clearance of corneal scar due to bullous keratopathy (BK). The infant

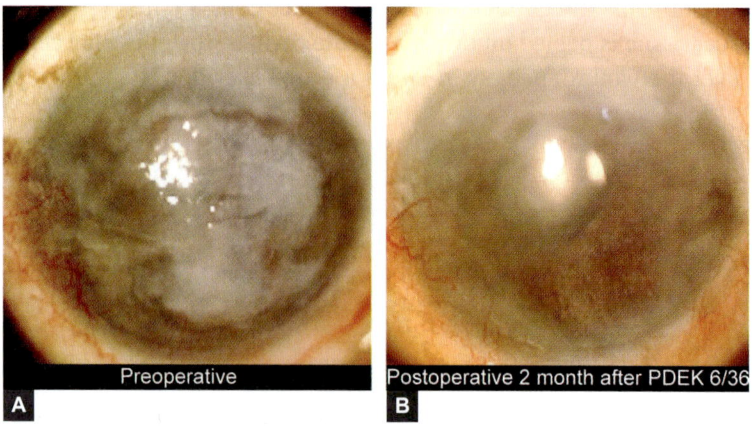

Figs. 21.2A and B: Same patient as Figs. 21.1A and B with pre- and postoperative. *Note*: The corneal clearance and vision has improved to 6/36.
(PDEK: Pre-Descemet's endothelial keratoplasty).

donor tissue is virtually rich in endothelial cell density count that probably translates into faster and better visual recovery (Figs. 21.3 to 21.5).

Adequate visualization of the intraocular structures is essential while handling complex cases of scarred cornea. Endoilluminator facilitates surgery as the scarred cornea when illuminated by an obliquely falling light allows better visualization and comprehension of graft orientation and positioning.[5]

Correction of any other associated intraocular condition like lens removal and intraocular lens (IOL) placement should be performed before PDEK procedure as doing so enhances the chances of graft survival and also helps to mitigate the issue of constant irritant that could probably be the cause of concern at a later stage. In cases associated with IOL decentration, subluxation or cases that require a secondary IOL fixation, glued IOL is performed in all cases followed by pupilloplasty that helps to narrow down the size of pupil.[6] This helps in adequate formation of anterior chamber (AC) and also prevents air diversion in the vitreous cavity.

DISCUSSION

Aphakic and pseudophakic BK is one of the major indications for corneal grafting in many developing countries[7-9] and many patients in developing

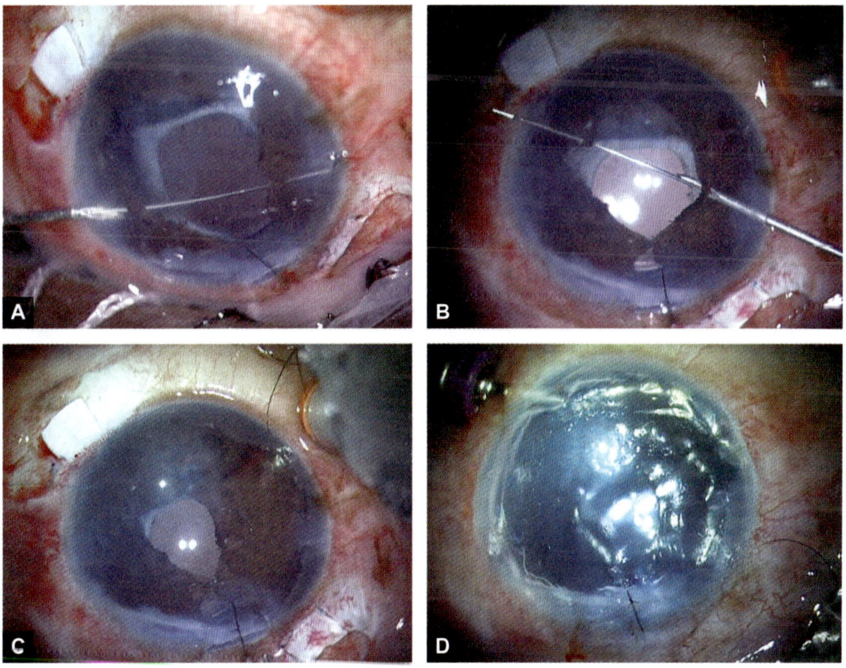

Figs. 21.3A to D: Scarred cornea treated with PDEK- Part 1. (A) Glued IOL done. Single pass 4 throw pupilloplasty being performed as pupil is dilated; (B) Single pass 4 throw pupilloplasty; (C) Pupil made small. This way the air in the AC remains there and the PDEK graft will not detach; (D) PDEK graft attached.

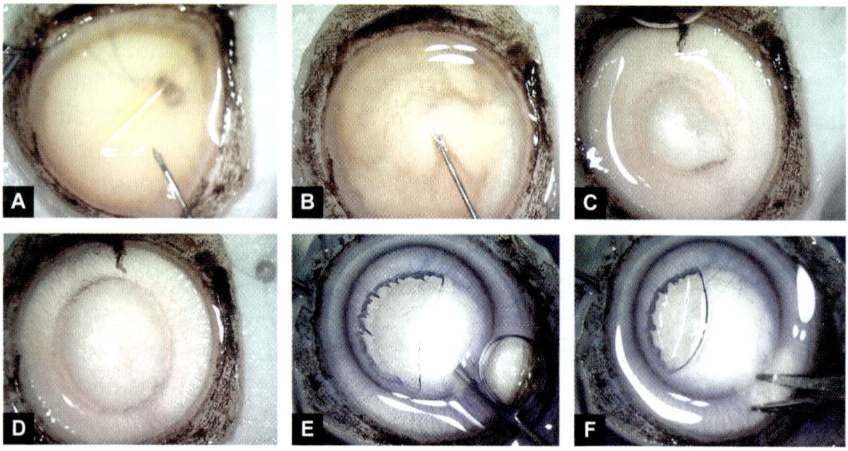

Figs. 21.4A to F: Preparation of young donor graft for PDEK to treat scarred cornea. (A) 30 G needle connected to a 5 mL syringe enters the donor cornea through the sclera; (B) Air injected into the donor cornea; (C) Type 1 big bubble forming; (D) Type 1 big bubble; (E) Knife entry into the bubble and trypan blue injected to stain; (F) PDEK graft dissected with scissor.

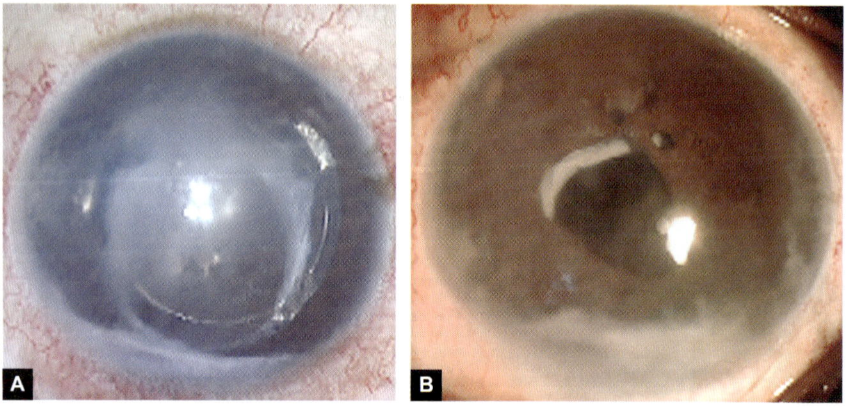

Figs. 21.5A and B: Pre and postoperative images of same patient shown in Fig 21.3. (A) Pre-operative showing scarred cornea; (B) Postoperative 2 months 6/12 vision after glued IOL single pass 4 throw pupilloplasty and PDEK.

countries like India do not seek surgical treatment until their bullous lesions are severe and the disease is advanced (Figs. 21.6 and 21.7).

The advantages of performing a PDEK in complex cases of BK is that PDEK requires a smaller size of incision rather than an open-sky condition and the integrity of the corneal surface in PDEK eyes is preserved without corneal incisions or sutures, eliminating the epithelium-related (such as epithelial defect and ulcer) and the suture-related complications (such as loose suture, infection, and neovascularization) of conventional PK.

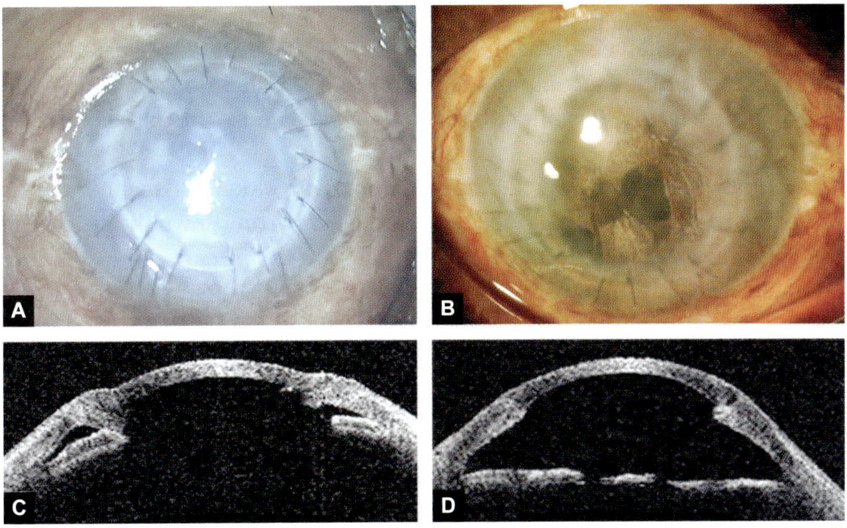

Figs. 21.6A to D: Scarred failed graft in a one eyed patient before and after PDEK and single pass 4 throw pupilloplasty. (A) Failed graft in a one eyed patient. Note the scarred cornea; (B) Postoperative after PDEK and Single pass 4 throw pupilloplasty; (C) Preoperative anterior segment OCT shows closed angle; (D) Postoperatove anterior segment OCT after single pass 4 throw pupilloplasty shows open angle.

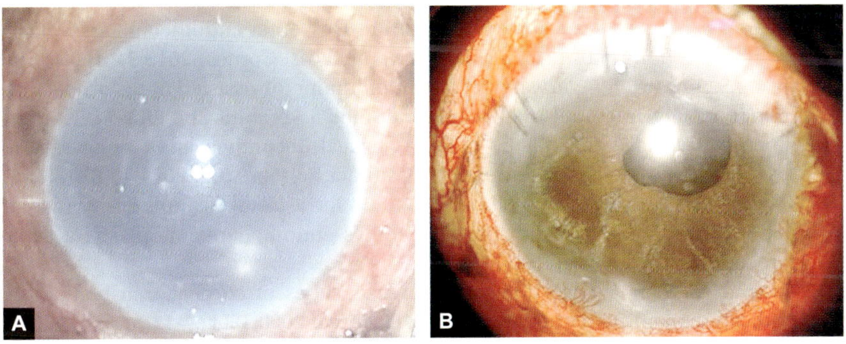

Figs. 21.7A and B: Pre- and postoperative images of a pseudophakic bullous keratopathy after PDEK.

However, if the BK eyes have severe subepithelial opacity and/or obvious stromal scar, we always scrap off the epithelium to enhance the intraoperative visualization of intraocular structures. This may often behave as superficial keratectomy. The corneal surface can be re-epithelialized in 3–4 days.

Although PDEK has unique advantages, it is a more technically challenging procedure in the treatment of complex BK as combined procedures (such as anterior vitrectomy, IOL removal, etc.) are necessary in eyes with intraocular comorbidities. Because PDEK is more difficult to perform than PK, the combined procedures will definitely challenge the surgeons skills even more.

Another problem challenging PDEK surgeons is the assessment of postoperative functional vision before PDEK surgery. Because complicated intraocular comorbidities accompany BK, a clear cornea does not guarantee good postoperative vision. It is difficult for surgeons to choose the perfect time for IOL implantation.

In our series, secondary IOL implantation with glued IOL technique was performed along with pupilloplasty that helps to narrow down the size of the iris diaphragm. This indirectly helps to maintain the integrity of AC and an adequate air fill in the postoperative period. PDEK is often performed as a second-stage procedure in cases with other comorbidities. PDEK combined with other intraocular surgeries is a feasible and effective procedure for complex BK with severe vision loss.

REFERENCES

1. Funderburgh JL, Mann MM, Funderburgh ML. Keratocyte phenotype mediates proteoglycan structure: a role for fibroblasts in corneal fibrosis. J Biol Chem. 2003;278(46):45629-37.
2. Wilson SE. Analysis of the keratocyte apoptosis, keratocyte proliferation, and myofibroblast transformation responses after photorefractive keratectomy and laser in situ keratomileusis. Trans Am Ophthalmol Soc. 2002;100:411-33.
3. Agarwal A, Dua HS, Narang P, et al. Pre-Descemet's endothelial keratoplasty (PDEK). Br J Ophthalmol. 2014;98(9):1181-85.
4. Agarwal A, Agarwal A, Narang P, et al. Pre-Descemet endothelial keratoplasty with infant donor corneas: a prospective analysis. Cornea. 2015;34(8):859-65.
5. Jacob S, Agarwal A, Agarwal A, et al. Endoilluminator-assisted transcorneal illumination for Descemet membrane endothelial keratoplasty: enhanced intraoperative visualization of the graft in corneal decompensation secondary to pseudophakic bullous keratopathy. J Cataract Refract Surg. 2014;40(8):1332-6.
6. Narang P, Agarwal A, Dua HS, et al. Glued intrascleral fixation of intraocular lens with pupilloplasty and pre-Descemet's endothelial keratoplasty: a triple procedure. Cornea. 2015;34(12):1627-31.
7. Maeno A, Naor J, Lee HM, et al. Three decades of corneal transplantation: indications and patient characteristics. Cornea. 2000;19(1):7-11.
8. Xie LX, Wang FH, Shi WY. Analysis of causes for penetrating keratoplasty at Shandong Eye Institute from 1997 to 2002. Zhonghua Yan Ke Za Zhi. 2006;42(8):704-8.
9. Chu W. The past twenty-five years in eye banking. Cornea. 2000;19(5):754-65.

CHAPTER 22

Cosmetic Iris Implant Complications: Managed by Triple Procedure of Cataract, SPFT Pupilloplasty and PDEK

Priya Narang, Amar Agarwal

INTRODUCTION

Anterior chamber angle supported iris implants were first described in 2004 for the treatment of oculocutaneous syndrome.[1] Subsequently, these artificial implants were marketed for iris color change in normal individuals solely for the purpose of cosmetic appearance. These implants were made of silicon and were available in single size with 15 mm diameter. Since then significant complications have been reported in the postoperative period that range from corneal degeneration to anterior chamber angle structure involvement with raised intraocular pressure (IOP), inflammation, uveitis, and cataract formation.[3-5] Significant complications have also been reported even during the explantation of these cosmetic iris implants with the requirement of secondary procedures for the correction of these defects.[3,4]

Several theories have been cited for the damage caused by these implants, the common reasoning being that as the peripheral edges of the implants are mounted in the anterior chamber angle they lead to constant friction and mechanical trauma to the corneal endothelium and the angle structures.[6] This leads to pigment dispersion and development of peripheral anterior synechias that eventually leads to raised IOP and development of glaucoma.

It is essential to remove the iris implants and surgical technique for atraumatic explantation of the cosmetic iris implants has been described to minimize the postoperative complications.

SURGICAL INTERVENTION

In our setup, after the removal of cosmetic iris implant in cases that are complicated with corneal decompensation with development of peripheral anterior synechiae (PAS) and cataract formation, we tend to perform a triple procedure of phacoemulsification with single-pass four-throw (SFT) pupilloplasty[7,8] and pre-Descemet's endothelial keratoplasty (PDEK)[9] procedure (Figs. 22.1 to 22.21).

After the procedure of phacoemulsification fluid infusion is introduced inside the eye with the help of trocar-anterior chamber maintainer (T-ACM).[10] SFT procedure is performed by passing a 10-0 prolene suture attached to the long arm of the needle through the proximal and distal iris leaflets.

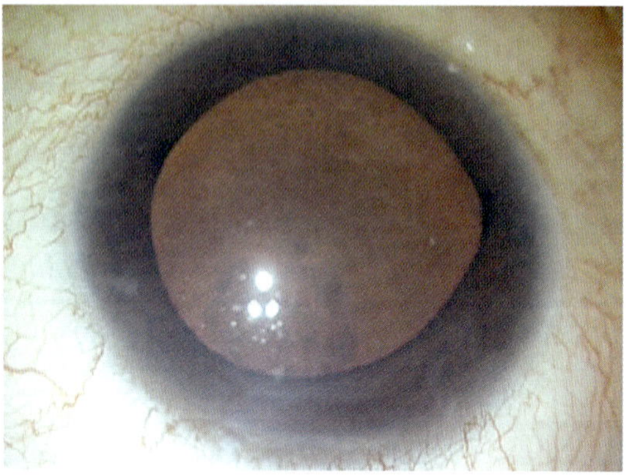

Fig. 22.1: Bullous keratopathy after iris cosmetic implant had been removed. Note the lens changes and also the pupil dilated with the iris stuck to the cornea. Intraocular pressure (IOP) was 40 mm Hg.

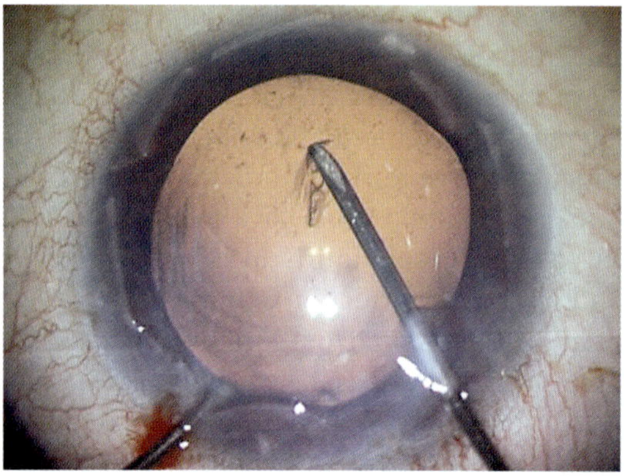

Fig. 22.2: Rhexis started.

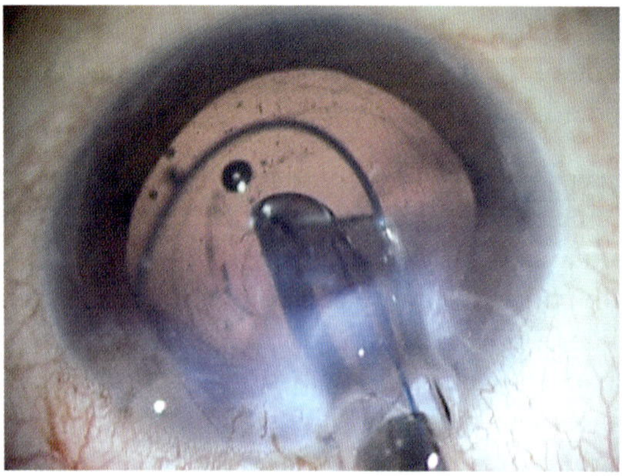

Fig. 22.3: Three piece foldable intraocular lens (IOL) implanted. An acrylic hydrophobic IOL is chosen (AMO) as IOL opacification does not occur later on which can happen with an acrylic hydrophilic IOL. A three piece is chosen also because it can be converted to a glued IOL if needed.

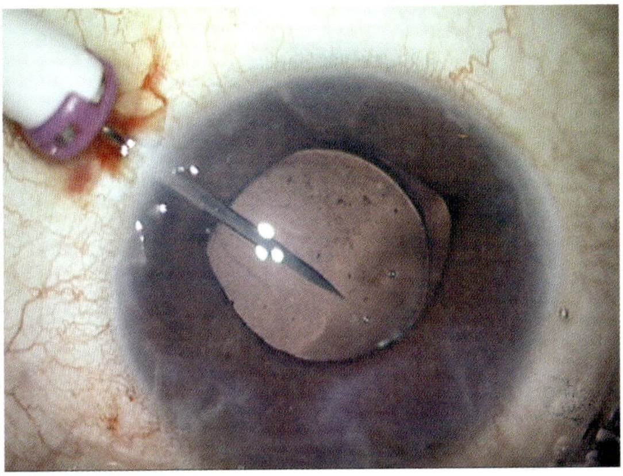

Fig. 22.4: Trocar anterior chamber (AC) maintainer fixed.

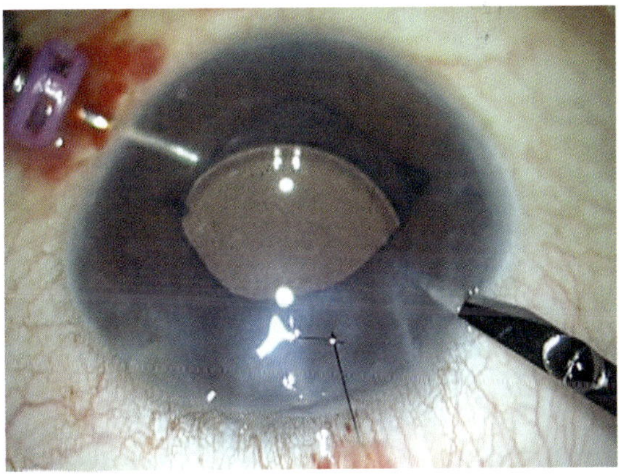

Fig. 22.5: Side port incision. Note the main incision is sutured.

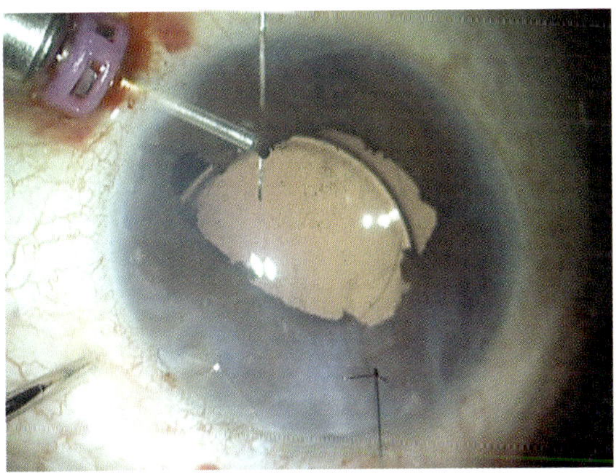

Fig. 22.6: Single-pass four-throw pupilloplasty started. Note the 10/0 straight needle Prolene suture passed through the cornea and then iris.

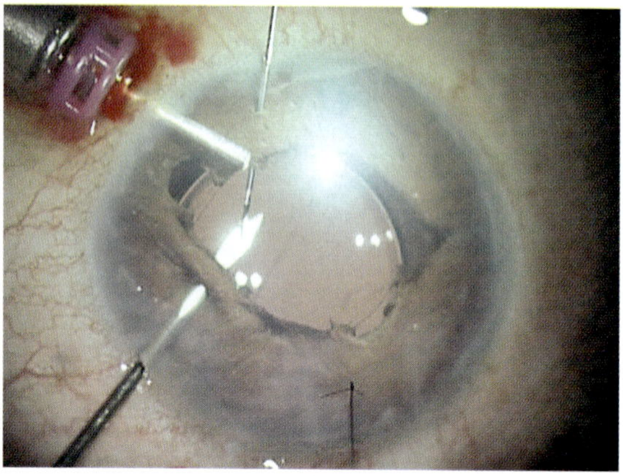

Fig. 22.7: 26 G needle passes through a paracentesis and then through the iris.

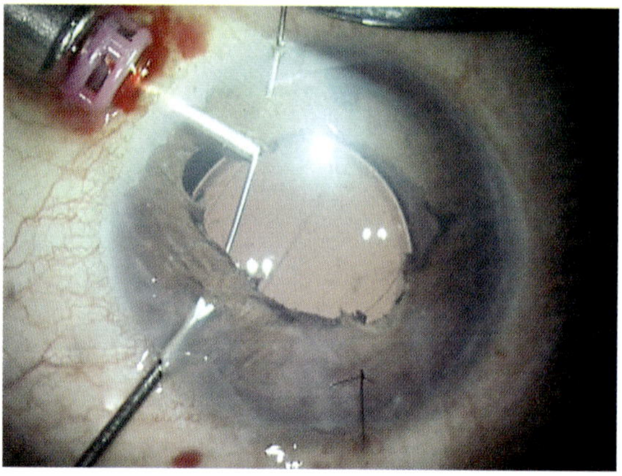

Fig. 22.8: Rail road technique. The 10/0 needle is passed into the 26 G needle.

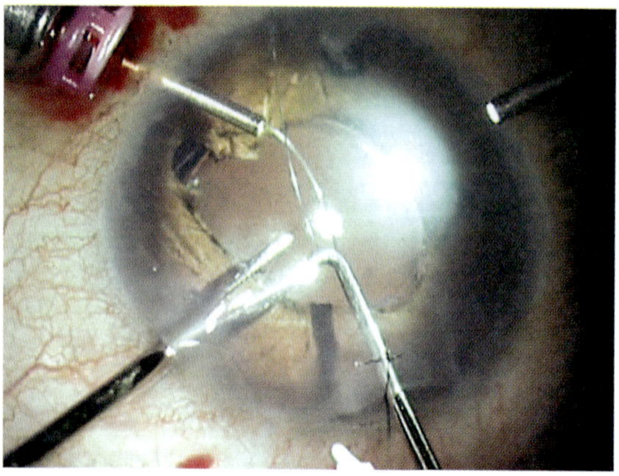

Fig. 22.9: Single pass loop created and brought out of the paracentesis.

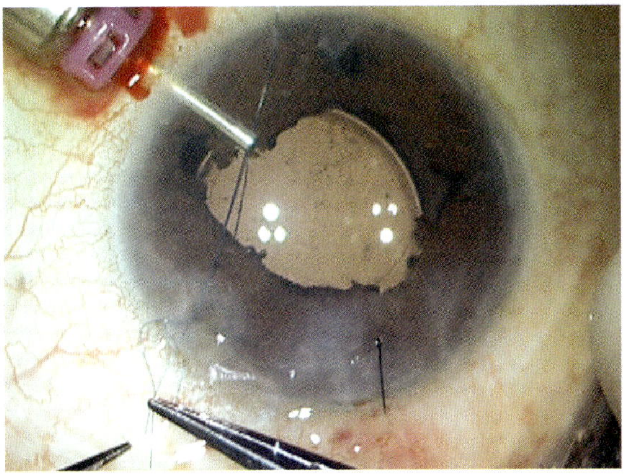

Fig. 22.10: Four throws.

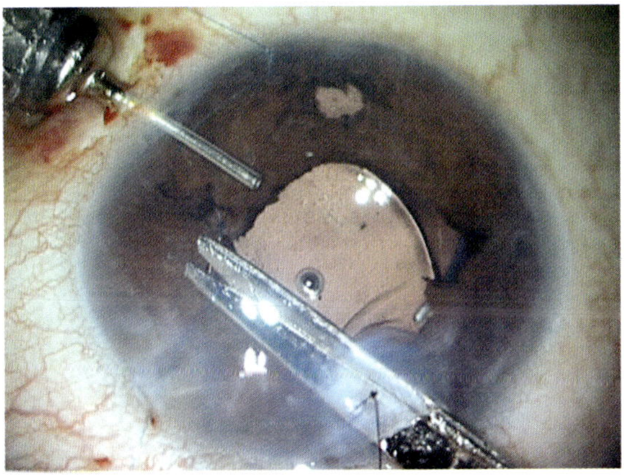

Fig. 22.11: Microscissor cuts the ends of the suture.

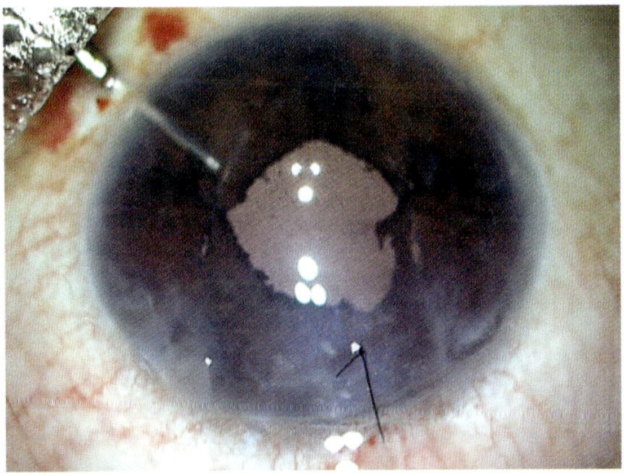

Fig. 22.12: Single-pass four-throw pupilloplasty completed. Note the pupil which was dilated has become small. The closed angle has now opened.

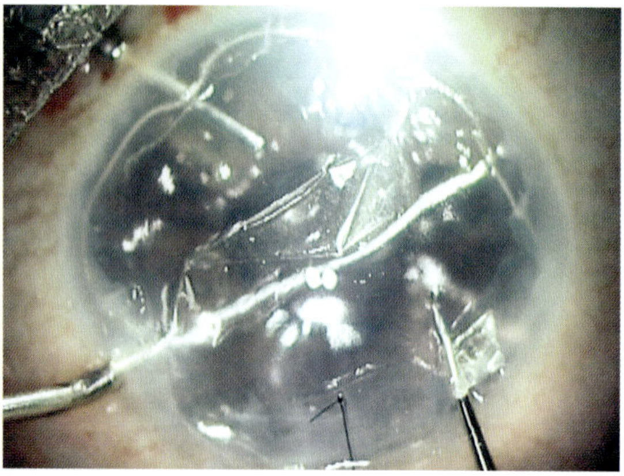

Fig. 22.13: Continuous air infused into the anterior chamber (AC) and descemetorhexis done.

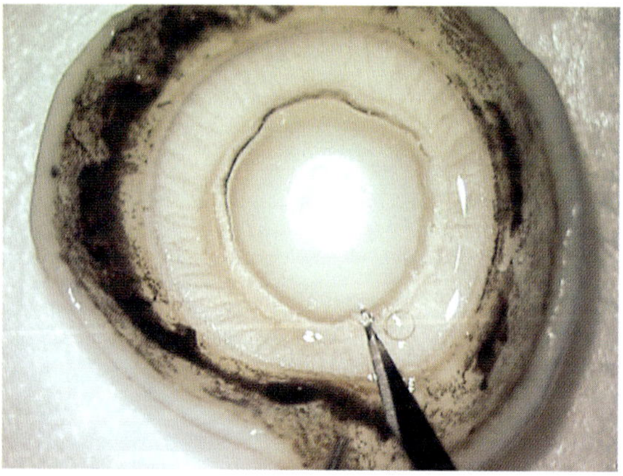

Fig. 22.14: Type 1 big bubble created in a young donor.

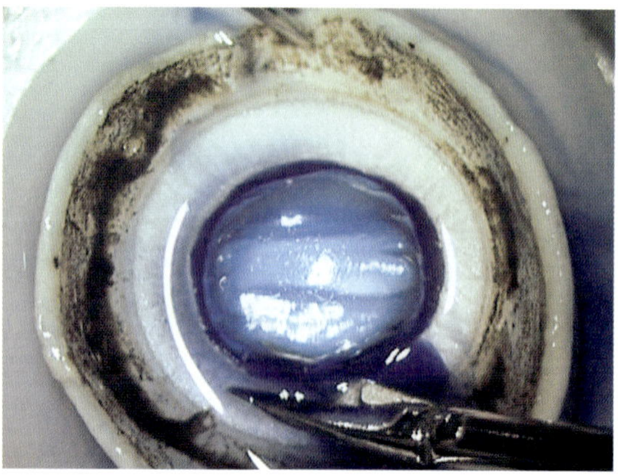

Fig. 22.15: Pre-Descemet's endothelial keratoplasty (PDEK) graft stained with trypan blue and dissected.

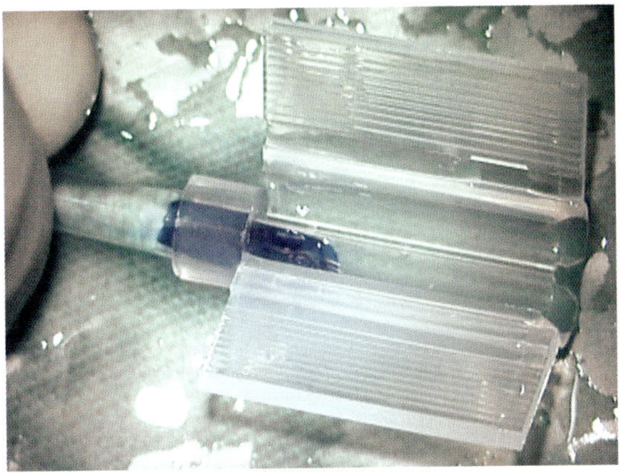

Fig. 22.16: Pre-Descemet's endothelial keratoplasty (PDEK) graft loaded in intraocular lens (IOL) injector.

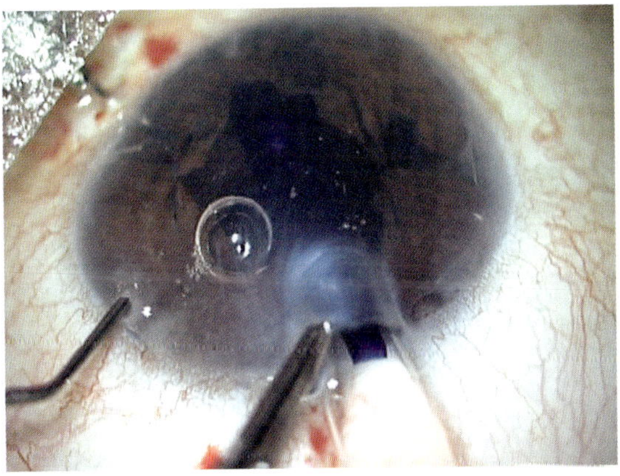

Fig. 22.17: Pre-Descemet's endothelial keratoplasty (PDEK) graft injected into the anterior chamber (AC).

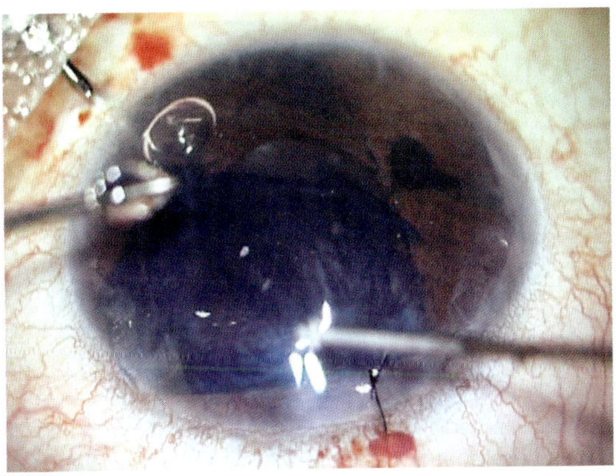

Fig. 22.18: Pre-Descemet's endothelial keratoplasty (PDEK) graft unrolled.

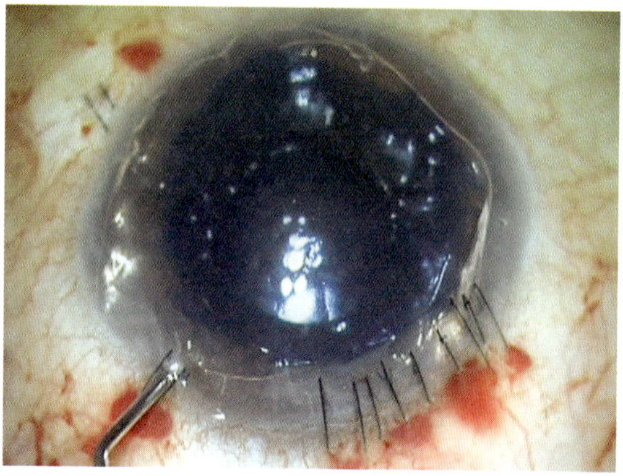

Fig. 22.19: Air injected under the graft and graft attached using air pump-assisted pre-Descemet's endothelial keratoplasty (PDEK) technique.

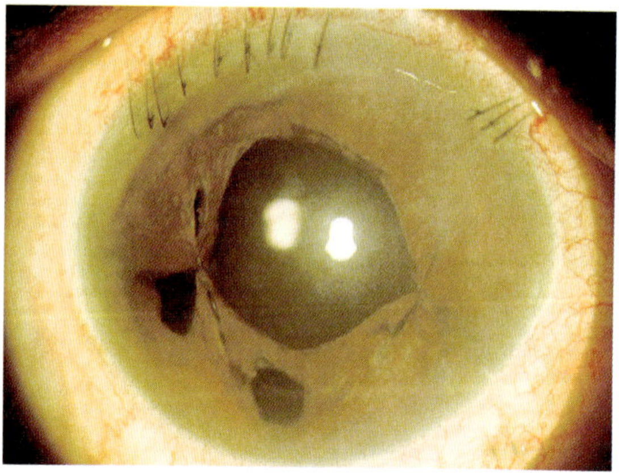

Fig. 22.20: One week postoperative 6/9. Intraocular pressure (IOP) was 12 mm Hg without medications.

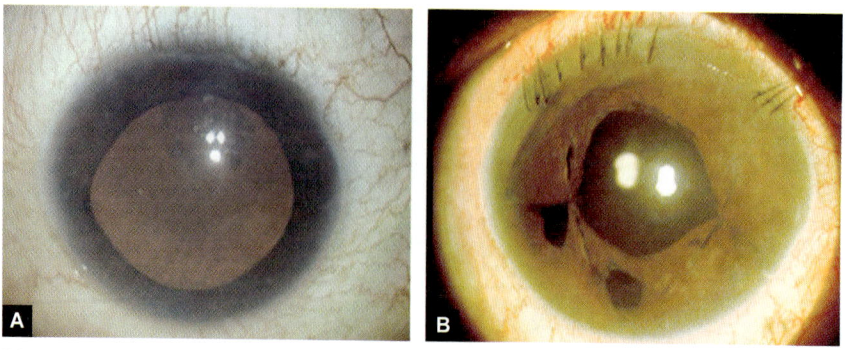

Figs. 22.21A and B: Pre- and postoperative of the iris cosmetic implant complication case with bullous keratopathy cataract and closed angle glaucoma. Postoperative 1 week vision 6/9.

A Sinskey's hook is passed through the paracentesis incision and a loop is withdrawn from the eye. The suture end is passed through the loop 4 times taking care to pass it in the same direction always. Once four-throws are taken through the loop, both the suture ends are pulled and this leads to sliding of the helical pattern inside the eye approximating both the iris leaflets. SFT is performed again in the opposite quadrant and this leads to the narrowing of the pupil size eventually creating a pull on the peripheral iris with breakage of PAS and opening of the anterior chamber angles.

The fluid infusion through T-ACM is stopped and air is infused inside the anterior chamber. Descemetorhexis is performed and the diseased endothelium—DM complex is removed. Air infusion is stopped; PDEK graft is then injected inside the AC and is gently unrolled using air and fluidics. Once the graft has totally unfolded; air is injected beneath the graft to provide sufficient air tamponade.

DISCUSSION

Apart from the techniques described for removal of the cosmetic iris implant,[6] various surgical procedures like trabeculectomy, goniosynechiolysis, Descemet's stripping automated endothelial keratoplasty (DSAEK), cataract extraction are advised in cases that are complicated with placement of cosmetic iris implants. Performing a triple procedure helps to restore the sanctity of eye and it also suffices well as a single stage procedure.

REFERENCES

1. Kahn DA. "Iris Diaphragm Implant (Newiris) in Oculocutaneous Albinism," poster presented at the Annual Meeting of the American Academy of Ophthalmology. Las Vegas, Nevada, USA, 2006.
2. Anderson JE, Grippo TM, Sbeity Z, et al. Serious complications of cosmetic NewColorIris implantation. Acta Ophthalmol. 2010;88:700-4.
3. Hoguet A, Ritterband D, Koplin R, et al. Serious ocular complications of cosmetic iris implants in 14 eyes. J Cataract Refract Surg. 2012;38:387-93.
4. Hull S, Jayaram H, Mearza AA. Complications and management of cosmetic anterior chamber iris implants. Cont Lens Anterior Eye. 2010;33:235-8.
5. Sikder S, Davis SW, Holz H, et al. Complications of NewColorIris implantation in phakic eyes: a review. Clin Ophthalmol. 2011;5:435-8.
6. Arjmand P, Gooi P, Ahmed II. Surgical technique for explantation of cosmetic anterior chamber iris implants. J Cataract Refract Surg. 2015;41:18-22.
7. Narang P, Agarwal A. Single-pass four-throw technique for pupilloplasty. Eur J Ophthalmol. 2017;27:506-8.
8. Narang P, Agarwal A. (2017). Single-pass four-throw (SFT) pupilloplasty for angle closure glaucoma. [online] Available from: https://www.eyeworld.org/single-pass-four-throw-sft-pupilloplasty-technique [Accessed September, 2017].
9. Agarwal A, Dua HS, Narang P, et al. Pre-Descemet's endothelial keratoplasty (PDEK). Br J Ophthalmol. 2014;98:1181-5.
10. Agarwal A, Narang P, Kumar DA, et al. Trocar anterior chamber maintainer: Improvised infusion technique. J Cataract Refract Surg. 2016;42:185-9.

CHAPTER 23

Optical Coherence Tomography Guided Pre-Descemet's Endothelial Keratoplasty

Soosan Jacob

INTRODUCTION

The challenge in performing both Descemet's membrane endothelial keratoplasty (DMEK)[1] as well as pre-Descemet's endothelial[2,3] keratoplasty (PDEK) lies in the thin nature of the donor tissue that hinders with proper identification of the orientation of the graft within the anterior chamber (AC). The graft tends to scroll up toward the Descemet's membrane (DM) because of the elasticity of the DM and it is therefore crucial to make sure that the scrolls face upward before unscrolling the graft. This can be challenging to ascertain because of the transparent nature of the graft and the difficulty can be compounded if visualization is poor secondary to an edematous cornea. Unintentional inverted grafts can cause iatrogenic primary graft failure in DMEK even in experienced hands.[4,5]

The author (SJ) described the endoilluminator-assisted DMEK (E-DMEK)[6] and the E-PDEK [7] techniques to identify graft orientation and to enhance visualization in DMEK and PDEK, respectively. However, other techniques such as the hand held slit lamp technique, Moutsouri's sign, S-stamp technique, punched orientation marks, optical coherence tomography (OCT)-guided determination, etc.

OPTICAL COHERENCE TOMOGRAPHY-GUIDED DMEK AND PDEK

Real-time intraoperative OCT is a new tool that can be used effectively to delineate structures better in three-dimension. The data can be integrated into the microscope so that the surgeon can see real-time OCT integrated into the microscope view itself. Foot pedal control gives the ability to control focus and area of scanning with the OCT. The OCT can be useful in vitreoretinal surgeries as well as in lamellar corneal surgeries. Hand held OCT is also now available which can be used intraoperatively for the required steps of surgery.

In endothelial keratoplasties, intraoperative OCT[8] is useful in various steps:

1. *Peripheral anterior synechiolysis*: OCT is useful for determining the presence of any peripheral anterior synechiae and confirming their release even through hazy, edematous corneas.

2. *Patency of pulsatility index (PI)*: The patency of the PI can be checked with the OCT in order to prevent postoperative pupillary block glaucoma.
3. *Completeness of host Descemetic stripping*: In case of any doubt, this can be verified through the OCT and any tags can be removed.
4. *Graft orientation within the cartridge*: This can be verified by looking at the direction of the edge curls through the OCT.
5. *Graft orientation*: Real-time verification of the orientation of the graft allows the advantage of definitively being able to determine that the right side of the graft is facing upward before floatation. This is done by verifying that the edges of the graft curl upward on OCT. This is applicable in both DMEK and PDEK (Fig. 23.1).
6. *Detection of edge folds and edge detachments post-floatation*: The presence or absence of any can also be determined and air pump-assisted PDEK technique[9] can be used for rectifying these.
7. *Presence of interface fluid after floatation*: Fluid pockets that can cause detachment postoperatively can be detected during surgery and if indicated, venting incisions can be made at these sites. OCT is also helpful in guiding the depth of venting incisions as well as verifying that all fluid has been removed through the venting incisions (Figs. 23.2A and B).
8. *Combined surgeries*: It is useful when combining with other surgeries such as a tube shunt placement or trimming/repositioning of an existent tube to intraoperatively determine the distance from the tube tip to the graft.
9. *Postoperative follow-up*: Graft attachment and resolution of edema can be tracked using the OCT. Edge detachments or shallow detachments can often be picked up easier with the OCT and it offers a repeatable way

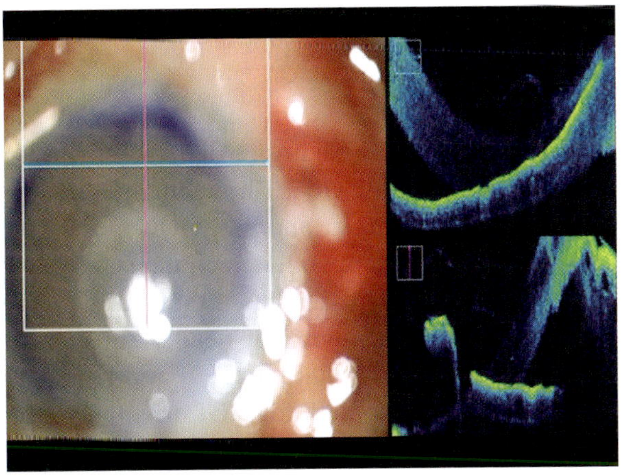

Fig. 23.1: Optical coherence tomography (OCT) view of a Descemet's membrane endothelial keratoplasty (DMEK) graft showing an inverted graft with scrolls facing downward.

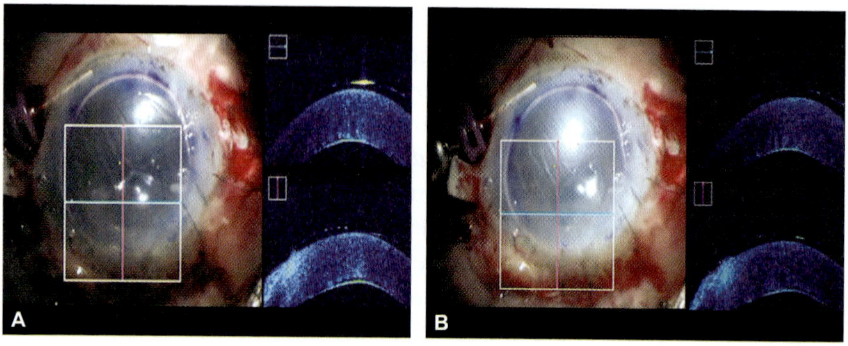

Figs. 23.2A and B: (A) Optical coherence tomography (OCT) at the end of surgery showing interface fluid; (B) With interface fluid drained.

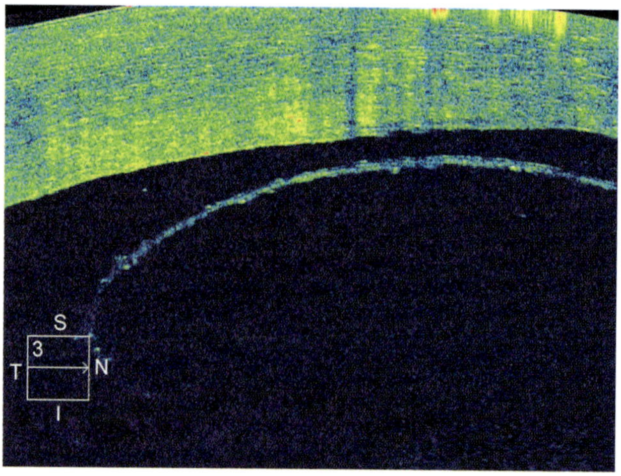

Fig. 23.3: An inverted pre-Descemet's endothelial keratoplasty (PDEK) graft seen postoperatively. Notice graft edge curling outward.

to measure resolution or increase in size of detachment. Graft thickness can also be measured with the OCT. Time domain OCT is helpful for an overall analysis up to the graft periphery whereas spectral domain OCT is helpful for detecting even minor graft detachments (Fig. 23.3).[10]

Disadvantages to the use of OCT include the need for expensive additional instrumentation and equipments; the need to constantly maintain the reticule onto the exactly correct position in X, Y, and Z axes. In addition, it may sometimes be difficult to maintaining OCT orientation and focus at the desired level as the eye moves with intraoperative maneuvers. Intraoperative inversion of images is also another issue that needs to be tackled before this mode of surgery can be seamlessly and effortlessly integrated into routine practice.

ENDOILLUMINATOR-ASSISTED DESCEMET'S MEMBRANE ENDOTHELIAL KERATOPLASTY

Endoilluminator has been used in cataract surgery for improving visualization for capsulorhexis[11] in white cataracts and in eyes with corneal opacities. Intracameral chandelier illumination fiber[12] has been used for Descemet's stripping automated endothelial keratoplasty (DSAEK). In the E-DMEK and E-PDEK techniques, an endoilluminator or vitreoretinal light pipe held externally throws light in an oblique direction on the graft. The light probe is held at an angle that allows good visualization and three-dimensional perception. Direction of scrolling of the graft edges and graft orientation are confirmed by visualizing the light reflecting off the edges of the graft. The entire graft can simultaneously be visualized in three-dimension in a sterile field throughout all important steps (Figs. 23.4A to C).

OTHER TECHNIQUES FOR CONFIRMING GRAFT ORIENTATION

Various other techniques have been described to determine graft orientation. The hand held slit lamp technique, Moutsouri's sign, punched out orientation marks and the S-stamp technique are other techniques used.

CONCLUSION

To conclude, OCT-guided surgery has various advantages. Definitive pre-floatation identification of orientation as well as the ability to be used for both DMEK and PDEK surgeries are major advantages together with the absence of the need to alter or stamp the graft as some other techniques require. It can be used even in cases with inadequately stained graft or in the presence of corneal edema. It is also not as dependent on graft position within the eye, depth of the anterior chamber or tightness of the scrolls. Though the OCT gives good depth perception and decreases the number of intracameral ma-

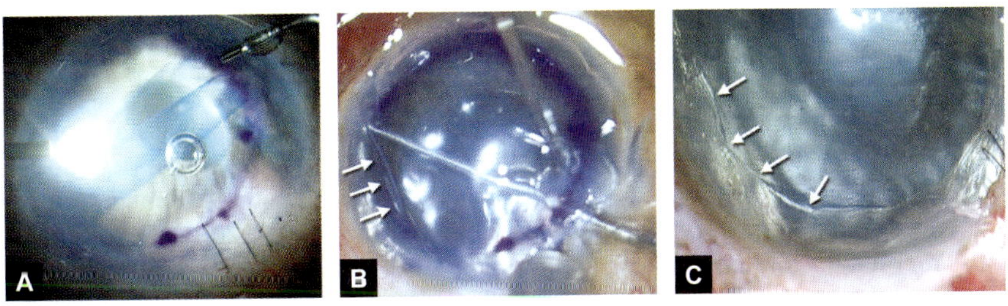

Figs. 23.4A to C: (A) Endoilluminator-assisted PDEK (E-PDEK) showing good comprehension of orientation of graft and ability to visualize graft in a non-touch technique from end to end; (B) Endoilluminator allows easy identification of edge folds at the end of surgery; (C) It also allows the entire margin of the graft to be easily visualized.

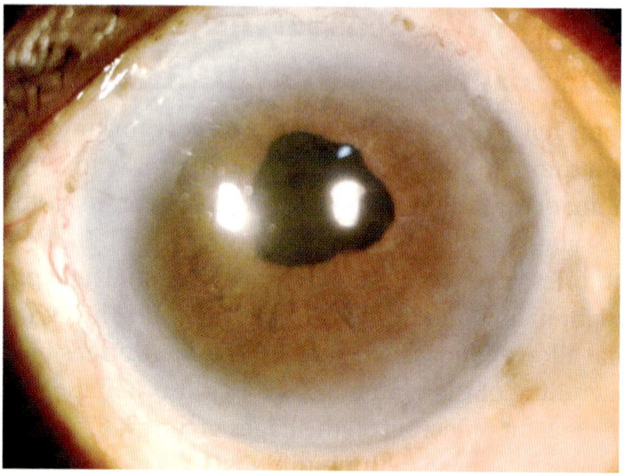

Fig. 23.5: Postoperative clear cornea after optical coherence tomography (OCT)-assisted endothelial keratoplasty.

neuvers required to confirm orientation, it still provides only a slit section of the graft and therefore does not give the instantaneous ability to see the entire graft from end-to-end in three-dimension. Microscope integrated OCT allows maintenance of sterility and seamless integration, however handheld OCT does not do either of these. Other major disadvantages are the need for expensive intraoperative equipment as well as distraction during surgery because of inversion of the OCT image, the need to keep focusing and aligning as well as an overload of data that may really not required. In the author's experience, the endoilluminator-assisted technique provides all the advantages of the OCT-guided technique in addition to being able to visualize the entire graft three-dimensionally at the same time even while performing other steps. It is also a much more economical and easily available alternative and aids in all steps by increasing depth perception by the surgeon (Figs. 23.4 and 23.5).

REFERENCES

1. Dapena I, Moutsouris K, Droutsas K, et al. Standardized "No-Touch" technique for Descemet membrane endothelial keratoplasty. Archives of Ophthalmology. 2011;129:88-94.
2. Agarwal A, Dua HS, Narang P, et al. Pre-Descemet's endothelial keratoplasty (PDEK). Br J Ophthalmol. 2014;98(9):1181-5.
3. Dua HS, Faraj LA, Said DG, et al. Human corneal anatomy redefined: a novel pre-Descemet's layer (Dua's layer). Ophthalmology. 2013;120:1778-85.
4. Yoeruek E, Hofmann J, Bartz-Schmidt KU. Histological and ultrastructural findings of corneal tissue after failed descemet membrane endothelial keratoplasty. Acta Ophthalmol. 2014;92:213-6.
5. Dirisamer M, Van Dijk K, Dapena I, et al. Prevention and management of graft detachment in descemet membrane endothelial keratoplasty. Arch Ophthalmol. 2012;130:280-91.

6. Jacob S, Agarwal A, Agarwal A, et al. Endoilluminator-assisted transcorneal illumination for Descemet membrane endothelial keratoplasty: enhanced intraoperative visualization of the graft in corneal decompensation secondary to pseudophakic bullous keratopathy. J Cataract Refract Surg. 2014;40:1332-6.
7. Jacob S, Agarwal A, Kumar DA. Endoilluminator-assisted Descemet membrane endothelial keratoplasty and endoilluminator-assisted pre-Descemet endothelial keratoplasty. Clin Ophthalmol. 2015;9:2123-5.
8. Saad A, Guilbert E, Grise-Dulac A, et al. Intraoperative OCT-assisted DMEK: 14 consecutive cases. Cornea. 2015;34:802-7.
9. Jacob S, Narasimhan S, Agarwal A, et al. Air pump-assisted graft centration, graft edge unfolding, and graft uncreasing in young donor graft pre-Descemet endothelial keratoplasty. Cornea. 2017;36:1009-13.
10. Siebelmann S, Gehlsen U, Le Blanc C, et al. Detection of graft detachments immediately following Descemet membrane endothelial keratoplasty (DMEK) comparing time domain and spectral domain OCT. Graefes Arch Clin Exp Ophthalmol. 2016;254:2431-7.
11. Mansour AM. Anterior capsulorhexis in hypermature cataracts. (letter). J Cataract Refract Surg. 1993;19:116-7.
12. Inoue T, Oshima Y, Hori Y, et al. Chandelier illumination for use during Descemet stripping automated endothelial keratoplasty in patients with advanced bullous keratopathy. Cornea. 2011;30 Suppl 1:S50-3.

Chapter 24

Eye Bank Preparation of Pre-Descemet's Endothelial Keratoplasty Grafts

Elizabeth Shen, Adam Fox, Patrick Conrick, Sumit Garg

INTRODUCTION

Tissue bank preparation of endothelial tissue is constantly evolving. The increase in Descemet's membrane endothelial keratoplasty (DMEK) procedures has been swiftly followed by improved strategies for DMEK preparation. Pneumatic dissection of tissue, widely used for deep anterior lamellar keratoplasty (DALK), has more recently become a time-saving, "no touch" alternative to the manual dissection traditionally used for DMEK preparation. It has also become the primary technique for developing pre-Descemet's endothelial keratoplasty (PDEK) grafts.

While DMEK strips only Descemet's membrane and endothelium from recipient stroma, the proposed advantage of PDEK lies in the preservation of the pre-Descemet's layer. The big bubble technique has enabled the eye bank community to obtain a graft that potentially combines the advantages of younger donor tissue with the better visual outcomes of DMEK. Other potential advantages of PDEK tissue include: higher endothelial cell counts (secondary to younger donors), grafts more resilient to tearing (due to the slightly thicker nature of the graft), and theoretically similar rates of rejection as compared to DMEK.

In a traditional DMEK preparation, a type-2 air bubble is injected which extends to the corneal periphery separating pre-Descemet's layer and Descemet's membrane. This yields a DMEK graft approximately 15 μm thick and 10 mm in diameter. For a PDEK graft, a type-1 air bubble is injected between posterior stroma and pre-Descemet's layer. This centralized bubble does not extend to the periphery, leaving peripheral tissue that is fused to the rest of the stroma. This yields a graft that is about 25–30 μm thick and 7–7.5 mm in diameter. The type of air bubble created depends on the cleavage plane at which air is injected and thus determines the type of graft.

TECHNIQUE

All selection criteria for DSAEK and DMEK tissue also apply to PDEK tissue selection, except for donor age. DMEK grafts require tissue to be from a donor in the fifth or sixth decade, whereas PDEK grafts can be taken from donors as young as 2 years of age or younger.

1. The donor sclerocorneal disks are placed endothelial side up and covered with viscoelastic, balanced salt solution or Optisol. Scoring Descemet's membrane at the limbus every few clock hours step is an optional step that may help avoid formation of a type-2 bubble. A 30 G needle is inserted approximately 2 mm from the limbus, bevel up, into the posterior stroma (Fig. 24.1).
2. The needle is advanced to the center, and air is injected until a big bubble is formed (Fig. 24.2).

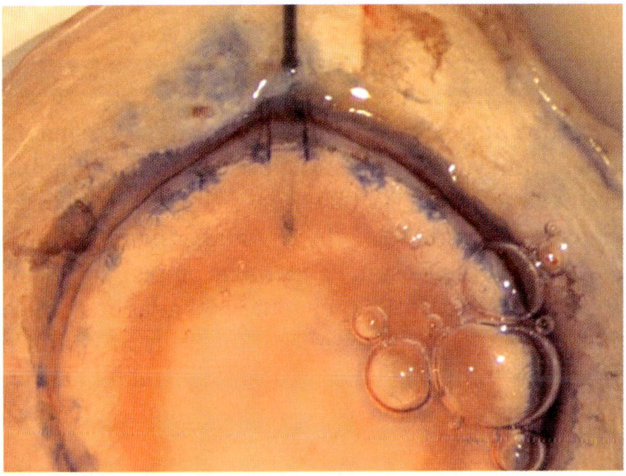

Fig. 24.1: Insertion of 30 G needle into posterior stroma of donor tissue.

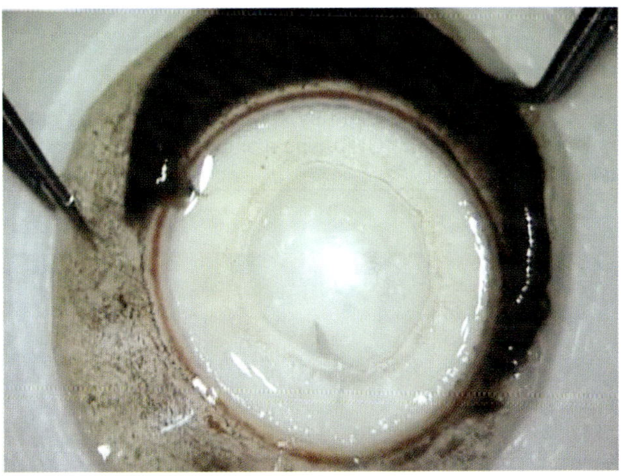

Fig. 24.2: Formation of a type-1 bubble by injecting air into the posterior stroma.

3. If the surgeon prefers to cut the graft, the bubble can be deflated and the tissue stored and delivered to the surgeon to be cut in the operating room. In this instance, trypan blue is typically applied prior to storage to visualize endothelial damage. Alternatively, if the surgeon prefers pre-cut tissue, the graft with the bubble is cut with scissors or trephinated by the eye bank prior to storage (Figs. 24.3A to C).
4. A hinge spanning approximately one clock hour is maintained to keep the graft in place (if scissors are used), and an S-stamp is applied to the pre-Descemet's side of the graft prior to storage (Figs. 24.4A and B). Note that the graft must be gently folded to expose the pre-Descemet's side and then folded back (Fig. 24.4C). The graft, stained with trypan blue, can then be grossly assessed for endothelial loss.

ENDOTHELIAL CELL LOSS

The primary disadvantage of a pneumatic dissection is the inability to check endothelial cell count with specular microscopy after the bubble is formed. Studies of eye bank-prepared DMEK tissues report an estimated endothelial cell loss of between 5% and 15%.[1-3] The few studies in the literature on PDEK suggest that endothelial cell loss in PDEK tissue preparation is no worse than what has been observed in DMEK preparation.[2,4] Variations in technique may affect endothelial cell loss. For example, one study of DMEK preparation examined variations in the big bubble technique and found that grafts that were left with an inflated bubble had a higher endothelial loss compared to

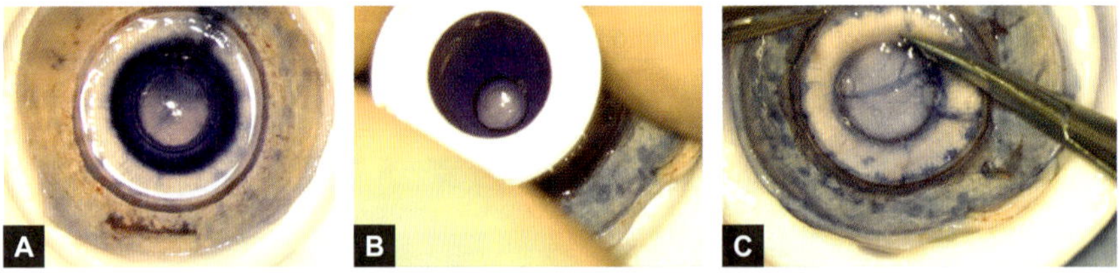

Figs. 24.3A to C: (A) Graft stained with trypan blue prior to being cut; (B) Trephination of the graft with bubble intact; (C) Cutting along the border of the graft outside the diameter of the bubble.

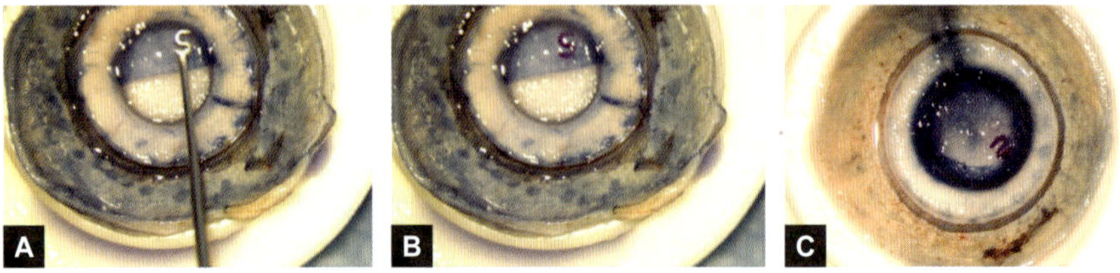

Figs. 24.4A to C: (A and B) S-stamp applied to the pre-Descemet's side of the graft and (C) The backwards S-stamp when visualized with endothelium side-up.

grafts in which the bubble was deflated prior to trephination.[3] Deflating the bubble may be one method to better preserve endothelial cell vitality.

Since PDEK preparation is still in its incipient stages, it is unknown exactly how much endothelial cell loss occurs. However, the ability to use donors from all ages is a significant advantage over DMEK preparation since tissue from younger donors has higher endothelial counts than older donors. Furthermore, grafts that are pre-cut could in theory be used for dual purposes: a PDEK graft and a DALK graft. Determining the best practices for handling and preserving precious corneal tissue is of utmost importance. The emergence of PDEK is yet another stride toward improving endothelial keratoplasty.

REFERENCES

1. Boynton GE, Woodward MA. Eye-bank preparation of endothelial tissue. Curr Opin Ophthalmol. 2014;25(4):319-24.
2. Altaan SL, Gupta A, Sidney LE, et al. Endothelial cell loss following tissue harvesting by pneumodissection for endothelial keratoplasty: an ex vivo study. Br J Ophthalmol. 2015;99:710-3.
3. Venzano D, Pagani P, Randazzo N, et al. Descemet membrane air-bubble separation in donor corneas. J Cataract Refract Surg. 2010;36(12):2022-7.
4. Busin M, Scorcia V, Patel AK, et al. Pneumatic dissection and storage of donor endothelial tissue for Descemet's membrane endothelial keratoplasty: a novel technique. Ophthalmology. 2010;117:1517-20.

CHAPTER 25

Pre-descemetocele

Priya Narang, Amar Agarwal

INTRODUCTION

Descemet's membrane (DM) is a thin, transparent, elastic sheet of tissue and the herniation or anterior bulging of an intact DM through a defect of the overlying corneal stromal and epithelial layers is known as descemetocele. The surgeon comes across descemetocele in cases of progressive corneal ulceration or degeneration that starts with a defect in the corneal epithelial layers and eventually progresses to involve the stroma with an intermediate stage of descemetocele followed eventually by corneal perforation.

During this sequence of events, a stage is attained where a layer of pre-Descemet's layer (PDL; Dua's layer)[1,2] covers the descemetocele.[1-9] This PDL is a distinct layer and we the authors believe that it provides mechanical strength and support to descemetocele and that during this stage where the PDL supports DM, descemetocele resists perforation and we tend to interpret this stage as a pre-descemetocele.

OPTICAL COHERENCE TOMOGRAPHY

We performed an optical coherence tomography (OCT) examination for demonstration of the existence of pre-Descemet's layer (PDL; Dua's layer) overlying a descemetocele and to demonstrate pre-descemetocele as a separate clinical entity.

CASE STUDY

A 50-year-old male patient with a previous history of corneal infection presented with progressive loss of vision in left eye. Upon examination, his vision was hand-movement perception and slit lamp examination revealed corneal ectasia with a bulge and thinning of central corneal layer suggestive of a descemetocele of 4 × 3 mm (Figs. 25.1A and B). Subsequent Fourier-domain OCT imaging showed thinning of the layers of cornea with the thickness of the ectatic part being 32 μ (Fig. 25.2).

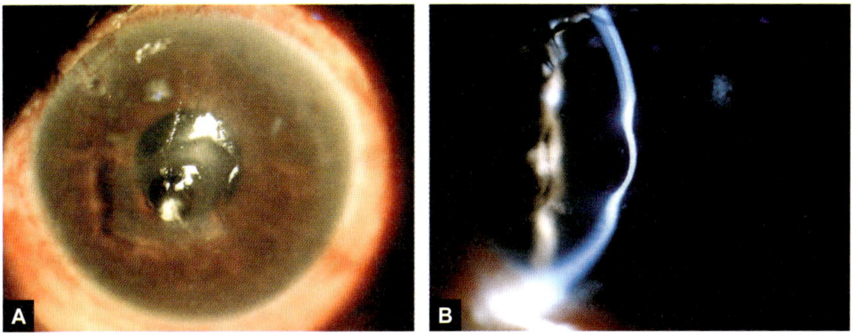

Figs. 25.1A and B: Pre-descematocele. (A) Clinical photo; (B) Slit lamp photo.

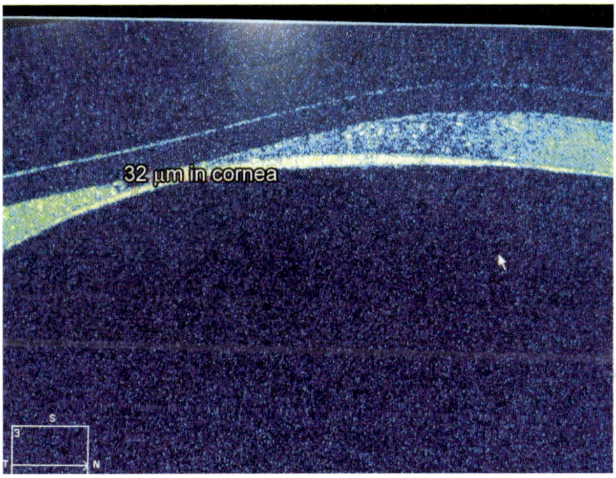

Fig. 25.2: Optical coherence tomography (OCT) showing the ectatic layers of pre-Descemet's layer along with Descemet's membrane.

DISCUSSION

Pre-Descemet's layer has been described as a distinct layer that sets it apart from the rest of stroma with a thickness that ranges from 6 μ to 15 μ.[1] DM represents a layer of 8–10 μ and is considered to be resistant to proteolysis. In clinical practice, it has been demonstrated that some descemetoceles resist perforation better than others. This is probably due to the presence of an additional layer of PDL that has been demonstrated to withstand a high pressure of 700 mm of Hg in donor corneas.[1] Many surgeons have attempted the triple procedure of DALK with phacoemulsification[4,5] and successful outcomes have been reported with the deep stromal dissection. The inherent weakness of DM to take pressure has been denoted clearly in a DALK study where the surgeons tried to perform a phacoemulsification after baring DM that resulted in DM rupture whereas after baring PDL they could successfully complete the procedure.[5]

Our OCT findings reveal that descemetoceles can be covered with PDL that offers resilience and delays the perforation of descemetocele. When the overlying PDL melts or dissolves, the descemetocele is more likely to perforate. The point of contention here is that PDL is a tough layer as compared to DM and DM has been known to rupture and give way in extreme conditions. We put forward a clinical entity of pre-descemetocele where we believe that all descemetoceles that are yet not perforated have an additional support of PDL and that the thickness of the descemetoceles should be closely monitored with OCT and a further progression towards thinning of the descemetocele membrane should prompt a surgeon for early surgical intervention.

Another clinical implication of the presence of PDL is that it does not signify an exigency and that surgeon has a reasonable time frame to arrange for a good donor graft. DALK can be used to treat descemetocele if PDL is detected on OCT. Baring a PDL allows surgeon to perform DALK at an early stage or else in advanced stage it would necessitate the surgeon to perform a penetrating keratoplasty (PK) procedure with its inherent side effects of irregular astigmatism, open sky procedure, and the possibility of endothelial rejection and a subsequent graft failure.

Various studies have been published that denote the existence of descemetocele in cases of corneal melting and measures to prevent the eye from perforation[6-8] but to the best of our knowledge, none of these studies have incorporated the application of OCT to assess the thickness of the residual corneal tissue that resists perforation.

The terminology "predescemetal corneal ulcer" has been used in past to denote deep corneal ulcers that have not yet ruptured.[9] Some surgeons have reported the evidence of presence of PDL in descemetoceles[2] and we the authors also suggest that this stage of descemetocele where a layer of PDL is detected on OCT should be labeled as a pre-descemetocele and not a descemetocele.

CONCLUSION

A descemetocele when covered with a PDL should be correctly designated as a pre-descemetocele. Loss of PDL leads to baring of DM that eventually ruptures. Further study is warranted to determine the progressive thinning of pre-descemetocele to a level of descemetocele that has a threat of impending perforation.

REFERENCES

1. Dua HS, Faraj LA, Said DG, et al. Human corneal anatomy redefined: a novel pre-Descemet's layer (Dua's layer). Ophthalmology. 2013;120(9):1778-85.
2. Dua HS, Faraj LA, Said DG, et al. "Dua's layer is not just residual stroma" Author reply. Ophthalmology. 2014;121:e25-6.

3. Agarwal A, Dua HS, Narang P, et al. Pre-Descemet's endothelial keratoplasty (PDEK). Br J Ophthalmol. 2014;98(9):1181-5.
4. Panda A, Sethi HS, Jain M, et al. Deep anterior lamellar keratoplasty with phacoemulsification. J Cataract Refract Surg. 2011;37(1):122-6.
5. Zaki AA, Elalfy MS, Said DG, et al. Deep anterior lamellar keratoplasty—triple procedure: a useful clinical application of the pre-Descemet's layer (Dua's layer). Eye (Lond). 2015;29(3):323-6.
6. Tong L, Tan DT, Abaño JM, et al. Deep anterior lamellar keratoplasty in a patient with descemetocele following gonococcal keratitis. Am J Ophthalmol. 2004;138(3):506-7.
7. Gabison EE, Doan S, Catanese M, et al. Modified deep anterior lamellar keratoplasty in the management of small and large epithelialized descemetoceles. Cornea. 2011;30(10):1179-82.
8. Sharma N, Kumar C, Mannan R, et al. Surgical technique of deep anterior lamellar keratoplasty in descemetoceles. Cornea. 2010;29(12):1448-51.
9. Küchle M, Seitz B, Langenbucher A, et al. Nonmechanical excimer laser penetrating keratoplasty for perforated or predescemetal corneal ulcers. Ophthalmology. 1999;106(11):2203-9.

Index

Page numbers followed by *f* refer to figure and *t* refer to table.

D

E

R

S

T

U

V

W

Y